MENOPAUSE WITHOUT MEDICINE

REVISED FIFTH EDITION

LINDA OJEDA, PH.D.

FOREWORD BY JEFFREY S. BLAND, PH.D.

Hunter House PUBLISHERS

Library of Congress Cataloging-in-Publication Data

Ojeda, Linda.
    Menopause without medicine / Linda Ojeda ; foreword by Jeffrey S. Bland.— Rev. 5th ed.
        p. cm.
    Includes bibliographical references and index.
    ISBN-13: 978-1-63026-787-2
    1. Menopause—Popular works. I. Title.
RG186.O325 2003
618.1'75—dc21   2003011025

Project Credits

Cover Design: Peri Poloni, Knockout Books
Book Design: Brian Dittmar Graphic Design
Book Production: Jinni Fontana
Copy Editor: Kelley Blewster
Proofreader: John David Marion
Indexer: Nancy D. Peterson
Acquisitions Editor: Jeanne Brondino
Editor: Alexandra Mummery
Publicist: Lisa E. Lee
Sales & Marketing Coordinator: Jo Anne Retzlaff
Customer Service Manager: Christina Sverdrup
Order Fulfillment: Lakdhon Lama
Administrator: Theresa Nelson
Computer Support: Peter Eichelberger
Publisher: Kiran S. Rana

Printed and Bound by Bang Printing, Brainerd, Minnesota

Manufactured in the United States of America

9 8 7 6 5   Fifth Edition   08 09 10 11 12

CONTENTS

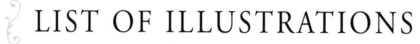

LIST OF ILLUSTRATIONS

Throughout the text, the superscript numbers refer to the Endnotes, which are located at the end of the book.

Most common health and medical terms used in the text are further defined in the Glossary.

ACKNOWLEDGMENTS

Writing a book is not a solitary endeavor. Many creative people contribute to making the work more than a collection of ideas and facts. The staff at Hunter House have pooled their talents and skills to help me produce something that I could not have accomplished alone. They have been delightful to work with, from the first edition to this extensive fifth revision.

I would like to express my heartfelt appreciation to my editor Kelley Blewster for her attention to detail and accuracy, her insights, original ideas, and helpful anecdotes. I thank Jeanne Brondino, friend and diplomat, for her understanding and smoothing out of rough spots even before the writing began. I am grateful to Alex Mummery for her editorial, organizational, and (most importantly) computer skills both on this edition and the last. Continued appreciation goes to the entire staff at Hunter House—Christina Sverdrup, Earlita Chenault, Jo Anne Retzlaff, and Lakdhon Lama—for helping to make this updated edition a work of which we can all be proud.

And a final thank you to my publisher and dear friend, Kiran Rana, who believed in my message long before it was in vogue.

I am indebted to the staff of the Professional Compounding Pharmacists of America (PCCA) for allowing me to attend their HRT symposium in Houston, Texas. The doctors, pharmacists, researchers, and organizers provided me with a wealth of information that saved me an enormous amount of time and energy while I learned about natural hormones. Dr. Mark Gonzalez, pharmacist and owner of Med Specialties Compounding Pharmacy in Yorba Linda, CA, continues to keep me informed of new research.

Honorable mentions go to my family, Roland, Jillian, Erik, Joey, and Jill; my sister Carol and my brother Ken; friends Karan, Marilyn, Linda, and Ursula who painstakingly listened to me and supported my efforts through the sometimes grueling writing process.

⤜ Important Note ⤛

The material in this book is intended to provide a review of natural therapies. Every effort has been made to provide accurate and dependable information. However, professionals in the field may have differing opinions, and change is always taking place. Any of the treatments described herein should be undertaken only under the guidance of a licensed health-care practitioner. The author, contributors, editors, publishers, and the experts quoted in the book cannot be held responsible for any error, omission, professional disagreement, outdated material, or adverse outcomes that derive from use of any of the treatments or information resources in this book, either in a program of self-care or under the care of a licensed practitioner.

FOREWORD

A virtual revolution has taken place in the field of applied clinical biochemistry over the past decade. This has come about as a result of our increased recognition of the important part that nutrition plays in health. The book you now hold in your hands, *Menopause Without Medicine*, is both a testament to and an agent of this revolution.

In the past, we considered genetic inheritance the major factor in human health. In recent years, however, we have learned much more about how various nutrients modulate human biology. While our genes dictate predispositions to specific problems, the nutritional environment and our lifestyle habits alter the genetic risk. In fact, these factors may be *more* important in determining the health patterns of midlife and later age than our genes.

As a result, I believe that understanding the basics of proper nutrition and the important role it plays in the aging process is vital for everyone.

Menopause Without Medicine is a well-researched, comprehensive health guide for women approaching or going through menopause. It offers them a program to ease the transition, as well as specific nutritional remedies for common menopausal symptoms. Dr. Ojeda addresses the crucial physical problems associated with menopause: hot flashes, vaginal dryness, and osteoporosis. She explains them in terms that are easy to understand and provides sound nutritional and lifestyle advice for counteracting or minimizing these conditions.

Our society, focused on youth, must grow to understand that old age is not a disease. The problems we associate with aging and menopause are not inevitable. Dr. Ojeda lays proper stress on the necessity of preparing the body in the early years so that later symptoms will be minimal. Because she has carefully evaluated many scientific and clinical studies, and collected in one place the best of what we currently know about relief for the symptoms of menopause, the information in *Menopause Without Medicine* is valuable to all women.

Equally important is the author's attitude, which maintains that women must take care of their health on all fronts: physical, mental, and emotional. Her book goes beyond the physical aspects of menopause to discuss the effects of cultural attitudes toward and the emotions associated with menopause. In writing about issues like self-image and beauty care, sexuality and depression, Dr. Ojeda addresses the real concerns of women who want to deal positively with all the changes that accompany the change.

Perhaps most important is Dr. Ojeda's purpose in writing this book: to empower women entering a new phase, to offer them hope and a greater measure of control over their lives. I believe *Menopause Without Medicine* is a book that can help most women in their quest for good health. It will certainly help all women to prepare for menopause with understanding, confidence, serenity, and even, it is to be hoped, joyful anticipation.

— Jeffrey S. Bland, Ph.D.
Founder and CEO of HealthComm International, Inc.
Author of *Nutraerobics, Your Health under Siege, The 20-Day Rejuvenation Diet Program,* and *Genetic Nutritioneering*

INTRODUCTION

Never say never. After writing the fourth edition of *Menopause Without Medicine*, I vowed it would be the last. I had gotten through menopause myself, had experienced each phase publicly, and I was ready to move on to new challenges. With heartfelt conviction I told my publisher that I could not return to this subject, that I had nothing to add, no more to contribute. Then, amidst major reconstruction on my home and pressing personal problems, something happened that changed my mind. Headlines hit the news that hormone replacement therapy (HRT) increased the risk of breast cancer and heart disease. Women and their doctors panicked, throwing out the pills that the day before had promised to curb their hot flashes, protect their hearts, and strengthen their bones. I could not understand the hoopla, especially among the medical community. The evidence of harm caused by certain kinds of HRT has been showing up for decades. For thirteen years I've cautioned women in previous editions of this book alone. But now, many researchers, scientists, and clinicians have denounced the hormone preparation that was abruptly withdrawn from the market, advising women to seek alternatives. (Not all hormones were condemned with this announcement; only the ones that most women take, a combination of synthetic estrogen plus progestins.)

Doctors are currently at a loss as to how best to advise women. I've been watching the morning TV shows, which feature the most learned medical authorities, and they say nothing that provides direction, nothing that gives hope. All in all, I find TV doctors and the major media extremely disappointing when it comes to offering real solutions. This morning, a doctor from the National Institutes of Health said that the bottom line is "we need to know more." I don't know about you, but I don't find that statement too helpful. When interviewed, the medical minds continue to rehash the dilemma but don't know where to go from there. What a shame they haven't investigated remedies outside their discipline. What a pity they offer women no answers.

All this is why I cannot remain in the shadows. In a glimpse of a moment I knew I had to complete what I had started so many years ago—long before menopause was a newsworthy topic. I feel compelled to reassure women that they indeed do have options. There are a slew of natural remedies—vitamins, herbs, and foods —that work to control menopausal symptoms. I've tried them and found them effective. Additionally, however, if these nonhormonal remedies prove ineffective for you, there are safer hormonal alternatives to the potentially cancer-producing hormones that have been foisted upon us by the drug companies. Research concerning natural (bioidentical) hormones remains in its infancy because multi-million-dollar drug companies cannot profit as heavily from natural products and therefore won't fund major studies on them. Still, independent research in the United States and Europe has shown that hormone preparations are not all equal, and that gentler versions not only minimize menopausal symptoms, but they also build bone and may actually protect against breast cancer. I advise you to read the research, investigate other sources, consult with a variety of health professionals, and decide for yourself—especially if you are not ready to give up your hormones.

⮞ A Little Personal History ⮜

Let me share with you a little personal history before I tackle these topics. Almost twenty years have passed since I first started poring over medical journals searching for information about menopause—a topic that, at the time, was largely ignored by the medical community. Only a handful of books could be found on the shelves, and even women's magazines omitted stories of the experiences and dilemmas women face during this major life transition. How times have changed! Walk into any bookstore today and check out the women's health section: The racks are crammed with books on all aspects of midlife, from physical to psychological, from experiential to spiritual. Menopause not only is out of the closet; it's the hottest topic of the new millennium.

I remember collecting data for the first edition of this book and eagerly sharing my findings with friends and acquaintances. I was startled to realize how uncomfortable people became at the mere mention of the "M" word. Responses ranged from nervous laughter and bewilderment to downright embarrassment. I learned to lower my voice when asked how I spent my day. Only in these past few years has the topic of menopause filtered into everyday conversation. My book preceded Gail Sheehy's *The Silent Passage* by a few years; it came out at a time when women were not yet comfortable complaining publicly about hot flashes and night sweats. It's hard to believe, but women in my mother's generation didn't even tell their best friends when they were entering "The Change." Fast forward two decades, and *Menopause: The Musical* plays off-Broadway and travels from coast to coast sharing the tale of menopausal misery while women become increasingly able to laugh at themselves and commiserate with others about their mutual experiences. Both women *and* men seem quite comfortable discussing hot flashes, mood swings, and hormone therapy. At the gym, in the office, in business meetings, in restaurants, and at parties, everyone has an opinion to offer or a story to tell.

Coinciding with the publication of the third edition of this book came my own real-life menopausal experience. The symptoms that were once technical terms took on an entirely different meaning: hot flashes, sleepless nights, irregular periods, heart flutters, weight gain, and the decision about hormones faced me head-on. I found myself turning to my own words, seeking remedies I'd discovered long ago. I also experimented with new foods, nutrients, and herbs that had come to my attention since the publication of the first two editions. No longer was *Menopause Without Medicine* just the product of my extensive research as a nutritionist; it ranked second to the Bible as my daily guide. And I can say with a new confidence that the recommendations in the book did work for me. Even though menopause is now behind me, I continue to follow the same dietary program of nutrients and soy that I recommend in these pages, and I still do the exercises presented in Appendix D.

As I entered the year 2000 and completed the fourth edition, I faced yet another stage in my life: postmenopause. Three years prior I'd celebrated my menopausal birthday (meaning I ended a full year without having a menstrual period) and parted with most of the bothersome symptoms, sighing with relief that I had made it through without relying on hormone replacement. Many of my friends who vowed with me to abstain from conventional hormone therapy had changed their minds once the symptoms took over the quality of their lives. I know they were riddled with guilt because they, too, wanted to ride it out without using drugs. Unfortunately, diet, herbs, and exercise aren't enough for everyone, and outside intervention is sometimes necessary. I continually reassured them that for some women hormone replacement is the best choice, and I have not changed my opinion. Be kind to yourself whatever decision you make.

Since I made it through menopause without the use of hormones, I never guessed that I would reconsider them as a possible treatment for me. Symptoms were no longer the issue; the health of my bones was. Since I fit the profile of a woman at risk for osteoporosis—petite, light-complexioned, and small-boned—and having undergone a DEXA test that indicated loss of bone to the point of osteopenia, I felt it was time to revisit my options. I was already exercising regularly, eating bone-building foods, and taking the requisite supplements, yet it wasn't enough to stave off osteoporosis. I was crushed, but I knew I had to do something. The choices before me were to take HRT (natural estrogen plus progesterone; I didn't consider synthetic hormones an option) or to try one of the nonhormonal drugs prescribed to treat osteoporosis. It didn't take long for me to eliminate the popular osteoporosis drugs; there were no long-term studies on their safety, and early reports indicated that the bone produced was inferior to normal bone. And then there were the drugs' nasty side effects, as is the case with many alien substances we introduce into our bodies. If my only other option had been synthetic estrogen plus

progestin, I would have done nothing. But there exists a solution few women know about: natural hormones that appear to be safer and yet are still effective for preventing loss of bone. Another factor that swayed me was a heart irregularity I have that is helped by estrogen. I decided to give HRT a try for one year, retest my bones, check my blood for the heart problem, and then reevaluate. The results of my DEXA test have arrived just in time to make publication. According to the report summary, there is a slight negative change compared to the previous X ray; however, it is not considered statistically significant. So I guess I'm holding my own. Still, I'm not entirely satisfied with these results. I think I can do better. After discussing the possibilities with my compounding pharmacist, we decided that I will take a saliva test to determine the exact status of my hormones—estrogen, progesterone, and testosterone. Even though I have no other symptoms to suggest they may be deficient, there is a possibility that one or all may require a boost. I'm also considering upping my supplements of calcium, magnesium, and vitamin D, possibly by 200 mg to 500 mg per day. And the final phase of my new and improved bone-building plan is to add a ten-pound weight that I will carry in a backpack when I walk the hills in my town. I'll give this regimen a year and then retest to determine how well the program is working.

Women Have Options

I have devoted an entire chapter in this new edition to describing the differences between synthetic hormones and natural, or bioidentical, hormones. The synthetic hormones that are now shunned by most doctors have been suspect for years. Because they are not recognized, utilized, and excreted by the female body in the way that the body's own hormones are, they build up inside the cells, potentially causing cancer, blood clots, and a host of other devastating side effects that have been downplayed in the brochures we've read at the doctor's office. They have also been overprescribed to women over forty who endure perimenopausal symptoms, many of whom could have managed well with herbs and nutrients. Furthermore, many medical doctors automatically handed out the same dosage to every woman over forty-five who visited their office, when smaller amounts could still have helped and been safer for the individual.

Natural hormone therapy differs completely from synthetic HRT. For starters, the hormones are called *bioidentical* because they exactly match the hormones our bodies make naturally. This means that they are recognized by the body and are therefore better utilized. Women who have switched to natural hormones from synthetic ones find them more tolerable, and with fewer to no side effects. Just like the synthetics, natural hormones are FDA-approved and are regulated by licensed compounding pharmacies. And just like the synthetics, a doctor must prescribe them. The difference is that natural hormones can be custom-made to fit your hormonal profile and your individual symptoms. In prescribing natural hormones, it is the goal of the health professional to bring your body back into hormonal balance by testing the levels of all your sex hormones (not just estrogen) and determining the smallest amount that will effectively treat your particular need, whether it be a reduction of symptoms or preventing further loss of bone. Using these preparations requires more time and effort from you, your doctor, and your pharmacist, but it's worth it to know that you're not taking too much of a hormone that you don't need. Even if you haven't heard of natural HRT, be aware that the treatment has been evolving for more than fifteen years in the United States and is used by millions of women here and in Europe.

Few women's health issues are as beset with confusion and controversy as developing an appropriate treatment for menopause. Just using the word *treatment* suggests that menopause is a disease requiring medical care, doctor's visits, and prescription drugs. The medicalization of menopause has given birth to a giant industry composed of products, drugs, books, and nutritional supplements. Big business has discovered a dynamic market in aging baby boomers. But before you are convinced by the well-designed advertisements of vibrant, healthy midlife women popping pills, consider the possibility that the drug companies selling those multicolored tablets for menopausal relief may not have your best interests at heart. I am not antidoctor, antimedicine, or antihormones. What I wish to emphasize is that a hierarchy of questions and treatments needs to be considered prior to taking any drug. First, how bad is the symptom? Feeling distress at menopause does not always indicate that something has gone awry. It could be a normal sign of transitioning hormones. Remember when you started your periods? For a few months you felt physically and emotionally out of sync, but your body adjusted and you eventually adapted to your new cycle. As you leave your periods in the past, you may experience discomfort. If it is minimal, and if you are relieved to know that some discomfort is normal, can you tolerate it without medication?

Second, are there natural, dietary, or lifestyle changes you can make to ease the symptoms? This book provides many alternatives that have been scientifically proven to work effectively for a wide variety of complaints. Nutritional and lifestyle alterations take time to pay off, but stick with them for a few months and you will see noticeable differences.

There are women for whom diet, exercise, stress reduction, and supplements aren't appropriate or do not work quickly enough. If your symptoms are intolerable and interfere with your work, relationships, and enjoyment of life, by all means get help. But even if you reach this point, you have options. You can ask for low-potency pills, take them only as long as necessary, and then slowly taper off—always in consultation with your health-care provider. Many women are never informed that hormone replacement therapy doesn't have to last forever.

There is a growing appreciation of the role of nutrition in determining one's level of health. Even staunchly traditional physicians now admit that diet and lifestyle play a major role in many of the major diseases. This was hardly the case ten years ago—but time lags always exist between theory, accumulated evidence, and public awareness. It took fifty years for the medical community to indisputably link cigarette smoking to lung cancer. Decades passed before the medical establishment accepted that increased cholesterol levels were linked to heart disease. Studies showing the benefits of vitamin E in the prevention of heart disease and the treatment of hot flashes go back to the 1940s. And yet I still hear physicians say they need more studies before they can endorse diet and nutritional supplements as a part of health care. Given the scientific evidence in support of nutritional supplements and the absence of risks surrounding them, waiting to inform the public that nutrients may save their lives seems irresponsible.

Nutritional and herbal remedies, as effective as they are and as much as they have been studied, fail to reach the consumer to the extent that hormones and other drugs do. Up until 2002, we were still led to believe that supplements ranked only slightly higher than snake oil and placebos. Doctors on talk shows condescendingly shook their heads when someone brought up the necessity and validity of supplementing one's diet with vitamins and herbs. We were warned more about the potential toxic effects of these concentrated nutrient sources than we were about the potential risks of prescription drugs. Then, just when we nutritionists thought all hope was gone, another long-awaited landmark study made front-page headlines. After many years of reviewing data presented in writing, the medical community endorsed vitamin supplements. In a complete reversal of policy, the prestigious *Journal of the American Medical Association* recommended that all adults should take a daily multivitamin to help stave off heart disease, cancer, and osteoporosis. I am frustrated that it took them so long to arrive at this conclusion but happy that it finally did happen. This fact was as true thirty years ago when I first spoke of widespread nutrient deficiency as it is today, but it took that many years to prove beyond a shadow of a doubt that few individuals are adequately nourished. I'm at a loss to count the number of health advisories that are familiar to researchers yet have failed to receive the medical blessing that, if acted upon, could increase both the quality of our lives and the quantity of our days.

The time is ripe for us to take action. A door has been cracked open that will allow us the opportunity to talk to our doctors about natural remedies and natural hormones. More and more we are seeing individuals taking responsibility for their own health care. According to a 1993 study, one in three Americans uses alternative therapies and pays for them out of pocket. The cost of health (sick) care has skyrocketed, and people are seeking less expensive methods of treatment. The concept of prevention is finally reaching public awareness and medical acceptance. It took three decades to convince doctors that vitamin supplements can prevent disease and encourage health; hopefully, we can help close the time gap with our knowledge and interest in finding safer remedies.

We baby boomers are the trailblazers for the next generation. We have changed women's roles in the workplace, family, and society. Now we must be advocates for our own health care. We can no longer complacently accept a drug or medical procedure that seems wrong to us, even if everyone else is using it. We must ask the difficult questions and stand up for what we think is right. We cannot remain passive about our health care, even if being proactive means doing more research on our own, getting second and third opinions, talking to our friends about their decisions, and moving beyond our sphere of comfort into alternative areas of healing. We must decide when traditional medicine isn't adequate and also when alternative medicine isn't working for us. We need to tell our physicians about any alternative treatments we are undertaking, both to avoid compromising either therapy and also to educate our physicians. As difficult as it is for us to assume a larger role in our health, it also can be a challenge for our traditionally trained doctors to admit they don't know everything. It is my hope that some day our allopathic doctors, chiropractors, Chinese medical doctors, and holistic healers will join forces and work with each other, respecting and complementing each other's unique capabilities. We must work to this end, but until then, we must remain our own best advocates.

Menopause is an exciting time—a time when we have gained a better sense of ourselves, an appreciation for the cycles of our lives, and a clearer perspective on the future. Although menopause is a universal experience, each woman goes through it in her own way and in her own time. There are many difficult decisions to make about your health, and I don't claim to have all the answers, but I do offer you some new ideas, suggestions, and thoughts on easing your immediate symptoms and improving your future years.

I want to encourage you to feel good about whatever decisions you make regarding your health and well-being during your midlife years. Maybe you decided

in advance not to take any drugs for your menopausal symptoms, but when the hot flashes kept you up for months, you reluctantly succumbed. Resist blaming yourself or blaming others for their choices. Rather, let us encourage each other, share our stories, learn, grow, and be happy that we live in a time when we are free to talk about women's health concerns and to pass this legacy on to our daughters.

An exciting avenue has opened up to us in the last several years—the Internet. It has brought so many special-interest groups together, and, speaking personally, it has placed me in contact with other women who are sharing their menopausal experiences. I have been fortunate to participate as a speaker and health educator on several Internet sites, to listen to women's conversations, and to hear other authors, doctors, and specialists in the field discuss the multitude of issues that arise during midlife. I encourage you to join in and hear what others have to offer, have your personal questions answered, and stay current with the latest information. The Internet is the best way I know to connect with other women and with authorities in this field. The websites I recommend that are related to women's issues and specifically to menopause are www.power-surge.com and www.families-first.com/hotflash. Tune in, learn more about medical and natural options, and share your questions and concerns with other wonderful menopausal women.

A few words about the way the book is organized: Part One deals with immediate concerns; it gives you the straight dope on hormones and offers help for relief of menopausal symptoms. If you are desperately seeking a natural solution to a distressing condition, you may want to start with the specific chapter dealing with your concern and begin your program there. Part Two deals more generally with preparing for your future health. Among other things, it examines risk factors for the common killers of postmenopausal women: heart disease and cancer. Becoming aware of the dietary and lifestyle factors that influence these diseases and taking action to prevent them are the best insurance you have for future healthy years. The title of Part Three, "Nutrition for Life: A Woman's Guide," is self-explanatory. The section details strategies for optimizing your health through a program of diet and supplementation that you can tailor to fit your own needs and lifestyle. In it, I have provided outlines, questionnaires, and charts to help you plan a course of action.

The years to come, I believe, will be the most fulfilling, rewarding, inspiring, and fun. I know this because every day I am more awake and alive to the reality of what life has to offer. It is my prayer that you, too, will see the second half as the part of life for which we have been preparing. Rehearsals are over; let the show begin.

— Linda Ojeda, Ph.D., January 2003

PART I

MENOPAUSE
SYMPTOMS AND REMEDIES

CHAPTER 1

MENOPAUSE

THE REALITY

*The woman who wants her second-chance years to be
the best of all has to work at shaping her future.*

— DR. JOYCE BROTHERS, *Better than Ever*

Our society today, the society in which most of us have grown up, is clearly youth oriented. As much as we would like to believe that vitality and beauty are possible at any age, magazine ads and television commercials glaringly remind us that the emphasis on young bodies still prevails. Given our aging population and the host of beautiful older role models who now grace the screen, political arena, and corporate sector, I am beginning to believe that trends might be shifting from the overwhelming focus on nubile, wrinkle-free bodies. Young feminine forms still dominate the newsstand, but more and more older models like Lauren Hutton, Beverly John, and Cheryl Tiegs, and actresses such as Susan Sarandon, Goldie Hawn, and Candice Bergen stare at us from the checkout stand. They appear confident and seemingly comfortable with their age. Sure, they're airbrushed, and their lines and wrinkles have been swept away with a soft-lens camera, but midlife women are no longer hidden from view. This is progress. Even twenty years ago, when I first started writing about menopause, you could not find one positive midlife role model on the cover of a national magazine. Menopausal women were characterized as pleasingly plump matrons who had lost interest in looking good and were given to frequent hysterical outbursts. They were never depicted as sexy (imagine your grandmother wearing Victoria's Secret lingerie and enjoying sex), and as for creativity and adventure and starting a new career, those aspects of life were never even presented as possibilities. Gladly, times are a-changing.

Historically, medical attitudes toward menopause mirrored the negative stereotypes. Many earlier medical texts listed menopause as a disease or an unnatural phenomenon. The terms most commonly used to describe it included *climacteric, endocrine starvation, involutionary years, female trouble,* and *living decay.* No wonder women dreaded the so-called change of life! Descriptions such as these significantly warped their attitudes and responses to menopause, especially if they were poorly informed, which most were. Up until two decades ago, few books had been written about menopause, so women did not know what to expect, other than what their male doctors told them. There were no seminars or talk-radio discussions, and few women shared their personal experiences with even the closest of friends. Lack of information and negative conditioning certainly contributed to the physical and psychological symptoms that many of us "older" women remember as the typical stereotype of the menopausal woman. How could midlife women in the 1960s feel good about growing older when writers and doctors were telling women that their lives, essentially, were no longer relevant?

Robert Wilson, in his supposedly profemale book *Feminine Forever*, titled one of his chapters "The Loss of Womanhood and the Loss of Good Health."[1] He described the menopausal woman as the equivalent of a eunuch: unbearable, suicidal, incapacitated, and incapable of rationally perceiving her situation. Equally degrading was the work of David Reuben, M.D., author of the popular *Everything You Always Wanted to Know about Sex.* This authority maintained that the essence of femininity is tied to a woman's ovaries; once the estrogen is virtually shut off, a woman comes as close as she can to being a man. Such a woman is not really a man, he explains, but she is no longer a functional woman; according to Reuben, menopausal women live in the "world of intersex."[2] This is absurd. A woman's femininity is not defined by the amount of estrogen in her body any more than a man's masculinity is measured by his testosterone output. But this is what women were led to believe at that time.

Menopause is no longer regarded solely as an estrogen deficiency and a medical disease that requires intervention. Rather, the accepted view of menopause is that it is a major cultural, psychological, and physiological milestone for women. Its definition is now broader in scope, with symptoms linked to the consequences of aging as well as hormonal imbalance. The implication still exists, however, that menopause is predominately a negative event, like divorce or loss of a job. Many experts agree that menopause is a biological marker for aging; it signifies the end of reproduction in a culture where sexuality and childbearing are equated with female fulfillment, and it signifies the beginning of old age in a culture that extols youthfulness. Some still cling to this view, but is it true for all women, some women, or just a handful of women? Or is it an obsolete model reflective of antiquated ideas?

≈ What Women Really Think about Menopause ≈

The North American Menopause Society (NAMS) wanted to find out exactly how women felt about their menopausal experiences. In 1998, NAMS developed a set of questions and, with help from the Gallup Organization, conducted 752 telephone interviews across the United States, using a randomly selected sample of postmenopausal women ages fifty to sixty-five. Although individual postmenopausal women surveyed held differing views of menopause, the majority (51 percent) reported being happiest and most fulfilled during this time of their lives, compared to when they were in their twenties (10 percent), thirties (17 percent), or forties (16 percent).[3] They reported that many areas of their lives had improved since menopause, including family and home life, sense of personal fulfillment, ability to focus on hobbies or other interests, relationship with spouse/partner, and friendships. Sixteen percent of women felt their sexual relationship had gotten better since menopause, while an equal number said it had worsened; however, more than half (51 percent) said it had remained unchanged.

Approximately three-quarters of women also reported making some type of lifestyle change at midlife, including changes in their nutritional or exercise habits, reducing alcohol intake, reducing stress levels, stopping smoking, taking more time for themselves, and using alternative and holistic treatments. One reason for women's positive experiences, according to Wulf Utian, M.D., executive director of NAMS, is that women are talking to each other about their experiences. Rather than looking to their mothers' generation for advice (since their mothers were uncomfortable discussing the subject), they look to friends and other women who are going through the same experience. "We see an increasing trend toward women supporting other women and guiding their peers and the next generation through the many phases of life," Dr. Utian said. "Menopausal women see themselves as role models, and seem to be very interested in helping other women, as well as improving their own health."[4]

The thought of menopause should not and need not produce anxiety. A study of other societies indicates that the stereotype of the distraught woman is not universal, that our negative reactions to common physiological processes, such as menstruation and menopause, are culturally engendered. In countries where age is venerated and elders enjoy respect for their experience and wisdom, older women seem to manifest fewer physical and psychological symptoms. For example, South African, Asian, and Arabic women, who, it is said, welcome the end of the childbearing years, are reported to have positive attitudes about the change of life. Where there are different predefined concepts, aging seems to be more natural, less confusing, and not overlaid with negative images.[5]

Mayan women in Mexico have been studied by researchers because they do not complain of the characteristic symptoms of menopause and do not suffer from osteoporosis and bone fractures. Endocrinologically, they are no different from women in the United States. In fact, estrogen levels in Mayan postmenopausal women were at or below the values expected for U.S. women. Something that *is* significantly different is their attitude. Mayan women welcome the transition, as they will be relieved of many household chores and regarded as respected elders. In addition, they will become free from the taboos associated with menstruation. Menstruating women are believed to carry an "evil wind" during their periods, so the cessation of periods raises a woman's status in the community.[6]

Menopause, like menarche, is natural. We experience hormonal changes at menopause, just as we did in our adolescence. Any lifetime change may be accompanied by uneasiness and disequilibrium; it is normal and it will pass. How smoothly a woman adapts to any transition depends largely on her overall health—that of her body, her mind, and her spirit.

Menopause Is Big Business

In the West, historically, the menopausal woman was regarded with pity and indifference. Because she complained of symptoms that were as yet unexplained, she was labeled a neurotic hypochondriac, then sedated and left to suffer in silence. I am sure no one regrets leaving behind those days of disbelief and intolerance. But what replaced the ignorance—namely, the medical model of midlife—may be equally destructive.

Women who are fifty-something are no longer ignored; they are actively courted. They are presently a prime target of the medical industry, drug companies, and other interests that can benefit from an aging population. And the market is growing: Fifty million baby boomers are going through menopause, entering at a rate of between two thousand and four thousand per day. By the year 2015, nearly one-half of the female population will be menopausal. Talk about global warming.

Industry-financed medical researchers inundate us with information about the benefits of treating all menopausal signs and symptoms, severe or insignificant, with hormones. The assumption that menopause is associated with chronic disease further encourages widespread use of prescription drugs. While earlier hormonal therapies were marketed only to physicians, major drug companies now directly target female consumers in the grocery-store magazines. Before they experience their first hint of oncoming menopause, women are already primed to run to the doctor for pills.

Menopause is now a big business, and we women consumers need to be alert to what we hear and read. The fact that there is a strong bias toward medicalizing menopause is obvious. Now that hormone replacement therapy (HRT) no longer commands the primary focus since its reputation has been tarnished, an abundance of prescription drugs are primed to fill the void and sell us treatments for osteoporosis, vaginal dryness, hot flashes, and heart disease. Our buying power is huge and we are going to be courted and cajoled into taking drugs that we may not need. Before you decide on a new medication, please do some homework. Check with a few health professionals who are not quick to medicate, check out the Internet, read the latest in research, talk to your friends who may be knowledgeable, and trust your own instincts about what is appropriate for your body. Just because a product is advertised on TV and just because thousands of women are taking it, that doesn't mean it is the best drug for you. Also, find out if a natural, less potentially harmful remedy exists for your symptom. Often it does.

☙ The Range of Symptoms ☙

I was raised in an era when normal female topics, such as menstruation and menopause, were not openly discussed even among close friends. Our bodies, we were led to believe, were too mysterious to understand and too base to mention. Our intimate parts were ignored as if they did not exist. Even today, unfortunately, these childhood attitudes linger, preventing many of us from confronting and accepting problems and feelings that cry out to be addressed.

Attitudes concerning the menopausal experience have changed in the last few years, and they continue to evolve as women read, learn, and discuss their individual experiences. In the mid-1990s, a questionnaire designed by Fredi Kronenberg, director of menopause research at the Center for Women's Health at Columbia-Presbyterian Medical Center, New York City, was given to readers of *Prevention* magazine.[7] The results of the two thousand randomly chosen respondents (fifteen thousand actually provided information) may help us understand and appreciate the menopausal experience. The results of this extensive questionnaire include the following:

⊙ Intensity of symptoms ranged from stormy to breezy. Fifty-eight percent considered the process more of an annoyance than a major life disruption, and more than half agreed the symptoms were, for the most part, mild.

⊚ The younger the woman is at the onset of menopause, the more difficult the experience. The average age at which women enter menopause is fifty years, and a woman who has, for example, postponed motherhood, thinking she still has ten years left, and then suddenly finds herself starting menopause, probably has both physical and psychological issues to confront.

⊚ Weight gain is not inevitable at fifty; however, 42 percent of respondents gained in excess of ten pounds. Current research indicates that this additional poundage is more a function of aging than of estrogen decline.

⊚ The fact that sleep problems were prevalent was not surprising. Sixty-two percent of the respondents reported that hot flashes kept them awake. Frequent urination, which is related to lower estrogen levels, may also keep women awake; aging itself has an effect on muscle tone, and illnesses, such as diabetes, impact bladder function.

⊚ The years prior to menopause, called *perimenopause*, seem to account for most of the annoying symptoms, such as severe hormonal fluctuations. Once a woman has stopped having periods for a year, things usually stabilize.

⊚ Good health habits correlated with a more positive menopausal experience. Exercising three or more times a week was associated with fewer symptoms and a generally better transition. It is unclear whether exercise reduced the stress of menopause or had other benefits, but the more stress a woman reported in her life, the more difficult her menopause.

⊚ The relationship between a positive menopausal experience and a low-fat diet was even stronger than that for exercise. Women who described their diet as primarily vegetarian generally reported fewer symptoms. Eating soy products, such as tofu, correlated strongly with fewer symptoms. It may be that women who eat soy and vegetable products enjoy a lifestyle that is healthier in other ways, but the benefit might also be attributed to the large amounts of phytohormones in soy. Certain plants contain estrogen-like substances, called *phytohormones*, that appear to provide just enough hormonal effect to prevent menopausal symptoms. In countries where women consume large amounts of soy products, menopausal symptoms are appreciably reduced or nonexistent.

⇒ Personality Types ⇐

It appears that women with certain personalities may tend to develop certain menopausal symptoms. Although the evidence is not conclusive, there is value in relaying this information, because it may apply to and help a number of women.

Researchers have found that certain personality types find it more traumatic to adjust to changes during the menopausal years. Gynecologist Sheldon Cherry finds that women with a history of emotional problems have the hardest time. These include women with chronic sexual difficulties, immature women with narcissistic tendencies, women whose erotic attractiveness was the chief element of their personal worth, childless women facing the undeniable loss of fertility, and married women who feel that their meaningful years are over.[8]

Several authorities have observed that the manner in which women react to the change may be related to how they perceive themselves as women. Particularly vulnerable, according to British physician Barbara Evans, are women who over the years have defined their femininity in terms of bodily functions—menstruation, pregnancy—and motherhood.[9] For them, menopause represents the end of their womanly identity; it removes the purpose of their existence.

Another all-too-common phenomenon is women who submerge their own desires, talents, and personal growth to live totally through their children's activities and accomplishments. It is no wonder that, when their children leave home, these women undergo an emotional trauma similar to experiencing the death of a loved one. They have lost the chief component of their identity as women and as contributing members of society. This "empty-nest syndrome" often results in depression. The midlife woman must search for a new identity in her relationship to her grown children.

The degree to which a woman accepts or fears growing older also affects the transition. The reality of getting older has to be dealt with at some time in our lives, and often this time coincides with or begins at menopause. Since we can't turn back the clock no matter how many antiaging products we consume or lather on our bodies, we need to find a way to accept growing old gracefully. I'm not at all opposed to using any cosmetic or procedure that helps us feel good about ourselves, but, more importantly, we need to look into our souls to find purpose and meaning in our new lives or we will never be happy with who we are.

If you find yourself struggling with these issues, read about other women who are also searching for a new frame of reference for themselves. I just finished reading *Getting Over Getting Older*, by Letty Cottin Pogrebin, and I found it an honest, humorous, and highly personal exploration into the perils and pleasures of aging. She tells the truth about her own body's aging—being unable to read the print in the telephone book, letting out the waistband in all her skirts, her shoe size enlarging, her bra straps leaving permanent indentations, sleep creases that make her skin look like crepe paper. I can identify. As much as I want to accept the increasing wisdom and deepening spirituality that supposedly comes with years, I'm not always thrilled about the trade-offs: poor short-term memory, sagging breasts, purple veins in my neck, and cottage cheese–looking thighs. Pogrebin asks the question we all need to address: "What good is it to turn fifty with an unwrinkled face if there's no light behind the eyes, no passion in the voice, no new ideas happening inside the head?"[10] Some of us have more difficulty getting to this point than others, and I agree that it is sad if we find ourselves preoccupied with the physical signs of aging and miss the things we might contribute to our families and the world. Research indicates that women who accept menopause as a natural passage in life are likely to get through it unscathed. For them, the transition is comparatively uncomplicated, uneventful, and relatively symptomless. In addition, women whose educational skills make more options available to them are reported to handle the change with relative ease.[11] Numerous studies indicate that women with professional interests, intellectual and creative outlets, and challenging responsibilities have an easier time during menopause. It is not clear exactly why active women appear to suffer less physical and emotional pain than their homebound sisters, but some theories pose that they have less time to focus on their symptoms, are generally more knowledgeable about the physiological details of menopause and about their own bodies, and have higher self-esteem.

Whether a woman's symptoms during menopause will be closely related to her personality type or feelings about herself cannot be predicted with any certainty. To portray such a complex psychophysiological process in black-and-white terms would be misleading. Each woman has a highly individual chemical makeup, genetic predisposition, and hormonal balance. Even the most secure, well-adjusted, and happy woman may experience emotional upheaval during menopause. Fortunately, the majority of women not only accept the multiple challenges of menopause, but find it to be the most enriching time of their lives.

Creating a Positive Attitude

Women entering menopause are approaching what can be the best years of their lives. The life span of the modern woman is currently seventy-eight to eighty-four years, and gerontologists anticipate that it will soon increase to beyond ninety. Even the conservative American Medical Association's Council on Medical Services boldly asserts that with intelligent living we could all live to be ninety or one hundred years old. This means that, before too many more decades have passed, the average woman may be living as many years after menopause as she lived before it. We need to be concerned with enhancing the quality of those years. Just think: If a woman has devoted the first half or third of her life to raising a family, she can still return to college, start a new career, travel, write the great American novel, learn French, or climb Mount Everest. We don't have to restrict ourselves to one career or one life path. Our options increase, especially when we are mentally and physically prepared to exercise them.

Even in light of the opportunities menopause opens up for us, we should not underestimate the emotional impact menopause has on many women. Psychologist Helene Deutsch calls the psychological experience of menopause the most trying time of a woman's life, and Juanita Williams agrees: "Although it is the manifest sign of the end of reproductive life, its symbolic meanings invest it with an importance which extends far beyond its biological definition."[12] Whether this applies to you is not something a textbook or expert can predict—only you can say. If menopause represents more than a physical change to you, find a support group where you are free to discuss your feelings openly, talk to your friends, or, if you don't have anyone to share your feelings with (or even if you do), check out the Internet site Power Surge (www.power-surge.com). Not only will you find the support of wonderful women there, but the information that you will glean from the various doctors and health professionals who contribute to the site is unsurpassed. What we think and believe not only determines our daily decisions, but it also establishes the entire direction of our life. Attitudes shape our future. If you have accepted an idea—from yourself, a teacher, parent, friend, an advertisement, or any other source—and if you are firmly convinced that idea is true, it has the same power over you as a hypnotist's words have over the hypnotist's subject.[13] We translate into physical reality the thoughts and attitudes we hold in our minds, no matter what they are.

Our attitudes toward menopause may have been engendered by our culture and our families, but they are not unchangeable. If our ideas are counterproductive, we can choose to acknowledge the fears and anxieties we harbor, alter them, and begin to reverse the obstacles in our lives. Whether you are fifty years old or twenty, take stock of your belief system and your general attitudes. If you feel you are valued only for your children's or husband's accomplishments, then few can know and acknowledge the real you. If you think that to be beautiful you must be young, then your mature years will hold little joy for you. If you are convinced that the quality of your life will vanish at fifty or sixty or seventy, then it will. If you believe that your health, looks, body, and mind all begin to deteriorate with the onset of menopause, then they probably will. But if, instead, you believe that your

best years are still ahead of you, that beauty increases with wisdom and experience, that your later years offer unparalleled freedom and opportunity for new creative endeavors, then that is the reality you will create.

We women are often experts at suppressing our innermost thoughts. We have learned through years of conditioning to keep up appearances and to insist that everything is fine when our bodies and souls silently scream the opposite. We try so hard to please our partners, children, parents, friends, and neighbors, and to be all they would like us to be, that we lose sight of who we are and what we believe. We try to become everything to everyone, yet end up being nothing to ourselves. We carry around vestiges of ancient traditions, obsolete fears, and borrowed beliefs, promising that someday when life is less hectic we will sort everything out, and we lose touch with our inner selves.

Menopause is a time when many women rediscover themselves, the self that somehow lost its way in the midst of raising a family, earning a living, and doing life. The process may not be easy, but the rewards of rediscovering yourself can make the journey tremendously worthwhile. Be kind to yourself as you travel this road, and allow your instincts to direct your course.

Now let's take a look at the physiological processes involved in the phenomenon called *menopause.*

⋟ Defining Menopause ⋞

The word *menopause* is derived from two Greek roots: *mens,* meaning monthly, and *pause,* meaning to stop. It refers to the cessation of menstruation and the termination of fertility, events that don't necessarily happen at the same time. The time of a woman's final menstrual period can only be determined retrospectively. When a woman has not had periods for one year, she is said to have passed through menopause and is officially *postmenopausal.*

The span of time before the final menstrual period is known as *perimenopause.* It may last as long as a few months to several years and is characterized by irregular periods and other symptoms, such as hot flashes, changes in sleeping patterns, fatigue, heart palpitations, vaginal dryness, mood swings, and weight gain. The number, degree, and intensity of symptoms vary from woman to woman.

Terminology describing the ovarian and hormonal transitions associated with menopause has changed in the past several years. At one time the term *climacteric,* considered the counterpart of puberty, referred to the entire menopausal process, from the first sign of premenopause to the last menstrual period. It is seldom seen in print anymore, and I personally don't miss it. The word connotes climax and

finality. While it is true that menstruation ceases, menopause is far from being the last chapter of a woman's life.

The term *change of life*, or *the change*, is more representative of the diversity of the entire midlife experience and its accompanying physical, emotional, and spiritual dimensions. These are vague terms, and appropriately so: Each woman defines them as she sees them applying to her individual life. Menopause is unique to each woman; even though some of the symptoms are the same, the number, intensity, and expression of symptoms vary from person to person.

When Will It Begin?

For most American women today, the termination of fertility usually takes place between forty-eight and fifty-two years of age. Interestingly, the mean age of menopause has increased by approximately four years over the past century, and gynecologists report that many women are now still menstruating well into their sixth decade.[14] Improved nutrition, healthier lifestyles, and modern medical advances are the most notable reasons for this increase in childbearing years. This news may be encouraging to women who have postponed having children.

Many factors influence whether menopause will arrive early or late, and these are discussed below.

Lifestyle. Several studies have examined the effect of lifestyle on the onset of menopause. Nutrition in particular appears to be a significant factor. An extensive survey conducted in New Guinea found that undernourished women start menopause around the age of forty-three, while those more adequately nourished do not begin until age forty-seven.[15] Research on large population groups indicates that European women, who supposedly engage in healthier habits than Americans, tend toward a later menopause.

Nature and nurture. Heredity must always be taken into account. There is some indication that women tend to follow in their mothers' footsteps: If the mother had a late menopause, the daughter's may be late as well. But is this nature or nurture? A growing number of scientists believe that the influence is cultural rather than genetic. Children tend to imitate their parents' habits: how much they exercise, how and what they eat, how they handle stress, and whether they smoke cigarettes or drink alcohol. These environmental factors may be at least as important as inherited tendencies.

Smoking. The data from two large, independent studies involving several countries have confirmed that smokers generally experience earlier menopause. There are two probable explanations |for this finding: First, nicotine, which acts on the central nervous system, may decrease the secretion of hormones; second, nicotine may activate liver-metabolizing enzymes that alter the metabolism of the sex-related hormones.[16]

Trauma. A traumatic experience may trigger early or premature menopause. Premature menopause occurs when periods stop permanently before the age of forty. Early menopause may start at any time before the normal age range of forty-eight to fifty-two. Prolonged stress or a crisis can temporarily halt the production of certain hormones, and the ovaries, responding to the lack of these hormones, may cease production of eggs and, subsequently, of estrogen and progesterone. Periods stop and typical menopausal symptoms appear. This *traumatic menopause* should not be confused with

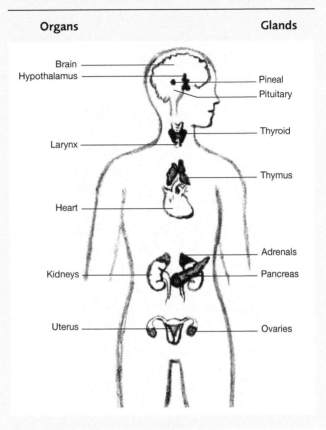

Figure 1. Glands and Organs in the Female Body

Organs — Glands

Brain
Hypothalamus
Larynx
Heart
Kidneys
Uterus

Pineal
Pituitary
Thyroid
Thymus
Adrenals
Pancreas
Ovaries

psychogenic amenorrhea, which is a temporary cessation of periods caused by tension, fatigue, exercise, low body weight, or malnutrition. If an underweight woman stops menstruating because of an inadequate amount of body fat, she will usually resume her normal cycle shortly after her weight returns to normal. In other words, psychogenic amenorrhea is most often temporary; this is not generally the case for women going through premature or traumatic menopause.

A continuously low body weight. Women who have been undernourished for long periods of time are likely to go through menopause several years earlier than the norm. If a woman's body weight remains unnaturally low to the point of anorexia, it is possible that the ovaries will shut down permanently, resulting in premature menopause. Women in their thirties, and even some in their twenties, have ended their childbearing years through self-starvation.

Oophorectomy and hysterectomy. When a woman's ovaries are irreparably damaged or when she has them surgically removed *(ovariectomy or oophorectomy)*, she will begin menopause immediately. This operation should not be confused with a *hysterectomy*, the removal of the uterus alone. Many women are under the impression that after a hysterectomy, the change is imminent. However, though the woman will no longer have periods or be capable of becoming pregnant, if one or both ovaries—or even if only part of one—are left intact, eggs and female hormones will continue to be produced until menopause occurs.[17] A hysterectomy can, however, result in an early menopause, perhaps even by as much as several years.[18] Early menopause is also a possibility whenever the blood circulation is cut off or compromised in any way, such as during sterilization by tubal ligation, or from damage caused by radiation treatment, chemotherapy, and certain diseases.

I would like to digress for a moment. There is considerable controversy today about unnecessary hysterectomy or ovariectomy. Because women have frequently accepted medical recommendations without asking questions or seeking second opinions, they have often been victims of unnecessary surgery. Studies estimate that from 15 percent to 60 percent of all hysterectomies and ovariectomies are unnecessary. Hysterectomies are the second most commonly performed major surgical operation for women in the United States, second only to cesarean section. By age sixty, 25 percent of American women consent to have their uteruses removed and 52 percent of these women elect to have their ovaries removed as well.[19] Are all these operations being performed for valid reasons? Many concerned health advocates think not.

The decision to have one's female organs removed is a serious one. Several books offer guidelines on when hysterectomies may be indicated and when they are normally performed but are not compulsory. If you are faced with making a decision about whether or not to undergo a hysterectomy, begin by gathering as much information as you can, both pro and con. For excellent discussions on this subject, I recommend *The New Our Bodies, Ourselves*, by the Boston Women's Health Book Collective, and *Sudden Menopause*, by Debbie DeAngelo, R.N.C. Ask your physician why surgery is indicated, what exactly is to be removed, what your alternatives are, and what the future implications are. Do not be afraid to ask these questions—it is *your* body. Once you are clear about the basis for the diagnosis, get a second opinion. Before you go ahead, make sure you are satisfied that this is the right choice for you. If surgery is unavoidable (and it may be your *only* option), prepare emotionally and nutritionally to minimize any aftereffects. A healthy mind and a strong body are the best guarantees for a smooth operation and a quick recovery.

Now, let's return to the factors that affect the onset of menopause. As discussed, when estrogen is diminished in any way, menopause is likely to begin early. The biological clock may also operate in reverse: Should the premenopausal supply of estrogen continue as usual, menopause will be delayed.

Drugs that induce menopause. Certain drugs act to block the effects of estrogen in the body. One of the most common of these is tamoxifen (brand name: Nolvadex), used to prevent the return of breast cancer and, in some cases, to reduce the risk of developing breast cancer in certain women with a high risk for the disease. It attaches to estrogen receptors in breast tissue, thus preventing estrogen

Factors That May Influence Timing of the Onset of Menopause	
Earlier	**Later**
genetics	genetics
stress	stress
drugs	drugs
underweight	overweight
damaged female organs	cancer of breast or uterus
hysterectomy	fibroids
tubal ligation	diabetes
smoking	
malnutrition	

from attaching to those same sites and inhibiting its action. Predictably, it also blocks the effects of estrogen in other ways, often resulting in menopause-like symptoms such as hot flashes, and, less frequently, menstrual irregularities and vaginal dryness.

Lupron and Synarel, two drugs used to treat endometriosis, work by suppressing menstruation. Therefore, they can cause menopausal side effects such as hot flashes, headaches, mood swings, decreased sex drive, vaginal dryness, and others. However, most treatment plans involving these drugs last only for up to six months, and when the drug is discontinued, estrogen levels usually return to normal and these symptoms subside.

Excess body fat. One common condition that can *delay* menopause is an excess of body fat. Overweight women menstruate longer than their thinner sisters because their bodies manufacture greater amounts of estrogen. Estrogen is produced not only in the ovaries, but also in the fatty tissues of the body from another hormone, androstenedione. The more fat a woman carries, the more estrogen she makes. I suppose this could be construed as one "natural" way to postpone menopause, but it is certainly not the wisest. For one thing, an overabundance of circulating estrogen increases the risk of estrogen-based cancers. Having a little extra padding is not a worry and may minimize symptoms, but, as in all things, more is not necessarily better.

Other physical problems. Certain diseases have been known to provoke the endocrine system into extending estrogen production. Although the evidence is not

conclusive, physicians have observed that women with cancer of the breast or uterus, women with fibroids, and women who are diabetic may experience menopause somewhat later than the average woman.

Who Experiences Symptoms?

It has been estimated that 75 to 80 percent of women passing through menopause experience one or more symptoms, but only 10 to 35 percent are affected strongly enough to seek professional help. While it is impossible to predict who will suffer severe symptoms, certain generalizations can be made.[20]

Characteristics of Women Likely to Pass Through Menopause Undisturbed

- relatively late onset of menstruation
- never been married
- never been pregnant
- gave birth after age forty
- relatively high income
- better educated

Characteristics of Women Likely to Suffer Severe Menopausal Symptoms

- premenstrual syndrome sufferer
- had premature menopause
- had artificial menopause (oophorectomy)

It is obvious from the above lists that physiology is only one piece of the menopausal puzzle—and probably the easiest part to understand. Why should women who have never been married or who have had a child after forty be less likely to experience menopausal symptoms? Is there another underlying common denominator—lifestyle, education, diet—that might explain these parallels? Future research must address these questions.

Generally, the rate at which estrogen levels drop influences the number and severity of symptoms. Usually, these follow one of the three following patterns:

Pattern A: Abrupt ending. This is the immediate cessation of menstrual periods, where periods stop without prior warning. It is fairly uncommon; in most cases, the ovaries stop functioning gradually. If the estrogen supply stops suddenly, the chances of experiencing symptoms are greater. However, not all women follow the norm. Menopause researcher Rosetta Reitz found a group whose periods stopped abruptly, yet who complained of relatively few symptoms.[21] She presumed these women had a high threshold for discomfort. This suggests that, while there are definable patterns, it is difficult to predict how any one woman will go through the change.

Pattern B: Gradual ending. This is a more common occurrence, involving a progressive decline in both the amount and duration of the menstrual flow. Typically, periods become shorter, are delayed, or are skipped; finally, they terminate altogether. A woman may not even be aware of the irregularity of her cycles. If the ovaries atrophy slowly, if the organs they stimulate are not hypersensitive, and if they continue to supply a sustaining amount of estrogen, symptoms are insignificant.[22]

Pattern C: Irregular ending. Irregular menstrual patterns are also relatively common. The flow may be sporadic; it may become heavier, lighter, or alternate monthly. The number of days between periods may increase or decrease. Some women may go an entire year without one period, and then, without warning, start menstruating again. Many "change-of-life babies" have been born because women thought they could no longer become pregnant and were thus safe. Doctors now urge women to continue birth control for two years after their last period.

Numerous researchers, searching for possible relationships among roles, behavior, and a tendency toward menopausal distress, have found that a psychological component is clearly involved in menopausal distress.[23] How much of a woman's discomfort is physical and how much is a response to cultural expectations and her own belief system is difficult to determine. Each woman's symptoms and physical reactions may be genuine and yet nothing like those of her friends.

⇒ The Menstrual Cycle ⇐

To have a good understanding of the ways in which a woman's body changes from age forty to age sixty, it helps to know how the menstrual cycle works. Even in this age of health consciousness and fitness, too many women do not know what occurs monthly in their bodies. Comprehending how your body works is critical to taking charge of your health and your life. Even if you believe you understand the process of menstruation, please read this section carefully—it may increase your body awareness.

The female menstrual cycle is the twenty-eight-day or twenty-nine-day period that repeats itself monthly for the duration of a woman's fertile life. It involves an interplay among the brain, the ovaries, and four primary hormones,

Figure 2. The Menstrual Cycle

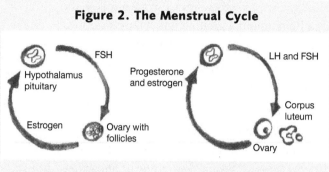

Phase I: Estrogenic

◉ Hypothalamus signals pituitary when hormones are at lowest point

◉ Pituitary sends FSH to ovaries

◉ One follicle matures as egg

◉ Estrogen level signals brain to secrete LH along with FSH

Phase II: Progesteronal

◉ With surge of LH, mature egg is released from ovary

◉ Remnant follicle (corpus luteum) produces progesterone and estrogen

◉ Follicle disintegrates, no longer produces hormones

◉ As hormones diminish, menstruation begins; uterine lining sloughs off

two secreted in the brain and two in the ovaries (see Figures 1 and 2). The release of these hormones is primarily for the purpose of stimulating the cells that line the uterus in preparation for a possible pregnancy. The uterine lining, or endometrium, is built up in the first phase of the cycle and shed during the menstrual period.

A cycle has no beginning or end, but for the purpose of explanation we will start with the physical stages of the menstrual cycle at the *hypothalamus*, an endocrine gland in the brain. Commonly referred to as the "master controller," the hypothalamus plays a key role in many basic bodily functions, such as regulating body temperature, water balance, metabolic rate, appetite, sleep patterns, and tolerance to stress. The hypothalamus sends a message in the form of a hormone to the *anterior pituitary gland*, another endocrine gland located just below the hypothalamus. The tiny pituitary responds to the message by secreting the first hormone of the cycle, called *follicle-stimulating hormone* (FSH). Like all endocrine hormones, FSH is a messenger traveling from one organ to act on another part of the body, in this case, the ovaries.

Within the ovaries are small sacs called *follicles* that contain eggs and the female hormone estrogen. Stimulation from FSH causes one of the follicles to grow, and as it does, estrogen is released. When a specific amount of estrogen is circulating in the bloodstream, the pituitary, again under instructions from the hypothalamus, secretes its second hormone, *luteinizing hormone* (LH). By this time, the egg is mature and ready to burst from the follicle.

The egg is expelled into the fallopian tubes and makes its way into the uterus. The actual release of the egg is called *ovulation*, and it marks roughly the halfway point in the cycle. Remaining behind in the ovary, the remnant follicle is now a functioning endocrine gland called the *corpus luteum*. It is the corpus luteum that

produces both estrogen and proges-terone, the second female hormone, which is dominant in the second half of the cycle. The varying levels of the four hormones active in a typical menstrual cycle are shown in Figure 3.

If the egg is fertilized by a sperm, it implants, or attaches to the lining of the uterus, and a special hormone called *chorionic gonado-tropin* is secreted. This hormone stimulates the continued secretion of estrogen and progesterone so that the developing embryo will be nourished. Without fertilization of the egg and continued hormonal production, the corpus luteum shrivels and dies, and estrogen and progesterone secretion drops. When both hormones reach their lowest point, the thickened uterine lining is sloughed off through the vaginal opening and menstrual flow begins. Low blood levels of estrogen and progesterone then begin to act as a signal to the brain to produce FSH, and the whole process starts again.

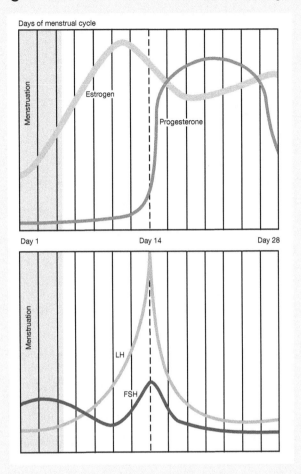

Figure 3. Hormone Levels in the Menstrual Cycle

During the cycle, estrogen's primary function is to increase the blood supply and thus thicken the endometrium, with the goal of creating a suitable environ-ment for the fertilization, implantation, and nutrition of the embryo. Progesterone further prepares the uterus for reception and development of the fertilized ovum by making available an adequate supply of nutrients.

⥲ Changes at Menopause ⥲

The first indication of approaching menopause is the onset of *anovulatory cycles*, that is, cycles in which ovulation does not take place. Ovarian function actually begins to decline several years prior to menopause. The follicles that inhabit the

27

Figure 4. Premenopausal Menstrual Cycles

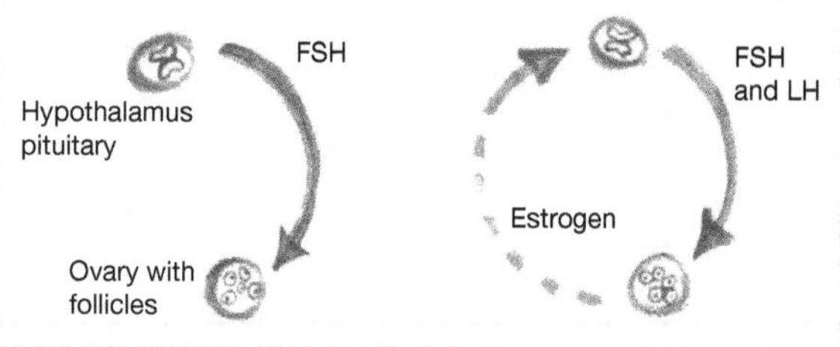

Phase I

- ⊚ Hypothalamus signals pituitary when hormones are low
- ⊚ Pituitary sends FSH to ovaries
- ⊚ Follicle does not respond

Phase II

- ⊚ Follicle may not grow sufficiently to produce egg
- ⊚ No progesterone produced
- ⊚ No period

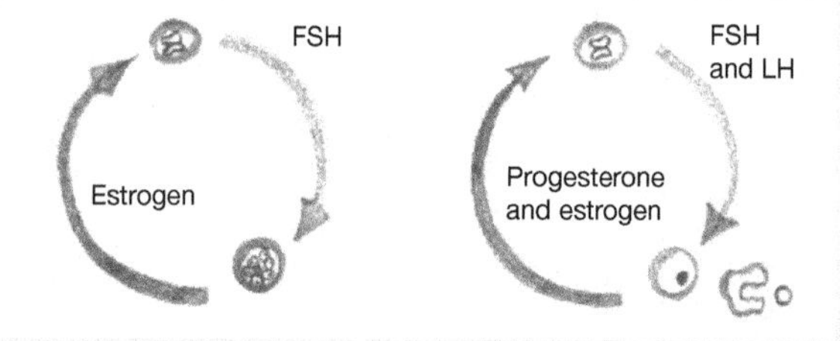

Phase I

- ⊚ Estrogen and progesterone still low
- ⊚ Hypothalamus signals pituitary to send more FSH
- ⊚ Follicle may or may not respond
- ⊚ If it does, estrogen is released

Phase II

- ⊚ Follicle may eventually produce egg
- ⊚ Estrogen and progesterone
- ⊚ Periods erratic

ovaries gradually diminish in number starting at birth, reducing from an initial 2 million potential eggs at birth to approximately 400,000 at menarche and about 25,000 at the beginning of perimenopause. With fewer follicles, some months may pass when menstruation does not occur. No follicle means no egg, no estrogen, no corpus luteum, no progesterone, and no period (see Figure 4). As the ovaries continue to reduce their production of estrogen and progesterone, the pituitary gland, in a desperate effort to stimulate the recalcitrant ovaries, pumps greater amounts of FSH and LH into the blood. FSH escalates, reaching levels thirteen times that of normal cycles, while LH levels rise approximately threefold.[24] As explained to me by gynecologist Larry Francis, this elevation of hormones is most commonly and easily used by physicians to test for the onset of menopause.

In the perimenopausal period, the levels of the brain hormones increase, while the ovarian hormone levels decrease. When the ovaries stop producing eggs, progesterone, which depends on a corpus luteum for production, is no longer secreted. Estrogen, however, can still be manufactured by the ovaries (although in smaller amounts), by the adrenal glands, and by extraglandular sources (including certain fat cells). During the premenopausal stage, the uterine lining is being stimulated exclusively by estrogen. With no periodic shedding of the uterine lining, the tissues continue to proliferate until the lining outgrows its blood-vessel supply. It may be several months before this happens; thus, periods are often missed or irregular. When the uterine lining does break down and disintegrate, it often comes off haphazardly, in uneven patches, resulting in a heavier than normal period.

Ultimately, the ovarian follicles no longer respond to the prodding of FSH and LH. Estrogen levels drop too low to cause growth in the uterine lining, menstruation ceases completely, and menopause begins. Although the mature ovary no longer ovulates, it has not ceased functioning altogether. In fact, the central region of the ovary is actively engaged in producing hormones that are converted into *estrone*, the form of estrogen that remains circulating in the blood after menopause. Tests have shown that some women show significant evidence of estrogenic activity more than twenty years after their last period.[25] Usually, the adrenal glands become the major source of postmenopausal estrogen. In fact, maintaining healthy adrenals may be one of the best ways to ensure continued estrogen production and a smoother transition.

Estrone is also converted in the body fat from another hormone, androstenedione. As was mentioned earlier, women with ample fat on their bodies not only experience menopause later because of higher estrogen levels, they also appear to suffer less discomfort than their thinner sisters. The conversion of androstenedione into estrone has been found to occur in the muscle, liver, kidney, brain, and possibly other unknown extraglandular sources.[26] Clearly, as the ovaries slow down, the production of estrogen diminishes, but the body readjusts, substituting other estrogen sources.

> ### Physiological Changes Following Menopause

Estrogen is of primary importance in the female life cycle. The amount of estrogen circulating in the body, its ratio to other hormones, and its rate of change and decline prior to menopause all have effects on physical health and emotional outlook. Estrogen acts directly on the uterus and influences other organs and tissues, such as the vulva, vagina, breasts, bones, hair, skin, heart, and central nervous system. As the level of estrogen decreases, substantial changes occur in the appearance

What Happens to the Hormones at Menopause

- Ovarian activity decreases.
  - Estrogen is produced in decreased amounts.
  - Progesterone is no longer secreted.
- Brain hormones temporarily increase.
  - FSH and LH are produced in greater amounts.
- Estrone is produced from various sources, including
  - adrenal glands
  - body fat
  - extraglandular sources
  - ovaries

and function of all these organs. This is not to say that every menopausal symptom is related to declining estrogen levels; some are connected to other diminishing hormones like progesterone and testosterone, and some are the natural results of aging. Postmenopausal women experience varying degrees of atrophic (shrinking and thinning) changes of the vagina, cervix, uterus, and ovaries. Most women can expect a decrease in the size of the cervix and uterus, accompanied by a reduction in cervical mucus. Some women become more prone to bacterial infections because of the decline in cervical secretions. The labia majora (larger skin folds of the vulva) become thinner, flatter, paler, and less elastic. The vaginal wall shortens and loses its muscle tone as well as some of its normal secretions, sometimes making intercourse uncomfortable or painful.

Structures around the reproductive organs suffer loss of muscle tone as a result of natural aging and lack of exercise. In the extreme state, the relaxed structures fall into other organs. For example, the uterus may fall, causing the cervix to rest on or even enter the vaginal wall. A sensation of heaviness in the vaginal area or the feeling that tissue is protruding outward may indicate a descending bladder, uterus, or rectum. Lack of muscle tone may also cause the urinary sphincter muscles to fail to contract satisfactorily, so that urine escapes when the individual laughs, sneezes, coughs, or lifts heavy objects. Uncontrollable urinary leaking (incontinence) can be prevented or relieved through special exercises, called Kegel exercises, described in Chapter 5.

Fat disappears from the breast tissue, reducing the breasts' size, shape, and firmness. Nipples tend to become smaller and less erect. Some women report decreased sexual stimulation from the breast, but whether this change is caused by physical or psychological reasons is undetermined. On the positive side, women who have been tormented by fibrocystic breast disease (lumpy, painful breasts) will be relieved to know that this discomfort usually subsides during or after menopause.

Aging also creates obvious changes in the hair and skin. Body hair may thin out in some women and increase in others. New growth on the upper lip and chin is ascribed to the reversed ratio of estrogen to androgen. While women always have the "male" hormone androgen in their systems, it is only after menopause that the hormone generally shows its presence in a physically discernible way.

Wrinkling and loss of skin tone are particularly noticeable around the face, neck, and hands. Characteristic "purse-string" wrinkles form around the mouth, and "crow's feet" develop at the corners of the eyes. Natural preventive measures, such as consuming a diet rich in antioxidants and moisturizing the skin with products that include glycolic acids, alpha hydroxy acids, and retin A, can minimize at least some of these fine aging lines.

For many years, women passively accepted the "matronly" image of aging: As women get older, their body configuration alters, fat redistributes, metabolism slows down, and there is a tendency to gain weight. This image is changing. With a little conscious effort, regular exercise, and fewer calories, women are working to maintain healthy, trim, and toned figures throughout their lives.

When hormone levels fall, the bones tend to lose density. Reduced estrogen activity has been directly related to accelerated bone loss, and diminishing progesterone as well as testosterone levels also may also play a part. Loss of bone mass is believed by many researchers to account for the prevalence of hip and vertebral fractures as well as the hunched-over posture of some older women. All women should be particularly aware that diet and exercise—especially in the early adult years—are keys to preventing this crippling disease, osteoporosis.

Physical Changes at Midlife

- Some atrophying of vagina, cervix, uterus, and ovaries takes place.
- Vaginal wall shortens, thins out, and loses muscle tone.
- Labia majora become thinner, paler, and less elastic.
- Supporting structures (sphincter muscles, bladder, rectum) lose muscle tone.
- Secretion of cervical mucus is reduced.
- Breast size, firmness, and shape changes.
- Body hair gets thinner in most women; in some, it increases.
- Wrinkling and loss of skin tone occur.
- Body fat is redistributed.
- Bone mass is lost.
- Metabolic rate slows.

Clearly, all the female hormones are vital to the female body. When we produce too much or too little, symptoms occur. However, even though more than fifty symptoms have been attributed to the endocrine changes that occur during the change—tiredness, nervousness, headaches, irritability, depression, insomnia, joint and muscle pain, dizziness, heart palpitation, breathlessness, and impatience, among others—a direct cause-and-effect relationship for each has not been clearly determined. Ovarian decline and diminished hormonal levels are hardly the only factors to consider. More important may be the overall health of the individual and her ability to adapt to the transitions taking place in her organ systems and in her life.

⇒ Diagnosing Perimenopause ⇐

The first signs of perimenopause appear as symptoms: heavy and irregular periods, hot flashes, night sweats, and urinary incontinence. If you're in your mid-forties or older and experiencing any of these conditions, you probably don't need verification that you're on the cusp of menopause. A younger woman, on the other hand, may want to check out her symptoms with clinical tests. Sometimes your doctor will order a blood test to determine FSH levels, because these levels characteristically remain high during perimenopause. Confusingly, this is not always true; FSH levels

may continue to fluctuate, so your reading may indicate normal even though you're definitely premenopausal. Blood tests for levels of estrogen and progesterone are also sometimes performed; however, most doctors find levels of these hormones so variable that they cannot reliably indicate a woman's status.

A product called the Menopause Home Test has been cleared by the FDA. It can help you and your health-care provider determine if you are in menopause by gauging the level of FSH in your body. Since the product enables you to track FSH levels over time rather than to get just one reading, it can be helpful in determining which form of therapy may be best for you. According to Judith Reichman, women's medical advisor for *The Today Show*, the Menopause Home Test is 99-percent accurate compared to blood tests performed by physicians. To get more information about this test, log on to www.power-surge.com.

The next chapter addresses the confusion over hormone therapy. Subsequent chapters discuss in more detail specific symptoms and problems associated with menopause. Remember that, for the most part, suffering through severe symptoms is neither normal nor necessary. In most cases, a commonsense approach to nutrition, regular exercise, and an otherwise healthy lifestyle are the only "medication" you will need.

CHAPTER 2

HORMONES

DISPELLING THE CONFUSION

*We are not spiritually unconnected from the drugs we take, or from the
pain and suffering that goes into their making.*

— ALICE WALKER

E very woman over fifty can tell you where she was when she heard the news
that certain hormone preparations increase the risk of breast cancer. The
study, known as the Women's Health Initiative (WHI), sponsored by the
National Institutes of Health and reported in the *Journal of the American
Medical Association*, was abruptly ended in 2002 when surprised researchers discovered that the risks of taking a particular combination of estrogen with progestin
outweighed the benefits. The widely anticipated study quashed the hopes of doctors who firmly believed in the medication's efficacy. Furthermore, the six million
American women who had been prescribed the particular hormone preparation
under scrutiny were forced to question the trust they had placed in the medical
establishment. Executives at Wyeth-Ayerst, the drug company that supplied pills
for the study and that sold its product to all these midlife women, also must have
been numbed as they watched the firm's stock plummet 24 percent in one day.

Until the fateful announcement, approximately 38 percent of U.S. women
between the ages of fifty and seventy-four used hormone replacement therapy
(HRT).[1] The majority of women on hormones took either Premarin, an estrogen-
only preparation, or Prempro, which is Premarin with the addition of progestin,
a synthetic form of progesterone. By 2000, forty-six million prescriptions of
Premarin made it the second most popular medication in the United States; it raked
in more than a billion dollars in sales for Wyeth-Ayerst.[2] Although Prempro's sales
were only about half of Premarin's staggering numbers, they had been growing
steadily—as had its manufacturer's profits.

A Brief History of HRT

Originally, the U.S. Food and Drug Administration approved the use of estrogen for the short-term relief of menopausal symptoms. Later, long-term use of estrogen for the prevention of osteoporosis was also approved, until the increased risk of endometrial cancer from estrogen-only preparations led to the addition of the second female hormone, progesterone. Because of the increased risk of endometrial cancer with unopposed estrogen therapy, it is the combination of estrogen and progesterone that is recommended for women who still have their uterus (that is, women who have not undergone a hysterectomy).

Widespread use of either estrogen or the combination of estrogen and progesterone continued to extend far beyond the FDA's original intent; doctors prescribed the drugs to treat conditions collectively couched under the umbrella of "quality-of-life symptoms." Women were swallowing hormones not only to stop hot flashes and to build their bones, but also to keep mentally sharp, lubricate the vaginal wall, and plump up their skin. HRT seemed to hold such promise that most doctors confidently encouraged their menopausal patients to take it for annoying symptoms and to protect their heart and bones. Several doctors tried to convince me that Premarin would be beneficial to my heart, even after I reminded them that the results from the Heart and Estrogen/Progestin Replacement Study (HERS) in 2000 told us this was not necessarily the case (for more on the HERS study, see Chapter 9). But these physicians were unwavering supporters of HRT and not about to bend.

That is, until the *Journal of the American Medical Association (JAMA)* report of July 2002 rocked their world. The prestigious journal asserted that HRT caused an increased risk of breast cancer significant enough that the huge Women's Health Initiative study was stopped immediately. Women and their doctors were at a loss about what to do. Some women discontinued treatment immediately, only to find their symptoms returning. Others chose to continue taking their pills, hoping they would miss becoming one of the unlucky ones to discover a lump in their breast. Still others turned to herbs and soy to treat their menopausal symptoms, while wondering about the health of their bones and trying to figure out what the studies meant for them. The answers are not clear-cut and probably won't be for several years, and they are definitely not the same for all women. More than ever, in order to make wise personal decisions, we need *all* the information—information that has been available but not widely promoted.

❧ A Closer Look at the WHI Study ❧

The WHI was not just another study in the long history of conflicting hormonal research. It was the *crème de la crème,* the gold standard of scientific evidence. It involved a large sampling of 16,608 healthy, ethnically diverse postmenopausal women between the ages of fifty and seventy-nine. It was designed to definitively answer nagging concerns about HRT. The women were divided into various study groups; members of one group took estrogen plus progestin (specifically, Prempro), and members of another group were given a look-alike dummy pill (placebo). As in all double-blind studies, the two groups were compared and evaluated; neither the women being studied nor the researchers they came into contact with knew whether they were in the group receiving the real drug or the group receiving placebo.

You know how the story ends. This long-awaited study that was scheduled to continue for three more years, until 2005, was ended abruptly when a routine data-monitoring board examining the results to date noticed that the accumulating numbers exceeded the upper limit of risk. According to acting director of the study Jacques E. Rossouw, "The breast cancer risk exceeded the predefined boundary for safety."[3] This meant that the same doctors who had so adamantly supported synthetic HRT were forced to notify women to stop taking it immediately.

The primary reason the WHI trial terminated prematurely was because the women taking Prempro showed an increased risk of invasive breast cancer. Even though researchers assure us that the risk to one individual woman is small for breast cancer, several other outcomes of the study forced the decision to terminate.

Specifically, the data showed the following additional risks per ten thousand person-years among women who took the estrogen-progestin combination:

- eight more invasive breast cancers

- seven more coronary heart disease events

- eight more strokes

- eight more pulmonary embolisms (PEs)

Risk reductions per ten thousand person-years among women who took the drug included the following:

- six fewer colorectal cancers

- five fewer hip fractures[4]

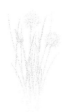

("Person-years" are similar in concept to "man-hours." Five thousand individuals who took the drug for two years would equal ten thousand person-years; likewise, ten thousand individuals who took the drug for one year would also equal ten thousand person-years.)

At first glance, these numbers don't seem particularly scary—unless, of course, you are one of the seven or eight additional women who contracted breast cancer, heart disease, stroke, or a PE. Statistics are cold and often difficult to grasp and personalize. *The John R. Lee, M.D., Medical Letter* clarifies these numbers and provides a greater appreciation for what they really mean. He points out that for the six million women who were using Prempro (a conservative estimate), the above numbers translate to approximately 4,800 more women who could expect to get breast cancer, 4,200 more who could expect to suffer from heart disease, and so on.[5] (This is assuming that the women in question only took the drug for one year, resulting in six million person-years. If they took it for longer—and note that the WHI study followed its subjects for an average of 5.2 years—then the numbers go proportionally higher.) I don't know about you, but this doesn't sound like a small risk to me.

An important point needs to be emphasized about this study. The trial tested only two drugs, Premarin and Prempro. (The above results were observed only for Prempro; the WHI study of the effects of Premarin continues.) However, everyone seems to be equating these two hormone combinations with all HRT therapies. They are not all the same. Differences do exist, and I will soon elaborate on them. Furthermore, the trial used only one single-dosing regimen (one tablet containing 0.625 mg conjugated equine estrogens, plus 2.5 mg medroxyprogesterone acetate, a form of progestin). We don't know if the results can be extrapolated to lower doses or to other formulations. Even the authors of the study acknowledge that it is possible that transdermal estradiol with progesterone (*not* progestin), which more closely mimics the normal physiology and metabolism of human sex hormones, may provide a different risk-benefit profile. The remainder of this chapter looks at different hormone preparations that are available and presently being used both in the United States and in Europe. One or more of these may offer a safer alternative than conventional HRT while proving more effective than herbal preparations.

One personal reflection: We have received a loud wake-up call. Until the unforgettable 2002 WHI report, doctors handed out samples of Prempro like candy and too many women casually took them without question. Safer alternatives for menopausal symptoms have been available and discussed for many years; this book, for one, was first published in 1989. I realize that many of you have mentioned

herbs, vitamins, and soy to your doctors, and that they in turn made you feel stupid and naïve. Now they will be forced to open their collective minds and pay attention to your alternative suggestions. This is a fantastic opportunity for us to voice our opinions. More women than I like to admit never questioned these courses of treatment, even in light of early reports about their possible risks. We need to take the time to learn all we can about our bodies and what we put in them. Hormones still may be an option for you, but before you make that decision, understand if and why you need them, which ones are the safest, and how to determine whether they are wrong or right for you. You must do your own homework; do not let one doctor or one TV celebrity convince you about what is best for you. Be your own advocate. Read, study, and compare, and then decide for yourself.

Estrogen

So how does a woman answer these questions for herself? How does she wade through all of the hype about hormones and find some real answers? This chapter can be a starting place. The rest of it is devoted to describing the different sex hormones that circulate in our bodies, as well as some of the options available for rebalancing them, if necessary, with different forms of hormone replacement therapy. The range of choices you have may surprise you. Many women are unaware that options exist for HRT beyond the synthetic drugs that have been doled out so readily for the past several decades.

Let's start by looking at the hormone most women think of first when they wonder how to counteract menopausal symptoms: estrogen.

QUESTIONING CONVENTIONAL ESTROGEN THERAPY

Premarin entered the market in 1949 as the first oral hormonal preparation; it continues to be one of the most prescribed drugs in the United States. It has dominated all the large-scale studies on HRT and thus provides us with considerable research into its benefits, risks, and side effects. Premarin is an oral compound known as conjugated equine estrogens (CEE). If you examine the word *equine*, you will realize it means "horse." In fact, the name *Pre-mar-in* tells you exactly what the drug is: pregnant mare's urine. There is no doubt that horse estrogen exerts estrogen-like effects in the human body and works quite well to reduce the symptoms of menopause; it is instrumental in preventing the further loss of bone and thus protecting women from osteoporosis. But it comes from the urine of a four-legged, pregnant animal sporting a tail. It is not native to female humans—female horses, sure; women, no.

Many women who are otherwise complacent about the source of the pill they have been consuming are incensed by the method in which this hormone is derived. If you are at all sensitive to animal cruelty, you, too, will be outraged. The pregnant mare is confined in a concrete stall, not much larger than her body size, for most of the eleven-month pregnancy. She is unable to turn around and barely gets to move while the urine is collected in a cup fastened to her body. After giving birth, she enjoys a few months of freedom before she is reimpregnated and returned to confinement. The foals are either discarded or kept as replacements for worn-out mares. For detailed information about this practice, log on to www.Menopause Online.com.

Premarin has been labeled "natural" because it comes from a living animal, but chemically it is unlike the hormones produced by women. Our bodies operate on three unique estrogens that are present in approximately the following ratio:

estriol, 60–90 percent

estrone, 10–20 percent

estradiol, 10–20 percent

(Read more about the human estrogen trio on page 40.) Contrast this with Premarin, which is a mixture of estrone (75–80 percent), equilin (5–6 percent), and estradiol, plus other horse estrogens (5–19 percent).[6] Notice the difference in both the kinds and the amounts of hormones. The estrogen found in the greatest amount in the human female body, estriol, is left completely out of the mix, and the proportion of estrone ranks far higher in Premarin than it occurs in women naturally. Equilin and other horse estrogens are not molecules we find anywhere in the human chemical makeup. They are specific to horses. We really don't know how equilin affects a woman's body, because the drug companies have not spent any money pursuing this question.

It is the opinion of a great many doctors and clinicians that the reason some women suffer horrendous side effects from Premarin is because it is foreign to a woman's body. Premarin is not metabolized in the body in the same way that human hormones are. A woman's body contains all the essential enzymes and cofactors it needs to process its native hormones when they are present in their natural proportions. The more potent hormones, such as estradiol, naturally break down into weaker "daughter" compounds. However, Premarin doesn't contain the necessary enzymes and cofactors to metabolize equilin, and as a result, the horse estrogen stays in a woman's body longer, producing a more potent and long-lasting effect on our estrogen receptors. Levels of equilin metabolites (products of metabolism) can remain elevated in the body for up to thirteen weeks or more after being

ingested, due to storage and slow release from the fat tissues.[7] Maybe it's not the hormones per se in HRT that increase the risk for breast cancer.

NATURAL ESTROGEN: A BETTER CHOICE

A fairly recent development in the management of menopausal symptoms is the growing interest in natural, or bioidentical, hormones. Because these hormones have not been subjected to the extensive research the synthetic ones have, you may be unaware that natural hormones exist and that they offer an alternative that appears to be safer and relatively free from side effects. Pharmaceutical companies have little incentive to invest their money in a product they can't exclusively patent, which is the case with natural hormones. It is estimated that it costs a pharmaceutical company between 300 and 500 million dollars to research and bring to market a new prescription drug. A drug company cannot patent a product unless its chemical formula is original. Since natural hormones are derived from natural materials, anyone can make them, so no one has the opportunity to monopolize the market. Anyone can produce them, so they are marketed at a much-reduced profit margin. Even so, natural hormones are FDA approved, just like the synthetics, and are available through a compounding pharmacy with a doctor's prescription (read more about compounding pharmacies later in the chapter). Healthcare providers who prescribe both synthetic and natural hormones report that women experience fewer side effects with the natural ones, and that once they switch away from synthetics, they never go back.

Considerable confusion abounds over the definition of the term *natural hormone*. Most people assume that a synthetic hormone is made in a lab, whereas a natural hormone originates directly from the wild or nature. This is not the case. Both are made in the lab, and even synthetics can be derived from natural products. The difference between the two is not their source—whether they come from soy, yam, or urine, or whether they were developed in a test tube. The primary distinction lies in their basic molecular arrangement. If the chemical structure of the product identically matches a woman's naturally occurring hormone, it is considered "natural." Simply stated, a natural hormone exactly replicates the human female hormone. Another, more precise label for "natural hormone" is "bioidentical hormone." Premarin has a chemical composition very close to that of a woman's natural hormone, but the two are not identical. Some estrogens that come from soy or from the Mexican yam claim to be natural, but if the chemical composition does not match that of a woman's natural hormone, then the estrogen is not truly natural and will not be accepted by the body as its own.

Some brand names of natural hormone preparations (estrogen only) include Estraderm, Estrace, Vivelle, and Climara.

THE HUMAN ESTROGEN TRIO

When we speak of the female hormone estrogen we refer to it in the singular; however, a woman's body manufactures a trio of estrogens that circulate in the body at all times. The three sisters, which function differently and at different stages in a woman's life, are estradiol, estrone, and estriol. Understanding how they differ can help us make a more informed decision about the products we decide to use.

Estradiol is produced mainly by the ovaries each month and is the estrogen most constant in our body throughout life. As the most powerful of the three, unopposed estradiol is most implicated in an increased risk for breast cancer. Estradiol is commonly, and sometimes exclusively, used in conventional hormone therapy.

Estrone is the estrogen associated with the menopausal woman. It is made in the adrenal glands and the ovaries and is also derived from body fat. Women who store more fat seem to complain less of menopausal symptoms because of the presence of greater amounts of this circulating estrogen in their bodies. Estrone functions like estradiol but is considered weaker in its effects. Some studies have found higher levels of circulating estrone in women with breast cancer.

Estriol is produced in the ovaries and the placenta during pregnancy and is the weakest of the three estrogens. It is a breakdown product of the other two and helps keep the body in equilibrium. Studies from the United States and Europe indicate that it is probably the safest of the three and holds much promise as a replacement for estradiol and equilin in HRT preparations. Estriol has been widely used by women in several European countries for the past fifty years, primarily for menopausal symptoms.

ESTRIOL: THE HOPE OF HRT

Recent studies have validated some of the anecdotal accounts that short-term use of estriol does relieve menopausal symptoms such as hot flashes, vaginal dryness, insomnia, and urinary tract infections.[8, 9] Whether women can take it long-term is still unanswered, but reports are hopeful. Additionally, its effects on the heart show promise, even though research addressing this issue is scant. One study showed that in women taking estriol, total cholesterol was lowered, HDL levels improved, and triglycerides came down (as contrasted with the effects of conjugated, or mixed, estrogens, which raised them).[10] Two decades ago a study reported in *JAMA* indicated that when women took between 2 and 8 mg/day of estriol for six months, it did not affect their blood pressure, weight, Pap smears, or mammograms.[11] What is still unknown is whether estriol prevents bone loss, as estradiol does. Some of the research looks promising; however, it is not consistent enough to make any claims at this time.

How estriol effects breast tissue is an ongoing debate that has yet to be resolved. Early studies led us to believe that estriol may be protective against breast cancer; in fact, it has actually been used as a treatment for breast cancer. An important study reported in 1966 showed that higher levels of estriol in the body correlated with remission of breast cancer.[12] It is still too soon to make any proclamations about the safety of estriol in relation to breast cancer, but one point is crystal clear: We need more research on this overlooked estrogen.

If estriol is safer, is effective in treating menopausal symptoms, and stands the test of time, why have so few studies on it been conducted? It has been over twenty years since this question was first posed to the medical community in the *Journal of the American Medical Association.* The author of the article, Alvin H. Follingstad, M.D., publicly complained about the lack of large clinical trials on estriol, which are needed for FDA approval.[13] Even at that time Dr. Follingstad felt enough presumptive and scientific evidence had been accumulated indicating that estriol is safer than estrone and estradiol, yet two decades later practitioners and women still wait. Without a doubt, more large-scale trials are needed to answer the questions about estriol, especially regarding its role in cancer. Until that happens, the existing research from Europe and the United States, scant though it may be, indicates that estriol is a better bet for hormone replacement than the options usually foisted upon us.

Increasingly, clinicians who practice "alternative" medicine are combining estriol with estradiol and estrone (both of which have been subjected to more research than estriol) for the prevention of osteoporosis and other menopausal symptoms. Jonathan Wright, M.D., a well-respected expert in nutritional medicine and a pioneer in the field of HRT, has developed a tri-estrogen formula containing all three estrogens in a balanced ratio closely replicating that in a woman's body: estriol (80 percent), estradiol (10 percent), and estrone (10 percent). He and others have been using this recipe for almost twenty years and have found that it very effectively relieves a variety of menopausal symptoms. All of the natural hormones used by Dr. Wright are derived from the Mexican wild yam (genus: *Diascorea*). He makes it a point to say that you can't get a significant amount of these hormones from eating the Mexican yam or from using creams derived from the yam directly, because the body lacks the requisite chemical cofactors required to convert the substances contained in these products into useful hormones. This must be accomplished in

Symptoms of Estrogen Deficiency	Symptoms of Estrogen Excess
◉ hot flashes	◉ mood swings (PMS)
◉ night sweats	◉ tender breasts
◉ vaginal dryness	◉ fibrocystic breasts
◉ foggy thinking	◉ water retention
◉ memory lapses	◉ nervousness/anxiety
◉ irritability	◉ irritability
◉ incontinence	◉ uterine fibroids
◉ bladder or vaginal infections	◉ weight gain in hips
◉ crying jags	◉ heavy menstrual bleeding
◉ depression	◉ severe headaches
◉ sleep disturbances	◉ recurrent vaginal yeast infections
◉ heart palpitations	◉ red flush on face
◉ decreased libido	◉ nausea
	◉ leg cramps

a laboratory. In his book *Natural Hormone Replacement*, Dr. Wright goes into greater detail, elaborating on the research and the usage of his formulation.[14]

Another option prescribed by some practitioners is a bi-estrogen formula combining estriol (80 percent) and estradiol (20 percent). The theory behind this blend is that menopausal women already have ample estrone in their bodies; concern continues that estrone may produce more unwanted metabolites and possibly bear a negative effect on breast tissue. Whichever recipe you consider, both are safer than products using either horse urine or 100 percent estradiol.

Both formulas are available through a compounding pharmacy, and either can be mixed with other hormones such as progesterone or testosterone. An experienced pharmacist, working with you and your doctor, can easily adjust the dosage according to your hormonal levels and symptoms. You also have a choice of delivery methods. Compounded products can be formulated to order in capsules, creams, lozenges, or suppositories.

DO YOU NEED ESTROGEN REPLACEMENT?

Unopposed estrogen therapy, also called *estrogen replacement therapy*, or *ERT*, may be unwise for some women who have a family history of breast cancer, blood clots, gallbladder disease, or migraines, or who themselves have high triglyceride levels. Additionally, estrogen alone is never a safe option for women who still have their uterus, due to the substantially increased risk it causes of endometrial cancer, which is cancer of the uterine lining. For women who have not undergone a hysterectomy, doctors prescribing hormone treatment always prescribe some form of estrogen plus progesterone. Considering these health risks, speak to your health provider about estrogen therapy even if you decide you want to take natural hormones.

Unbearable menopausal symptoms are often what drive women to use hormones. When we're out of balance, we will try almost anything to feel normal again. Conventional wisdom tells us that once perimenopause hits and we experience symptoms, we must boost estrogen to balance our dwindling levels. However, this is not always the case. Our bodies may be struggling to find a new equilibrium and in doing so actually may be producing too much estrogen rather than too little. Anything can happen during these perimenopausal years, and to blame all our symptoms on declining estrogen levels is an oversimplification of what may be occurring. Moreover, if we increase the estrogen dosage in an already estrogen-rich body, symptoms may get worse rather than better. To help you evaluate whether you have too little or too much circulating estrogen, consider the lists of symptoms found in the box on the previous page. You may find yourself with symptoms from both lists, which indicates that your perimenopause symptoms are not just about estrogen deficiency.

⇒ Progesterone ⇐

Progesterone is the "other" female hormone that women require monthly to maintain hormonal balance. It is synthesized in the body from cholesterol—as are all the steroid hormones—and is influential in the second half of the menstrual cycle, following ovulation. It also can be produced in the adrenal glands and the placenta during the first trimester of pregnancy. Progesterone is just as necessary to the female reproductive system as estrogen, but it has a completely different set of functions. It is unique in that it is a precursor to other hormones and can create and help to balance estrogen, testosterone, and cortisol, the stress hormone. It is involved in thyroid function and blood-sugar metabolism; it communicates with the central nervous system and stimulates bone growth. Most people think that estrogen is the female hormone that protects our bones. While it is true that estrogen helps prevent or slow bone loss, it is actually progesterone that initiates the building-up process.

QUESTIONING SYNTHETIC PROGESTINS

For the treatment of menopausal symptoms, synthetic progesterones, correctly known as *progestins*, are often added to estrogen to counter problems associated

Do You Need Supplemental Progesterone?

Whether or not you need supplemental progesterone depends on your blood levels of the hormone as well as on your symptoms. The following lists offer clues to help you decide:

Symptoms of Progesterone Deficiency

- premenstrual migraine
- PMS
- irregular or excessive menstrual bleeding
- anxiety

Symptoms of Imbalance (Decreased Progesterone/Excess Estrogen)

- bloating
- irregular periods
- mood swings
- weight gain (especially in the stomach area)
- premenstrual headaches
- painful breasts
- cold hands and feet
- decreased sex drive

Symptoms of Excess Progesterone

- sleepiness
- dizziness
- depression

with using estrogen alone. It is generally accepted that the combination of both hormones protects the endometrial lining, reducing the risk of uterine cancer.[15] Women who have had a hysterectomy and who opt for hormonal treatment most likely take only estrogen since they have no uterine lining to protect. Although this is the standard treatment, many health professionals disagree with offering any woman—whether or not she has an intact uterus—only one hormone and not the other, because our bodies naturally produce both estrogen and progesterone. Splitting up the pair can lead to imbalance, symptoms, and possibly greater problems years later.

Synthetic progestins may protect the uterus, but as part of the HRT duo they come with a high price tag: an increased risk for breast cancer and other serious conditions. As discussed earlier in the chapter, the definitive results of the WHI concluded that conventional HRT (specifically, the drug Prempro) increased the risk of breast cancer, heart attacks, stroke, and pulmonary embolism. When the news broke in the summer of 2002, doctors and women gasped at the results. But I'm left wondering why they had this reaction. Just two years prior, the National Cancer Institute reported in the *Journal of the American Medical Association* that women who used HRT sustained an even greater risk for developing breast cancer than women taking estrogen alone (read more about this study in Chapter 10).[16] Stacks of research papers preceded that one, and several books have been written warning women of this link. A study from the University of Southern California arrived at the same conclusion: There is strong evidence that the addition of a progestin to HRT markedly enhances the risk of breast cancer.[17] Folks, this is not new information.

Taking natural progesterone rather than a synthetic product is just as vital as taking natural estrogen. Clearly, an undeniable difference exists between what is native to the human body and what is not. Progestins are chemically altered hormones and therefore do not behave like the ones our bodies manufacture. These progesterone look-alikes exert a more powerful influence because they are treated by the body as foreign substances and metabolized into substances whose effects on the body haven't yet been studied. Progestins occupy progesterone receptor sites and thus interfere with the production of natural progesterone and its ability to balance deficiencies or excesses of other steroid hormones. Finally, it has been known for some time that adding progestin to estrogen negates the cardio-protective effects of estrogen, which is not the case with natural progesterone.[18]

Most women on conventional HRT who are prescribed a progestin get it in the form of medroxyprogesterone acetate (brand names: Provera and Cycrin), which is the substance added to Premarin to make Prempro. Some women do just fine taking Premarin—but add Provera or Cycrin and they report a litany of symptoms. Side effects including depression, moodiness, breast tenderness and enlargement, increased appetite, abdominal cramps, and headaches are the complaints that usually turn women off from HRT. Other considerations are the medical conditions that may affect a woman's tolerance to progestins; these include asthma, blood clots (or history of), cancer (or history of), changes in vaginal bleeding, diabetes, epilepsy, heart or circulatory disease, high blood cholesterol, kidney disease, liver or gallbladder disease, mental depression (or history of), migraine headaches, and stroke (or history of).[19] Furthermore, progestin must not be used during pregnancy or during pregnancy tests because it might harm the fetus; however, natural progesterone is frequently used to treat infertility.

NATURAL PROGESTERONE

As discussed in the earlier section on estrogen, most of the hormonal treatments on the market are synthetic, but a growing number of doctors believe that if natural products were used, the medical risks and side effects of HRT would be considerably lessened. Research utilizing hormones from natural sources is sparse, but preliminary studies show that natural hormones offer the same benefits as synthetic analogs but with fewer side effects. As with natural estrogen, the natural form of progesterone is derived from soybeans or yams, but what defines it as "natural," or "bioidentical," isn't its source but rather the chemical structure of the hormone. It must exactly match the molecular configuration found in a woman's own body.

The bioidentical version of progesterone outshines progestins in every area. It helps to balance estrogen as well as other sex hormones; it is utilized more efficiently and leaves the body quickly, like our own hormones; and side effects often experienced with synthetics—such as fluid retention, breast tenderness, depression,

and weight gain—are nonexistent.[20] Natural progesterone is also well-tolerated. In a study of oral micronized progesterone tablets, dizziness and sleepiness were listed as the only side effects, and they could be suppressed by taking the pills at bedtime.[21]

Natural progesterone is also superior to progestins when it comes to the heart. The famous PEPI (Postmenopausal Estrogen/Progestin Interventions) study showed that the adverse effects of synthetic progestins on blood fats and cholesterol levels were eliminated with natural progesterone.[22] Progesterone is key to building bone. John Lee, M.D., one of the pioneers who has tested natural progesterone in a clinical setting, has treated postmenopausal women with a natural progesterone cream plus a dietary program that includes vitamin and mineral supplements and moderate exercise. He found true reversal of osteoporosis even in patients who did not use estrogen supplements.[23] Other studies using progesterone cream have not shown such success, but the skin cream isn't the only way to administer progesterone if you are deficient. We eagerly await more research in this area.

A large body of evidence is building that indicates progesterone protects the breast from cancer. Since excess stimulation from estrogen has been implicated in breast cancer, it stands to reason that balancing estrogen with natural progesterone may diminish the risk. A study from almost forty years ago found that there was, indeed, a relationship between low progesterone levels and the incidence of breast cancer.[24]

Natural progesterone can be taken orally (as oral micronized progesterone), topically as a cream (transdermally), vaginally, or by injection. Oral preparations are typically prescribed in one of two ways: For women who still menstruate, it is often given in doses of 200 mg, taken for twelve to fourteen days per month; for menopausal women, it is usually prescribed in doses of 100 mg, to be taken daily. A compounding pharmacy can combine progesterone with estrogen into one capsule in a "tri-est" (containing all three forms of estrogen) or "bi-est" (containing two forms of estrogen) formula. A natural oral progesterone is commercially available under the brand name Prometrium; it can be found in most retail pharmacies. Individuals who are allergic to peanuts should be aware that Prometrium is mixed in a peanut-oil base.

Natural progesterone is also mass-marketed as a gel called Crinone, which is administered vaginally. This form of delivery has the advantage of being absorbed faster than tablets, creams, and even injections. Two major reasons why women discontinue HRT are uterine bleeding and psychological side effects. When two groups of menopausal women used two different forms of 4 percent Crinone vaginal gel (controlled-release and sustained-release), both groups found they did not

Creams Containing More Than 400 mg Progesterone per Ounce of Cream

Brand Name	Manufacturer	Progesterone mg per oz of cream
Angel Care	Angel Care USA	579–648*
Balance Cream	Vitality LifeChoice	470–517*
DermaGest	Broadmoore Labs	510
EssPro 7	Young Living Essential	548
Femarone 17	Wise Essentials	536
Fem-Gest	Bio-Nutritional Formulas	431
Renascence Progesterone	Marpé International	1,586
Maxine's Feminique	Country Life	443
NatraGest	Broadmoore Labs	446
Procreme	THG Health Products	489
Procreme Plus	THG Health Products	926
Progesterone Cream Max	Jason Natural Cosmetics	480
ProL'eve	Brain Garden	542
SupraGest	Health Alternatives West	452
Wild Yam Crème W/Prog	Wise Woman Essentials	525

* Ranges represent different amounts found in different lot numbers.

[Aeron LifeCycles Clinical Laboratory certifies that the progesterone cream products listed above contain the stated amount of progesterone. They produce the list as a service to consumers interested in knowing the progesterone content of topical creams and lotions. Manufacturers pay a fee to be included in Aeron's certification program. Aeron does not manufacture, sponsor, or advocate the use of any particular product.]

(Source: Aeron LifeCycles Clinical Laboratory website, www.aeron.com/pic.htm. June 2003)

suffer from these side effects, which are commonly encountered with synthetic progestins.[25] While not all women find a vaginal gel an appealing alternative, the good news is you don't have to use it every day to receive equivalent benefits.

Natural progesterone creams are growing in popularity and are now available over the counter in some pharmacies and health-food stores. Many doctors prefer the topical or transdermal creams because they offer a high degree of bioavailability; in other words, they are easily absorbed into the bloodstream and utilized. They are generally applied to the skin twice a day in 1/4-teaspoon doses, for a total of 1/2 teaspoon per day, which supplies 26 mg of progesterone. This number sounds minute in comparison to the levels of oral micronized progesterone typically prescribed, but because it is absorbed more quickly, the dosage doesn't need to be as high to provide equivalent blood levels. Some women feel the effects of progesterone cream in less than a week, but in those who are extremely deficient in the hormone it may take two to three months before optimum levels are restored.

Note: There are a number of progesterone creams on the market, but not all of them contain real progesterone, so buyer beware. Creams that contain wild yam extract (diosgenin) have no effect on the level of progesterone in your body. Look for U.S. Pharmacopeia (U.S.P.) progesterone products containing at least 400 mg of natural progesterone per ounce of cream. Aeron LifeCycles Clinical Laboratory has evaluated a number of commercial cream products with potential hormonal activity for progesterone content. A table summarizing them can be found on the previous page.

⇒ Testosterone ⇐

Testosterone is typically thought of as only a male hormone, but women produce it as well—in the ovaries, adrenal glands, and corpus luteum. Even though there is no clear decline of testosterone levels with natural menopause as there is after a hysterectomy, some women show signs of testosterone deficiency and experience a wide variety of symptoms; these include decreased sex drive, loss of energy, and a diminished sense of well-being. Several studies show that when testosterone is combined with estrogen as a menopausal replacement, several important benefits are observed. The combo therapy, called *estrogen-androgen replacement,* is currently approved in the United States for postmenopausal women who have failed to achieve relief of their hot flashes by taking estrogen alone. It is also prescribed for improving sexual function due to decreased libido. Strong evidence exists that it may reduce and possibly even reverse the development of osteoporosis.[26] In a study reported in 1987, women who had undergone surgical menopause and who took estrogen coupled with testosterone were compared to women taking estrogen alone; the women on the combination therapy reported better appetite, more energy, and a heightened sense of well-being.[27] Data also show benefits to the skin: increased thickness, collagen content, and suppleness.[28]

Some women's testosterone levels decline even before menopause. This phenomenon is possibly due to lack of testosterone production from the ovaries or to the declining production of two other steroid hormones from the adrenal glands, androstenedione and DHEA. Many women are unaware that testosterone receptors are found all over our bodies, especially close to areas considered strictly female. They're found in the breast nipples, in the vagina, and even in the clitoris. Testosterone stimulates growth of pubic hair and underarm hair when we enter puberty. When it's produced in inadequate amounts, we are less interested in sex, not easily aroused, and don't really enjoy it when and if it happens. If taking estrogen fails to restore your libido, perhaps your testosterone levels are below normal. The range should be between 30 and 60 ng/dl (nanograms per deciliter). Many conditions may account for declining testos-terone levels: birth control pills, ovariectomy, childbirth, chemotherapy, surgery, endometri-osis, depression, adrenal stress, and normal aging.[29]

Precautions should be taken when sup-plementing with testosterone, because using a too-high dose can result in women developing masculine tendencies that include acne, deep-ened voice, facial and body hair, and male-pattern baldness. (I'm reminded of a cartoon I saw that pictured a hairy, muscle-bound woman getting a shot from her doctor. The caption read, "I think we need to cut down on your dosage.") However, clinical evidence indi-cates that these changes are infrequent and are readily reversible once the dosage is reduced or the treatment stopped. One more caveat: Oral methyltestosterone (the type used in clinical trials) also adversely affects lipid levels by increasing total cholesterol and lowering HDLs. It is clearly not a drug you should take without sufficient reason, especially if your lipid levels fall within an unhealthy range.

OPTIONS FOR DELIVERY

A testosterone-and-estrogen combination tablet is made by Solvay Pharmaceuticals under the brand name Estratest. Most of the clinical studies conducted with this compound used conjugated estrogen. Natural testosterone is also available and can be compounded into a capsule with other hormones or made separately; for either option, you will need a doctor's prescription.

DHEA and DHEA-S

Dihydroepiandrosterone (DHEA) and its sulfated counterpart (DHEA-S) are androgens, like testosterone. In women, they are produced by the adrenal glands and the ovaries. DHEA works with the other steroid hormones in many interre-lated ways; in fact, it can be metabolized in the body into both testosterone and

---

Do You Need Supplemental Testosterone?

Examine the following lists of symptoms—and, if necessary, discuss them with your health-care provider—as a starting place for determining whether you need testosterone replacement. If you show signs of testosterone deficiency, or if you already have osteoporosis, it is a good idea to have your blood levels tested (read more about testing later in this chapter). For someone with a genuine deficiency, supplemental natural testosterone may be an option.

Symptoms of Testosterone Deficiency
- decreased libido
- lack of sexual enjoyment
- thinning pubic hair
- decreased energy
- decreased sense of well-being

Symptoms of Testosterone Overdose
- increased facial hair
- male-pattern baldness
- lowered voice
- acne
- mood disturbances

estrogen (estrone and estradiol). As a backup source of the hormone, all but 5 percent of DHEA is bound to a sulfur molecule circulating in the blood; this form (DHEA-S) can easily be converted into its active form when needed. Even though blood concentrations of DHEA and DHEA-S are higher in adult men and women than those of any other steroid (except cholesterol), the physiological role of the hormone is only vaguely understood. Most of the research on DHEA comes from animal studies, but, increasingly, human studies are confirming the findings that it is an important hormone that plays a key role in women's health.

A recent Canadian study described for the first time the medically important beneficial effects of DHEA when it was administered to postmenopausal women for twelve months. Most noteworthy, the authors state, was the stimulation of bone mineral density by DHEA. The observation of both a decrease in bone resorption and an increase in bone formation raises the hope of regaining, at least partially, the bone lost during the peri- or postmenopausal years. Furthermore, the addition of androgens was found in this study and others to effectively relieve hot flashes in women who had unsatisfactory results with estrogen alone. Another observation of major importance was that in this one-year span, there was no stimulatory effect of DHEA on the endometrium, as there was with estrogen alone.[30]

The literature indicates that DHEA touches on almost all aspects of health. It is a powerful immune-system stimulant; it can improve metabolism, energy level, mood, memory, and sexual function. Decreased levels of DHEA and DHEA-S have been attributed to chronic degenerative diseases. Levels do decline with age and with the onset of diseases such as cancer, diabetes, and heart disease. The question remains whether the reduced DHEA levels cause these conditions or are a result of the aging process. It has been shown that seniors who maintain a higher level of DHEA do experience a longer and healthier life. Additionally, when people take DHEA supplements, they tend to experience increased energy, a better ability to handle stress, improved quality of sleep, improved mood, and a general feeling of well-being.

Based on the studies that were then available, I reported in previous editions of this book that DHEA may be deleterious to women's hearts. Recent studies, however, show a positive cholesterol profile, including decreased blood cholesterol, triglycerides, and other lipoprotein components for up to twelve months while taking DHEA. It should be mentioned that Premarin and other conjugated equine estrogens raise triglyceride levels and also play havoc with the insulin response. Recent research shows that DHEA has another advantage over the equine estrogens: an inhibitory effect on insulin levels and glucose metabolism.[31]

DHEA supplements are widely available over the counter in health-food stores and markets, but before rushing out to pick up a bottle consider that these substances are hormones and not to be taken indiscriminately. Most doctors recommend that you first have your hormone levels tested to make sure that you need supplements (read more about hormone testing below). Dr. John Lee recommends that you also test your cortisol levels at the same time, because if your cortisol level is low, DHEA supplementation may be less effective and may reduce an already low blood-sugar level.[32] In this case, lifestyle modifications (diet, nutritional supplements, increased amounts of sleep, stress reduction) are more appropriate than supplementing with DHEA. Follow up every three months with additional hormone testing to make sure that the dosage you are taking is effective and not excessive. An average dose for women is between 5 and 25 mg per day. DHEA is found in tablets, sublingual tinctures, or transdermal creams. Especially if you decide to try DHEA supplementation without guidance from a health-care provider, which is *not* my recommendation, start with the smallest dose. Look for pharmaceutical-grade products, and avoid anything labeled "DHEA precursors" made from wild yam; they are not going to be broken down into a usable form in your body.

Signs that indicate a too-high dose of DHEA include increased facial hair, acne, male-pattern baldness, and abdominal obesity. These are reversible when you stop using the supplement. While DHEA can be an effective treatment for some women, proper dosage is important. Too much DHEA over a period of time can increase your risk of diabetes and heart disease; therefore, consult with a health professional, and test your blood or saliva levels prior to beginning your program.

⋙ Testing Your Hormone Levels ⋘

Before embarking on any hormonal replacement program, it is a good idea to undergo a baseline test to measure the levels in your body of all of the specific hormones you plan to use. By doing this you will find out which specific hormones are low and which are not. Then you and your doctor can better determine the dosages you need. There is an easy way to test hormone levels at home by testing your saliva. Standardized saliva hormone testing is the best way to tell what is happening hormonally in a woman's body. Unlike a blood test, which typically measures total hormone levels, the saliva test measures the amount in the blood of *free* hormone, or the part that is biologically active. Because hormones are bound to specific proteins in the blood, it is difficult to obtain an accurate measurement with a blood test. John Kells, president of Aeron LifeCycles Clinical Laboratory, a pioneer in saliva testing, explains, "When you test in saliva, you get a precise

accounting of the free hormones that are circulating through your body and inter-acting with your hormone receptors. You know what your hormones are doing for you right now."[33] Once you have either started replacement therapy or have begun integrating phytohormones (plant hormones) into your diet, you can retest your hormone levels to determine if your program is actually working. (Information on saliva testing and further suggested reading about natural hormones are found in Resources.)

The Compounding Pharmacist, Your Doctor, and You

Just as all women are different, natural hormonal preparations are not generic; that is, they don't all come in one dose, shape, or size. They must be custom-designed according to your specific hormonal deficiencies and individual symptoms. This is the job of the compounding pharmacist. Compounding pharmacists go beyond counting and dispensing multicolored pills; they make exactly the right combina-tion of hormones in the proper dosage that affords you the greatest benefit with the least number of side effects. It's not always easy finding a formulating pharmacist specializing in natural hormones who will work with you and your doctor, but it's getting easier to do so, as women are increasingly demanding safer hormones.

Some mail-order pharmacies specialize in women's health and will send you and your doctor informational packets on natural hormones. Women's Interna-tional, Madison, and Bajamar are three such companies I've worked with. If you would rather find a compounding pharmacy in your area, contact the International Academy of Compounding Pharmacists at (800) 927-4227 (its website can be found at www.iacprx.com). This organization will gladly help you. I have met some of the people involved with the organization and found them extremely helpful.

When introducing to your doctor the topic of switching to natural hor-mones, be aware that you may get any number of reactions. Because I've moved so often in the past five years, I've had several family doctors. I've met with reac-tions ranging from skepticism to intimidation to, thankfully, acceptance. Once I decided that I probably did need supplemental hormones, I called a compounding pharmacist in my area and asked the pharmacist to recommend a doctor. After I visited the doctor and underwent all the appropriate tests (blood and saliva), she and I decided on an oral tablet containing bi-est (two forms of estrogen) plus pro-gesterone. Because my prescription was already established, when I had to change doctors again, it was much easier convincing the new doctor that this was what I planned to do. But I would have switched doctors in a heartbeat had he disagreed.

As you consider what, if any, form of hormone therapy you need, avail yourself of the many medically oriented Internet sites. At most of them, you can get helpful information, listen to doctors being interviewed, and chat with other menopausal women. The all-time best, in my opinion, is the award-winning Power Surge website (www.power-surge.com). Tell the moderator, who goes by the moniker "Dearest," that I sent you.

≈ In Conclusion ≈

All women going through menopause will find that their hormones fluctuate as they establish a new equilibrium. This doesn't mean that all women will have symptoms or that all women will require hormonal replacement. Many will be able to control hot flashes and mood swings with herbs and soy milk. But some won't. And for those women whose lives are intolerable because of symptoms, or for those grappling with how best to prevent bone loss, taking hormones may be a viable course of action.

You may be afraid to try hormones because of the Women's Health Initiative findings of 2002. But be reminded that the hormones used in the study, Premarin and Prempro, do not represent all compounds. It bears repeating that *not* all hormones are the same. Christiane Northrup, M.D., succinctly sums it up in her newsletter. She writes, "Hormone replacement doesn't have to be risky if you use the right hormone, at the right dose, for the right reasons, for the right length of time."[34] No medication is without risk if it is the wrong one for you. Use your symptoms as a guide, monitor regularly, and work with your health-care professional in the decision-making process.

Here's one more piece of wisdom that is easily overlooked: Rely on your intuition. It speaks louder and clearer during this phase of your life than it ever has before. Slow down and pay attention to it.

CHAPTER 3

HOT FLASHES

A flush is anything but a flash.

— JOHN W. STUDD, MRCOG, KINGS COLLEGE HOSPITAL, LONDON

The most characteristic complaint of menopausal women is the bothersome hot flash, more correctly called *hot flush*. Up to 80 percent of women experience them to some degree, with up to 40 percent suffering enough to seek medical attention. Some women never have a hot flash, most are inconvenienced for a year or two, but for a few, flashes may persist as long as five or even ten years.

Hot flashes usually begin when one's menstrual periods are still regular or are just starting to fluctuate. They are often one of the first indications that menopause is approaching. Generally, they are most uncomfortable in the first stages of perimenopause, gradually decreasing in frequency and intensity as the body adapts to the hormonal changes.

Descriptions of a hot flash are as varied as the personalities of the women having them. Mine started with an immediate surge of heat enveloping my body from head to foot, as if someone had suddenly turned the thermostat way up. It happened regularly every night and in the early mornings for about three months, then gradually tapered off. The discomfort was minimal, but the interrupted sleep made me grouchy and groggy. It felt like a permanent case of jet lag. A friend described a wave of heat that began in her face and neck and worked down to her chest. She turned scarlet, perspired profusely, then shivered for several minutes. Changing her nightgown and sheets was a nightly ritual. Her experience seemed to take a great toll on her emotional health. Crying spells, panic attacks, and eating binges also disrupted her daily activities.

Flashes differ in duration, frequency, and intensity. Episodes may be brief—two to three minutes—but can also linger up to an hour. They can come several times a day or night, or only once or twice a week.

In itself, the hot flash is harmless. Nevertheless, as the body's temperature control system vacillates between very hot and cool, other body systems are strained as well. When flashes occur too often, they may be accompanied by unexpected and even frightening side effects: loss of sleep, fatigue, weakness, dizziness, a racing pulse, heart palpitations, headaches, itchy skin, and numbness in the hands and arms. These symptoms can catch you unawares and can trigger concern, as thoughts of more serious causes for them race through your mind.

What Causes Hot Flashes?

The hot flash is still not fully understood; researchers have only recently determined that measurable hormonal changes take place during a flash. Diminished estrogen levels are somehow responsible, but exactly in what way remains a bit unclear. Withdrawal of estrogen causes an increase in the levels of the hormones FSH and LH. The brain center that secretes these hormones, the hypothalamus, directs many body functions, including body temperature, sleep patterns, metabolic rate, mood, and reaction to stress. The higher the levels of FSH and LH, the more the blood vessels dilate, or enlarge, which increases blood flow to the skin, raising its temperature.

Hot Flash Triggers

- hot weather, hot drinks, warm clothing
- caffeine (coffee, tea, chocolate, colas)
- exercise (especially if you are not in good shape)
- vigorous lovemaking
- drugs of all kinds, alcohol
- large meals, meals eaten too quickly, spicy foods
- stress

Levels of other hormones and body chemicals also seem to fluctuate in response to altered estrogen levels and may participate in triggering a hot flash. Two neurotransmitters, epinephrine and norepinephrine, interact with the hypothalamus and help control dilation and contraction of blood vessels. The brain's natural mood controllers, beta-endorphins, drop in response to lowered estrogen and progesterone levels and may also be involved. Hormones do not operate in a vacuum. A rise or fall in any one of them creates a cascading interplay that can affect any number of bodily functions.

Who Will Have Hot Flashes?

The fact that hot flashes are somehow related to changing estrogen levels is undisputed. A sharp drop in estrogen can lead to severe symptoms. Women who have had their ovaries surgically removed report immediate and unpleasant hot flashes. Nonsurgical damage to the ovaries may also reduce hormonal output and increase

the likelihood of hot flashes. Because smoking diminishes hormone production and inhibits circulation, smokers can expect to suffer more than nonsmokers.

A gradual decline in estrogen results in fewer flashes. Women with more body fat complain less than smaller, thinner women, because fat cells produce more of certain a type of estrogen, estrone. The goal of nutritional support in counteracting menopausal symptoms is to accomplish this without burdening the body with excess estrogen and excess weight. A nutrient-rich diet can provide an optimum environment that will support your organs and glands so they will make the correct amount of hormones needed during this transition.

Hot flashes do not appear to be universal. In the Japanese culture, for example, they are rarely mentioned, and there is no word that refers precisely to this menopausal sign.[1] Since Japanese is a language in which extremely subtle distinctions are made about body states of all kinds, the absence of such a word indicates its lack of significance. The Maya in Mexico don't report hot flashes either.[2] Several studies suggest that this absence of hot flashes may be linked to diet. One common denominator among cultures in which menopausal symptoms are few or nonexistent is that the women consume higher levels of estrogen-containing foods. Even though their endocrine systems operate in the same way as those of Western women, the additional hormonal support provided by their diets minimizes or prevents symptoms.[3] Their positive outlook about growing older should also be considered as another possible factor.

Treating Hot Flashes Naturally

You don't have to be menopausal to experience a hot flash. Waves of heat may hit anyone, of any age, who engages in behavior that forces the system that regulates temperature to step up its activity.

Several ways exist to treat hot flashes naturally. The rest of this section explores some of these natural therapies.

EXERCISE

Treatments that stabilize the autonomic nervous system (which controls involuntary responses) may help in tempering hot flashes. Regular and moderate exercise, for instance, will decrease FSH and LH levels, reducing and possibly even eliminating symptoms.[4] The hypothalamus regulates the menstrual cycle, body temperature, and the autonomic nervous system. During menopause, when the hypothalamus becomes supersensitive to outside signals, exercise can stabilize it and help to restore more normal hormonal levels.

A 1990 study of seventy-nine menopausal women showed that moderate and even severe symptoms of hot flashes and sweating were reduced in both frequency and severity with exercise.[5] Of note to midlife women who would rather have a root canal than join a gym is that the women in this study exercised three to four hours a week—not an unreasonable commitment of time.

Exercise is considerably more effective, however, if it is begun well in advance of menopause. If your body is not conditioned, an increase in unfamiliar activity may stimulate the very response you are trying to avoid. Keeping the body in good working order enables it to handle discomfort with greater ease. To minimize midlife and aging symptoms, increase your physical activity level.

DEEP BREATHING

Relaxation methods that consciously relax both the mind and the body have been shown to reduce hot flashes. In a pilot study of thirty-three postmenopausal women who reported having at least five hot flashes a day, it was found that slow, deep breathing alone reduced the incidence of hot flashes by about 50 percent.[6] Researchers concluded that women who are unable to receive hormone replacement therapy might benefit from this technique.

It makes sense. If stress is a trigger for flashes, then activities that can reduce the surge of hormones related to anxiety would be beneficial. Many books describe relaxation and deep-breathing techniques. My favorite is the classic by Herbert Benson, M.D., *The Relaxation Response* (reissued 1990). If you can't wait to purchase the book and want to start practicing relaxation and deep-breathing exercises immediately, here is a summary of the basic breathing technique: Sit in a comfortable position. Close your eyes and relax all your muscles. Slowly breathe in and out through your nose, becoming aware of each breath. It sounds easy, but distractions may continually infiltrate your thoughts, breaking the mood. Attempt to disregard these intrusions and to keep breathing deeply for ten to twenty minutes.

DIET

Good dietary habits and additional nutritional support can often help in preventing and treating hot flashes. Hormones are formed from the building blocks of food, and if even one nutritional element is missing, a hormonal deficiency or imbalance may result. Preventing a physical ailment is always preferable to curing it, so nurturing the organs and glands with the right foods should be a primary goal throughout life. (Part Three of this book is devoted to helping you develop a nutrition plan for life.)

REDUCING SWEETS AND TREATS

Reducing minimally nutritive foods is crucial for menopausal women. After-dinner sweets, specialty coffees, and dinner wines, as comforting as they are, do not serve menopausal women well. If you are already well into menopause, you may have noticed that your favorite treats are not as well tolerated now as they were a few years ago. The same coffee and chocolate at night that delighted you earlier in life may now keep you up until dawn, producing nightmares, a racing heartbeat, and hot flashes. Pay attention to and avoid foods that are no longer worth the momentary pleasure.

Overdosing on sweets is especially aggravating to the body during menopause. A high sugar intake stresses the adrenal gland and pancreas at a time when both need to be in good working order. London University's John Yudkin, in his book *Sweet and Dangerous,* warns against the ill effects refined sugar can have on the hormones. A high-sugar diet, he reports, can cause a striking increase in the level of adrenal cortical hormone. It can slow the rate of transport of hormonal chemicals by as much as two-thirds, even in one week.[7] Sometimes just regulating your sugar intake may control uncomfortable hot flashes. Over the long term, high sugar intake may cumulatively weaken the adrenal glands so that estrogen is not converted efficiently. Remember, at menopause the adrenal glands take over the production of estrogen; when they can make this change smoothly, symptoms are less intense and less frequent.

Blood-sugar fluctuation, or hypoglycemia, is clearly a factor in the experience of hot flashes.[8] If your first sign of approaching menopause is a hot flash, stop and consider your diet. In fact, do more than think about it: Write down what you eat for a week or two. This may strike you as unnecessary, but a poll by the Human Nutrition Research Center found that over 80 percent of the population either under- or overestimates its food intake. It appears that few of us are clear about the calories, sugar, salt, fat, and nutrients we consume daily, and tracking our diet can be enlightening.

PHYTOHORMONES: PLANTS THAT HEAL

Much excitement concerning phytohormones has been generated in the women's-health community over the last several years. These are substances in plant foods that elicit a hormonal response. Before hormone replacement therapy was developed, traditional cultures used certain foods and herbs to treat a range of female complaints. Research today confirms that many menopausal women who avoid experiencing hot flashes have a plant-based or primarily vegetarian diet. We now

know that some plants and common foods, herbs, and spices contain natural substances that help the body produce its own native estrogen and progesterone. These phytohormones are also called *adaptogens*, because they work within the system to balance hormonal levels, raising them if they are too low and lowering them if they are too high.

Phytohormones, also called *phytosterols*, are structurally and functionally similar to steroid hormones. While the plant hormones do not actually contain human hormones, they do encourage their production within the body. Because plant hormones act systemically, they treat a broad range of conditions, such as hot flashes, vaginal dryness, menstrual irregularities, and fibroid tumors. They appear to improve blood flow to female organs, keep arteries clear, and offer protection from cancer.

Plant hormones have a centuries-old safety record. Compared with commercially prepared drugs, their potency is miniscule. Still, they effectively stimulate a woman's body to produce the

Natural Sources of Phytohormones	
alfalfa	oats
anise	orchard grass
apples	palmetto grass
barley	parsley
bluegrass	peas
carrots	pomegranates
cherries	potatoes
coffee	rape seed
date palms	red beans
fennel	rice
French beans	rye
garlic	sage
green beans	sesame
hops	soybeans
licorice	wheat

Source: Rami Kaldas and Hugh Claud, *"Reproductive and General Metabolic Effects of Phytoestrogen in Mammals,"* Reproductive Toxicology 3.2 (1989): 81–89.

hormones she needs, without causing toxic side effects (assuming safe dosage levels are used). Much like the body's natural secretions, phytohormones keep arterial pathways clear and help elevate HDLs (high-density lipoproteins, a.k.a. "good cholesterol," the type of cholesterol that removes excessive cholesterol from the blood).[9] Unlike synthetic estrogen, phytoestrogens appear to have no downside. Whereas the synthetic form carries with it an increased risk of breast cancer, plant-based estrogen effectively inhibits mammary tumors.[10]

Phytohormones abound in nature. There are hundreds—perhaps even thousands—within the cells of plant foods we eat every day. Phytohormones have long been sipped in teas and tinctures to relieve a range of symptoms. And foods such as soybeans and yams form the basis of medicinal hormones used to treat menstrual as well as menopausal discomfort. Some research suggests that natural estrogen and progesterone taken in pill form are as effective as the synthetic versions, yet offer fewer side effects and less long-term risk. (For more about natural versus synthetic hormones, see Chapter 2.)

Soy Studies

Soy, in particular, has often been demonstrated to ease menopausal discomfort. The component of soy most beneficial to women's health appears to be isoflavones (phytohormones with estrogen-like properties). Soy, the best source of isoflavones, is basic to the Asian diet. Asians may ingest up to 150 mg per day of isoflavones, as well as significant amounts of other plant-estrogen sources, such as legumes, cereals, and grains. Most experiments or trials use pure extracts of a particular isoflavone, but recent studies have used soy products to assess the effects of soy on hot flashes, vaginal cell changes, and some heart-related conditions, such as blood pressure and cholesterol levels. Six human studies, reviewed by researchers at the Second International Symposium on the Role of Soy in Preventing and Treating Chronic Disease (held in Brussels, Belgium, in September 1996), found at least a slight decline in the rate of hot flashes, and three of these found a significant drop.[11] One of them, from Melbourne, Australia, showed a 40 percent reduction in hot flashes when women consumed 40 grams of soy flour each day for twelve weeks. Similar results were found in the United Kingdom (using 80 mg of isoflavones for two months) and in Italy (using 60 mg of isolated soy protein with 76 mg of isoflavones).[12]

A 1998 U.S. study supports these findings. In a double-blind, placebo-controlled study, more than a hundred postmenopausal women, ages forty-eight to sixty-one, were divided into two groups. Each day for three months, one group was given a placebo, and the other was given 60 grams of isolated soy protein. The number of hot flashes and night sweats experienced by the women receiving the soy was reduced by 45 percent over the test period, compared to 30 percent in the placebo group.[13]

Some studies of soy's effects find no significant difference in relief from hot flashes between the group receiving soy and the placebo group. Several factors could influence this finding. First, the placebo effect may be very strong; in other words, perhaps women in the nontreatment groups felt better simply because they expected to. Second, some women may be more sensitive to soy than others. Finally, perhaps the dosages in some of the studies were inadequate to elicit a response.

How Much Soy Do You Need?

Dietary phytohormone intake from all sources—not just soy—differs dramatically among populations. People who eat a vegetarian diet take in about 345 mg to 400 mg per day, compared to the 80 mg a day of people consuming a more Western diet.[14] Studies show that vegetarians also suffer much less from hot flashes and other menopausal symptoms. So, there is a strong probability that if women eat more

plant foods rich in natural hormones, hot flashes and other menopausal symptoms will lessen.

Clinical tests show that the highest amounts of these natural compounds are found in soy products. Although no minimum daily requirements have yet been established for soy protein (or isoflavone) intake, studies do provide clues as to what amount effectively reduces menopausal symptoms. Some experts recommend as little as 50 mg of isoflavones per day, or two servings of soy, depending on the food's isoflavone content. For most women, such a low dose will probably not adequately calm raging hot flashes. A panel of experts agrees that the accepted dosage is the amount that is found in the traditional Asian diet, which ranges from 100 to 160 mg of soy isoflavones per day.[15] Specifically for the treatment of hot flashes, an article published in a prestigious medical journal recorded benefits from supplementing with a similar range: between 150 and 200 mg.[16] Most researchers are in accord that it is not necessary to ingest more than these amounts. In other words, if the highest dose noted here fails to quell your symptoms, adding more will not help.

It can be difficult to determine with accuracy the isoflavone content of one's diet. This is because isoflavone levels in the soybean itself vary; furthermore, different brands of soy foods contain different levels of isoflavones. Some food companies now list isoflavone content on their packages, but you should recognize that the information may be inexact. There are wide discrepancies among otherwise similar foods. With that caveat, the table in the box above lists approximate isoflavone content of some soy foods. (See Chapter 7 for more on soy research.)

It is always prudent to derive nutrients from foods first, but if you cannot incorporate the recommended amount of soy isoflavones into your diet, don't get discouraged. More and more companies are developing soy-based drinks and snack products high in isoflavone content. Physicians Laboratories, makers of Revival brand soy products, is one of the largest and most extensively researched of such companies. The Revival products, developed by medical doctors and used at Johns Hopkins and Memorial Sloan-Kettering hospitals, have been patented and are now being tested in double-blind, placebo-controlled clinical trials in many other U.S. hospitals. Revival offers soy shakes that provide up to 160 mg of isoflavones in a single serving, yogurt-covered soy nuts, and soy protein bars. Revival also offers teas

Isoflavone Content of Selected Soy Products

Food	Isoflavone (mg)
1/2 cup cooked soybeans	150
1/4 cup roasted soynuts	60
1/2 cup edamame (green soybeans)	50
1 cup soy milk	20–40
1/2 cup tofu or tempeh	35
1/4 cup soy flour	25
6 oz soy yogurt	25

and "coffees," which are made from organic, fresh-roasted soybeans instead of coffee beans (these "coffees" provide 10 to 20 mg of isoflavones per serving). Revival's products are made from the heart of the soybean, which is quite concentrated in soy proteins and isoflavones. That's why only one serving contains five or six times as much isoflavone as a single serving of traditional soy foods. The beans have been mechanically (rather than chemically) dehulled, then baked and ground up.

These products use the soybean as food, and thus are an alternative to pills containing isoflavone extract for women who resist the use of drugs. However, I must emphasize that getting as much soy (and other plant hormones) as possible from a diet of whole foods is vital. Don't assume that living on processed soy drinks and bars while ignoring the rest of your diet will keep you healthy. Your body is a living organism designed to optimally nourish itself from the foods of the earth in forms close to their original, natural state. Still, processed soy supplements may be a viable backup system for you. Revival products are not sold in retail outlets. Contact the company directly at (800) 500-8053, or visit its website at www.revivalsoy.com.

Some great books that contain recipes for soy foods are *The Simple Soybean and Your Health*, by Mark and Virginia Messina; *Estrogen: The Natural Way*, by Nina Shandler; *The Healing Power of Soy*, by Carol Ann Rinzler; and *Super Soy: The Miracle Bean*, by Ruth Winter. (Other practical ideas for adding soy to your diet are found in Chapter 15 of this book.)

Consuming more grains, fruits, and vegetables—with special emphasis on those high in phytohormones—may take you through menopause more smoothly. Remember, natural remedies do take time; noticeable results may require three or four months.

NUTRIENTS AND HERBS THAT SUPPRESS HOT FLASHES

Vitamin E. Clinical studies have shown certain nutrients to be effective in treating hot flashes. The most widely recommended is vitamin E. Medical journals first published studies of vitamin E as a treatment for hot flashes in the late 1940s. However, with the advent of estrogen therapy and tranquilizers, nutritional solutions were largely forgotten. More money could be made from a drug than from an unpatentable natural product. Only when it became clear that not all women were safe candidates for hormonal therapy did researchers dust off their books to rediscover this already proven alternative.

Studies in the late 1940s tested women who could not be treated with estrogen because they had estrogen-based tumors. All the women suffered from unremitting hot flashes and mood changes. After taking a regimen of vitamin E, the women

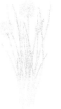

experienced either complete relief or marked improvement—without side effects.[17] Other early studies confirmed this finding.

Vitamin E is a hormone normalizer. Tests indicate that when vitamin E is low, the body's levels of FSH and LH increase. Since these hormones already tend to be overabundant in menopausal women, a shortage of vitamin E could exacerbate the situation. Vitamin E appears to have a stabilizing effect on estrogen levels, increasing the hormone output in women who are deficient and lowering it in those who are prone to excess. Adequate doses can buffer the hormonal ebbs and flows that occur during the change, relieving associated symptoms. Other menopausal symptoms that are helped by supplemental vitamin E include nervousness, fatigue, insomnia, dizziness, heart palpitations, shortness of breath, and vaginal dryness.[18]

Many nutritionists agree that the increase of refined foods in our diet, coupled with the absence of whole grains, nuts, and seeds, has led to a dangerous decline in dietary vitamin E. To compound the problem, vitamin E is destroyed when it is exposed to air, heated, frozen, or stored. While most of us experience only minor shortages of vitamin E that rarely degenerate into a classic "deficiency disease," the weakness engendered on the deeper, cellular level by a diet of mostly refined foods makes us susceptible to a host of symptoms, some of which appear to be directly related to menopause.

For relief of hot flashes, Doctors Barbara and Gideon Seaman recommend starting with 100 IU of vitamin E per day and gradually increasing the dosage over a few weeks to a few months until you experience results.[19] It may take up to 1,200 IU daily before reduction in the frequency or intensity of hot flashes is apparent.

Vitamin E should be complemented with the mineral selenium, as studies show that the two operate synergistically; that is, their combined effect is greater than that of either taken alone.

Note: If you have high blood pressure, diabetes, or a rheumatic heart condition, do not take more than 30 IU of vitamin E without first checking with your physician.

As a fat-soluble nutrient, vitamin E is absorbed from the intestinal tract only in the presence of fat. To ensure absorption, take vitamin E with a meal incorporating some fat—not, for example, with grapefruit and coffee. You can also aid its digestibility and utilization by taking it with lecithin, a fat that, incidentally, has been reported to reduce the incidence of hot flashes.

Good sources of vitamin E include sunflower seeds, almonds, crab, sweet potatoes, fish, wheat germ, and whole-wheat bread. (For the precise amount of this nutrient contained in certain foods, consult Appendix C.)

Bioflavonoids. Bioflavonoids function as weak estrogens and can be taken with vitamin C to relieve hot flashes and vaginal dryness. Like vitamin E, these vitamin-like substances have been successfully used in cancer patients for whom estrogen replacement therapy is contraindicated. Dosages range from 500 mg to 2,000 mg per day, and they are absorbed better when taken in divided doses.

There are over two hundred bioflavonoids, including rutin, hesperidin, and quercetin; hesperidin is recommended by some as being especially useful for menopausal complaints. The best dietary sources are the white pulp beneath the peel of citrus fruits; the skin of grapes, cherries, and berries; leafy vegetables; and wine.

Black cohosh. Also known by other names—such as "squaw root," because of its medicinal use by American Indian women, and *Cimicifuga racemosa*, its scientific label—this plant extract is widely used in Germany as an alternative to HRT. The word *black* in its name derives from the color of the part of the plant that is used medicinally, the rhizome (an underground rootlike section of a plant). *Cohosh* is the Algonquin Indian word for "rough," referring to the plant's texture.

Several independent studies carried out at different times over four decades have consistently demonstrated that a standardized extract of black cohosh relieves menopausal symptoms, including hot flashes, depression, and vaginal atrophy, within four to twelve weeks. Although black cohosh extract was thought to produce an estrogen-like effect, recent research indicates that this assumption can no longer be upheld. Chemicals from the plant extract do indeed attach to estrogen receptor sites in tissue, but researchers say the herb actually acts as a blockade of the receptor, rather than as a true estrogen substitute.[20]

Black cohosh acts as a hormone normalizer. It is important to note that although it relieves the symptoms of menopause, it does not offer estrogen's apparent benefits in preventing and treating heart disease and osteoporosis. Nor, however, does it carry estrogen's possible increased risk of breast cancer. All things considered, black cohosh is most helpful for the perimenopausal woman at low risk of heart disease and osteoporosis who desires management of her menopausal symptoms.

Germany's drug regulatory agency, Commission E, limits the use of black cohosh to six months, as hard information about long-term effects is still lacking. Short-term side effects may include gastrointestinal disturbances, weight problems, and headaches, especially with doses higher than indicated. The product Remifemin, distributed by the company Enzymatic Therapy, is a common, standardized form of black cohosh. (*Standardized* means that the amount of plant extract in each dosage is consistent.) The best results occur with a daily dosage of 160 to 300 mg. Take two 40-mg capsules or tablets twice a day.

Other herbal remedies. In the mid-1800s, Lydia Pinkham concocted a vegetable compound to cure female maladies. For over a hundred years, her company sold her natural potion as an alternative to medical prescriptions. Women have long passed down tried-and-true herbal remedies, but until recently, modern medicine held that these recipes merely provided a placebo effect for the "hysterical" woman. No longer. Herbs that were once considered worthless are now being studied for the treatment of many ailments.

Not surprisingly, the herbs found most effective for menopausal complaints are similar to those in Lydia Pinkham's original formula. These herbs, known to be natural sources of estrogenic substances, act on the pituitary and adrenal glands to stabilize the menstrual cycle. They include fenugreek, gotu kola, sarsaparilla, licorice root, and wild yam root. Nan Koehler, a botanist and herbalist, suggests making a tea with one of these herbs combined with another herb high in minerals, such as dandelion leaf, alfalfa, or borage.

Ginseng. Ginseng, a popular and potent herb, has been studied for five thousand years; millions of people the world over praise its stimulating qualities. In several countries it is used for temperature imbalances, such as chronic sweating, heat stress, and hot flashes. It is said to exert a "normalizing" action on the pituitary gland, as well as to help in rebuilding tissues, stimulating energy, enhancing physical and mental performance, regulating blood pressure, reducing cholesterol, and generally rejuvenating the body, strengthening it against the debilitating effects of stress. Ginseng is also believed to increase estrogen levels and is recommended for women during menopause.

Ginseng is available in many forms, some more energizing than others. The primary active agents in ginseng, called *ginsenosides*, are found in different proportions, depending on where and how the ginseng is grown. Some forms tend to stimulate the body; others relax and cool it.

Oriental cultivated ginseng, also called *panax*, is of the energy-producing variety and is commonly available in health-food stores in capsules, extracts, and teas. Siberian ginseng, often labeled just "ginseng," is not a true ginseng but is a related plant with the same energy-enhancing properties. Studies show that the Siberian extract improves the performance of long-distance runners, demonstrating its strengthening and endurance-building properties. American ginseng offers more of the cooling properties and is better for regulating the temperature-control system.

Unlike most vitamins and herbs, ginseng is most effective when taken on an empty stomach. Dosage varies, so follow the package directions. You can drop

the capsules into hot water to make a soothing tea. It is best not to take ginseng with vitamin C or a food high in vitamin C, since ascorbic acid tends to neutralize it. None of the tests to which modern scientists have subjected this ancient medicinal herb have shown it to have a single deleterious side effect.[21]

Vitex (vitex agnus-castus). Vitex, also known as *chaste tree* or *chasteberry*, is regarded throughout Europe as *the* herb for menopause, PMS, and uterine fibroid cysts. It profoundly stimulates pituitary function, altering LH and FSH secretions. Using vitex regularly for a few months will increase your natural levels of progesterone and help control hot flashes, depression, and a dry vagina. One caution: It is not to be taken with birth control pills.

Like most herbs, vitex comes in many varieties. The packaging will list the appropriate dosage, usually one capsule up to three times daily, or 10 to 30 drops of extract in juice or water up to three times daily. For optimum benefit, take it for at least three months, as herbs and nutrients restore balance to the body slowly and gently.

Herbs can be taken individually or in concert with others. Black cohosh, sage, dong quai, wild yam, and sarsaparilla combine well with vitex. Some mixtures may be labeled as "menopausal formulas." Experiment until you find one that works for you.

Natural Remedies for Hot Flashes

- Exercise moderately and regularly.
- Use deep-breathing or relaxation techniques.
- Eliminate triggers: sugar, coffee, alcohol, spicy foods, hot drinks, warm clothes.
- Maintain a constant blood-sugar level:
  - Eat every four to five hours.
  - Watch concentrated sugar, caffeine, and alcohol.
  - Don't overeat.
- Include one or more of the following in your daily diet:
  - vitamin E (800–1,200 IU, divided into one to three doses), mixed tocopherols preferred
  - selenium (15–50 mcg)
  - lecithin (6–12 capsules, divided into one to three doses)
  - vitamin C with bioflavonoids (1,000–3,000 mg spread throughout the day)
  - herbs: ginseng, vitex, black cohosh, sage, sarsaparilla, licorice root, wild yam root, dong quai, yarrow

---

Bioidentical Hormones Reduce Hot Flashes

Conventional hormone therapy will quickly eliminate hot flashes, but given the risks associated with it, it should be considered only as a last resort. Fewer studies exist on the more gentle bioidentical hormones (sometimes called *natural hormones*), but there is sufficient evidence that both estriol and natural progesterone are just as effective as conventional HRT in reducing both the number and severity of hot flashes.

Estriol, the weakest of the estrogens, has been shown to dramatically decrease hot flashes and many other symptoms associated with menopause when used in doses of 2–8 mg/day.[22] Several research papers have suggested that estriol does not stimulate growth in the cells of the uterus and breast; however, others remind us that no long-term trials have been conducted, so continuous use of estriol in high doses remains questionable.

Estrogen has historically been the primary treatment for hot flashes, but an increasing number of studies indicate that natural, or bioidentical, progesterone (as well as its synthetic counterpart, progestin) shares a similar effect. In one randomized, placebo-controlled study, researchers noted an 83 percent improvement in hot-flash symptoms among women using a transdermal progesterone cream in a 20-mg dose, as compared to a 19 percent improvement among the placebo group.[23] While estriol requires a prescription, progesterone cream is an over-the-counter product and can be found in health-food stores or pharmacies. (See Chapter 2 for a detailed discussion of natural and synthetic hormone therapies, including estriol and progesterone creams.)

⇒ Where Do I Start? ⇐

If you are bothered by incessant hot flashes, start by eliminating foods that are obvious triggers. Check your diet to see if you are promoting blood-sugar extremes. Fasting all day and overindulging at night can be just as devastating to the body as gulping down four cups of coffee and two chocolate-filled croissants. Check to be sure that your diet contains adequate amounts of the nutrients mentioned. If not, add foods that incorporate these substances, or supplement as indicated. When supplementing, try one nutrient or herb at a time so as not to overwhelm the body. That way, if you have an allergic reaction, the source will be obvious.

Your body is unique, and your program will be individual as well. Just because vitamin E worked for your friend does not mean it will remedy your flashes. Robert C. Atkins, author of *Dr. Atkins' Nutritional Breakthrough* and other books, describes the determined endeavors required to find the right natural remedy: "While vitamin E in 800 IU worked for one woman, another tried vitamin E, diet, ginseng, dong quai and still didn't feel better until lecithin was added to her regimen."[24] If food, diet, and exercise fail to adequately control your hot flashes and they are interfering with your quality of life, consider the bioidentical hormones, particularly estriol and natural progesterone.

CHAPTER 4

FATIGUE

Female fatigue is the most common "Silent Disease" of women.

— ELIZABETH WEISS, *Female Fatigue*

How often do you say that you feel tired and listless, that you lack energy at the end of the day? Such complaints come not only from menopausal women, but also from women of all ages. Most exasperating is the fact that in the majority of cases, doctors report no physiological basis for these symptoms. Boredom, stress, depression, and psychosomatic tendencies are often suggested as explanations for fatigue. This may be accurate, but let's consider some equally valid possibilities.

Excessive fatigue during perimenopause is usually caused by interruptions in sleep due to hot flashes or other disturbances triggered by hormonal irregularities. Lack of continuous, restful sleep tends to wear one down both physically and emotionally. Once the hormones stabilize, sleep patterns and energy generally return to normal. If you feel the hours you spend sleeping are adequate, but the tiredness still lingers, look to other possibilities.

Energy levels depend on many factors, some psychological, some physiological. Four culprits stand out among the functional causes of undiagnosed, persistent fatigue: low blood sugar, anemia, underactive thyroid, and tired adrenal glands. Each condition can be the result of several factors; the most likely but least often considered are the nutritional ones. In other words, these conditions can often be created and treated by the foods we do or don't eat.

Remember, as our organs age, they lose resilience. Many foods we once devoured with relish gradually become toxic to our bodies. Our glandular system needs to be treated with greater care and respect with each passing birthday.

Low Blood Sugar

Almost all of us experience the late-morning or midafternoon "droops" and regard it as a normal part of our daily routine. If we haven't eaten in several hours, it is not especially surprising that we feel tired and weak, have a headache, cannot think clearly, lose our temper, and crave sweets. We may be inclined to ignore these symptoms, but we should not. Our body is communicating something to us: We are being warned of a metabolic imbalance that, if left unchecked, could lead to far greater problems.

The metabolic irregularity to which I refer is called *hypoglycemia*, or, more commonly, low blood sugar. Hypoglycemia results from an imbalance in the body's sugar-regulating mechanism that prevents the maintenance of a stable level of sugar in the blood. The body breaks down carbohydrates (starches and sugars) into glucose, the fuel with which we operate. If too much glucose is circulating in the body, the excess is taken out of the blood with the help of the hormone insulin and is stored in the liver as glycogen. As the fuel is used up in daily activity, glycogen is gradually converted back into glucose, thus maintaining a stable blood-sugar level.

When the system is flooded with sugar, this equilibrium is disrupted and the body goes into a tailspin. Nearly every organ and gland must work overtime in a furious attempt to bring the blood-sugar level back to normal. For a while we feel ready to take on the problems of the world, but the elation is short-lived. The pancreas, reacting to what it perceives as an emergency, pours extra insulin into the bloodstream, which withdraws the sugar from the blood and restores equilibrium. In its exuberance, the overcompensating pancreas usually withdraws too much sugar, causing the blood-sugar level to drop dangerously low. We now experience fatigue, weakness, shakiness, loss of coordination, headaches, hostility, and a craving for more sugar. To ease these unsettling feelings and to "calm our nerves," we grab a cookie, cola, cigarette, or cup of coffee. This may provide momentary relief, but the pancreas overreacts again, and the cycle continues, up and down, day after day, year after year. Ultimately, the glands and the organs weaken.

For the most part, hypoglycemia is self-induced. By persistently eating highly refined carbohydrates such as concentrated sugars and white bread, drinking endless cups of coffee, and smoking cigarettes, we upset the delicate blood-sugar mechanism. Years of abuse render many of the endocrine glands ineffective. As a result, the adrenal and pituitary glands, pancreas, and liver may all produce decreased amounts of hormones no matter how much they are stimulated. Eventually, even minor stresses (such as large helpings of cake or ice cream) turn into major events, as the body, worn out from misuse, overreacts or refuses to respond.

The human biochemical system is not adapted to handle large amounts of concentrated sugar. Not only is refined sugar devoid of nutritional value, but also it leaches the body's vitamin and mineral reserves in the effort made to digest it. All carbohydrates require certain nutrients to be metabolized, the most important of which are the B-complex vitamins. Without adequate amounts of these vitamins, sugar ferments in the digestive tract and is converted into acetic acid and alcohol. Too much sugar, coupled with too few B vitamins, results in overacidity, gross nutritional imbalances, and low blood sugar.

I am not suggesting complete self-denial or a lifetime without chocolate cake. Realistically, if you can get by without sugar for five days out of seven, you are doing very well; six days out of seven is excellent. Remember, the older your body is, the less able it is to bounce back from dietary indiscretions. Be good to your-self—decrease your sugar intake and increase your ratio of sugar-free to sugar-indulgent days. On the days when you have that special treat, supplement with a B-complex vitamin. The ill effects will be reduced, and symptoms may be more moderate.

Many of us who were brought up on dessert after every meal have a hard time believing that sugar is all that harmful. The facts, unfortunately, are clear. Refined carbohydrates in general, and refined sugar in particular, have been implicated in a wide array of health problems, from obesity, diabetes, coronary thrombosis, and tooth decay, to high blood pressure, menstrual cramps, premenstrual syndrome, cancer, and mental disturbances. In countries where people live primarily on whole foods, many of these problems are nonexistent. When refined sugar and refined carbohydrates are introduced into these countries, the "diseases of civilization" emerge within ten years.

SUGAR AND "RAGING HORMONES"

Eating too much sugar is probably the greatest crime we women perpetrate against our bodies. When we are bored, anxious, happy, or depressed, we eat. Even women who restrain their urges three weeks a month may succumb two days before their periods and head straight for the nearest chocolate bar. It is not surprising that we suffer anxiety mixed with fatigue when we choose to subject our bodies to this roller-coaster existence.

Many men—and especially the male-dominated medical establishment—use an expression to explain the turbulent feelings supposedly experienced by women in connection with life transitions and menstrual events: "raging hormones." This absurd expression has been used to dismiss all female complaints. While our hormone levels do vary at different stages in our lives, whether or not they "rage" may relate to factors other than the female cycle. A blood-sugar imbalance resulting from stress or improper diet could easily trigger a mood swing. And if that is so, then men, too, can suffer from "raging hormones." I might add that many women have shared with me that they cannot relate to symptoms stemming from hormonal shifts. Their periods didn't cause them discomfort, and their menopause came and

went without fanfare. This is yet another reminder that we women are not all alike and don't like to be categorized as if we were.

DIAGNOSING HYPOGLYCEMIA

One of the best ways to determine if you suffer from a low blood-sugar level is to look at your symptoms. The body is always giving off signals, nudging you when something is awry. Fatigue may be the most common warning of an erratic blood-sugar level, but it's not the only one. Scan the following list of symptoms of low blood sugar to see how many of them apply to you:

- sudden feelings of nervousness, a sensation of "going crazy"
- periods of irritability for no reason
- spurts of energy after meals, followed by quick exhaustion
- sudden feelings of faintness or dizziness
- periodic bouts of depression
- sudden headaches
- temporary feelings of forgetfulness and confusion
- unprovoked anxiety and worry
- feelings of internal trembling
- heart palpitations
- rapid pulse not accompanying exercise
- abnormally antisocial feelings
- indecisiveness
- crying spells
- unexplained phobias
- frequent nightmares
- cravings for sweets
- indigestion, gas, colitis

Hypoglycemia is a disease with many causes, including a number of genetic, functional, and dietary imbalances. Because it is known to imitate other disease states and symptoms, it can be subtle and difficult to diagnose, thus making a

comprehensive examination, as well as a six-hour glucose-tolerance test, essential for identifying severe problems. Even the sophisticated blood glucose test is sometimes misleading; a person may fall well within the normal range (60–100 mg/dl) and still experience symptoms. Barbara Edelstein, M.D., finds in her practice that when blood sugar drops suddenly, even though not to a critical level, some women get very anxious, burst into tears, feel shaky, or become confused.[1]

If your doctor does not find anything wrong with you even though you experience many of the listed symptoms, it might be wise to seek out a nutritionist or a nutrition-oriented physician. Many orthodox physicians are not trained to recognize nutritional imbalances. Richard Brennan, founder of the International Academy of Preventive Medicine, claims that "despite hypoglycemia's seriousness, nine out of ten physicians who come into contact with the disease misdiagnose it."[2] Most physicians, when confronted with problems stemming from nutritional inadequacies, fail to treat the problem; they treat only the symptoms. Often—and I think this is especially true in the case of women—they dismiss the patient as a hypochondriac. My daughter, who did not suffer from hypoglycemia but from another serious medical condition, was encouraged to take Prozac and was given other bogus treatments and drugs before she found a qualified physician who diagnosed her correctly. Sadly, this occurred only after she'd endured years of excruciating pain.

SUGAR ADDICTION

The frequent and urgent craving for sugar has been compared to an addiction. William Dufty, a self-proclaimed former "sugar addict," writes in his book *Sugar Blues* that the only difference between a sugar habit and narcotic addiction is one of degree: "Sugar takes a little longer, from a matter of minutes in the case of a simple sugar like alcohol, to a matter of years in sugars of other kinds."[3] This may seem a bit of an exaggeration, but try going two days without your nightly raid on the refrigerator or your afternoon pick-me-up, and then think about it.

Through the years I've heard many doctors scoff at William Dufty for equating sweet attacks to overindulging on alcohol. Now, however, almost thirty years since he first proposed this possibility, his theory is gaining recognition and acceptance. Kathleen DesMaisons, Ph.D., has continued the pioneering work of earlier researchers in addictive nutrition and was actually awarded the very first doctoral degree in this specialty. According to Dr. DesMaisons in her book, *The Sugar Addict's Total Recovery Program*, "When you are a sugar addict, saying no is *not* an issue of willpower."[4] Your craving for cake and candy is profoundly affected by what and when you eat and by your brain chemistry at the time of craving. It's real. Your biochemistry can drive you straight to the grocery store for another box of cookies. It's as if you can't help yourself.

People who are driven to foods laden with white sugar and white flour are said to be "carbohydrate sensitive," which is not exactly the same as hypoglycemic. The woman with classic low blood sugar will always feel better almost immediately after eating. This may nor may not be the case with someone who's sugar sensitive. It's possible such an individual won't be at all satisfied or content with what she ate. Eating the wrong kind of food sometimes triggers a chain reaction of increasing blood sugar and insulin levels and may set the person off on a carbo binge. It may also directly affect her behavior and mood. Let's say you forget breakfast and later grab a bagel and diet soda. Soon afterward, you may feel depressed, short-tempered, forgetful, or unusually wired. In the longer term you may also experience extreme cravings, battle your weight, and struggle with eating disorders. All of these symptoms signal an acute sensitivity to simple carbohydrates, resulting in an imbalance of blood sugar and the brain chemicals serotonin and beta-endorphins.

Many of us know and love the familiar rush of beta-endorphins we experience after a sweaty workout. We relish the feelings of relaxation and satisfaction produced by those chemicals. Sugar-sensitive people unconsciously try to mimic that euphoric response by eating sugary foods. After you devour a gooey dessert, ask yourself if it's better than sex, better than your promotion at work, better than the hundred-dollar blouse you found on sale for twenty-five dollars. If so, then your beta-endorphins are overstimulated. You don't just feel good; you're ecstatic. Technically, your body is attempting to compensate for lower endorphin levels by upregulating or opening up more beta-endorphin receptors. The more opened receptors, the greater the impact or reward. But—here's the downside—the harder the fall when the sugar rush wears off. Furthermore, low serotonin levels make you feel depressed, lowering your resistance so that your plan to pass up the double mocha chocolate with whipped cream is doomed for failure.

If something in the last few paragraphs resonates with you, please pick up Dr. DesMaisons' book. Although I incorporate many of her suggestions in my recommendations for controlling blood sugar (below), she has much more to offer, including advice for keeping a journal to foster the awareness that will enable you to make lifelong adjustments to your daily diet. She also includes practical tips for detoxing yourself from sugar (no, you don't have to abstain entirely), for ordering meals when eating out, and for getting support when you need it.

DIETARY RECOMMENDATIONS FOR CONTROLLING BLOOD SUGAR

Blood-sugar imbalances can be controlled through a dietary program that reestablishes biochemical balance. Since many factors can raise or lower the blood-sugar level, it is important to treat the whole person. Minor imbalances can be controlled through diet, but in extreme situations, additional nutrient supplements may be needed.

To reverse high blood-sugar levels and to relieve fatigue, your diet must be designed for a slow release of insulin from the pancreas, ensuring a steady release of glucose into the blood throughout the day. The foods you will need to emphasize to create such a program are proteins (meat, fish, cheese, eggs, tofu/tempeh, seeds, and nuts) and complex carbohydrates (vegetables, beans, whole-grain breads and cereals, and some fruits). A small percentage of people with volatile blood-sugar regulatory problems may have to limit their intake of carbohydrates; they seem to operate best by emphasizing primarily protein-rich foods. Experiment and see what works best for you.

Specifically, you must integrate protein into each meal and snack. Don't think that this has to be a high-protein diet; rather, it's a protein-*sufficient* diet designed to maintain blood-sugar levels. Small portions adequately suffice. Ways to jack up your protein would be to add peanut butter, lox, or an egg to your whole-wheat toast; put soy or cow's milk or yogurt on your cereal; lather cream cheese on your morning bagel; fill your tortillas with chicken, beans, or cheese; sprinkle shrimp and pine nuts on your lightly cooked pasta. Marie Callendar, she of the famous pie restaurants, must have been hypoglycemic; on her menus she recommends, "An apple pie without cheese is like a kiss without a squeeze." Words to live by.

Your best carbo choices are vegetables, because they consist primarily of water and thus will not trigger an insulin response. Whole-grain breads and pastas, along with legumes, come next in the recommended list. Don't go crazy with larger portion sizes, and limit extras like jam and fruits. Removing white sugar and flour (even artificial sweeteners) from your diet calms down sugar cravings by balancing brain hormones. If you do "need" a little something extra, take it immediately after a meal, rather than by itself; you will experience less of a rush and, hence, less of a drain on your system. For me, because of the distress I feel minutes afterward, it's no longer worth it to sample a cookie between meals. I'm even experiencing difficulty taking communion. My stomach feels acidic, my body weak, and my brain muddled until I eat protein or a real meal.

Smaller, more frequent meals are recommended, as well as the elimination of concentrated sugars (even fruit juice, for sensitive people), caffeine, cigarettes, marijuana, and certain medications. A long list of prescription drugs can play havoc

with your blood-sugar levels and may create puzzling symptoms. Some medications that may send your sugar levels in either direction are anabolic steroids, estrogen, cortisone, lithium, thiazide, barbiturates, sulfonamides, and beta-blockers. If you take any prescriptions, ask your doctor about the possible effects they have on blood-sugar levels.

OTHER FACTORS THAT AFFECT BLOOD SUGAR

More factors than just the foods you eat can affect your blood-sugar level. The most significant of these are discussed in this section.

Stress

Stress in any form—physical, emotional, chemical, or nutritional—overworks the adrenal glands and can create blood-sugar imbalances. Specific medical conditions that stress the body and can precipitate or exacerbate hypoglycemia include pregnancy, lactation, cancer, tumors, chronic infection, and glandular malfunction. Be on the alert if you have any of these conditions. Since we cannot avoid all emotional stressors, and we often cannot escape environmental chemical stresses, we should learn to deal with those conditions over which we *do* have control: the physical and nutritional factors. We can physically strengthen our bodies through exercise, and we can nourish them with healthful foods and supplements, tipping the balance in favor of regeneration rather than degeneration. And let's not underestimate the recuperative power of meditation and relaxation therapy, biofeedback, water immersion, and massage.

Caffeine

Sugar is not the only factor to consider if your blood-sugar level is erratic. Coffee, chocolate, colas, and certain teas contain caffeine, which plays havoc with the body's sugar mechanism. Caffeine stimulates the adrenal cortex to produce more adrenaline, which in turn induces the liver to break down glycogen into glucose. Many people are unaware that caffeine is hidden in many soft drinks and in common over-the-counter medications such as Anacin, Excedrin, Midol, and appetite suppressants.

Alcohol

Alcohol is a central-nervous depressant, so drinking too much can increase fatigue and exacerbate depression. It can intensify hot flashes and insomnia, so menopausal women who are already experiencing these symptoms might limit wine consumption with dinner for a while. Physicians who have studied alcoholism believe that hypoglycemia may be a prime causative factor in this addiction.[5]

Cigarettes

Cigarettes change the rate at which the body handles food. A clinical experiment found that women who smoke more than fifteen cigarettes a day are apt to be fatigued as a result of the amount of nicotine their bodies are required to metabolize. Although the harmful effects of smoking can be partly offset through nutrient supplements, it is far better to end the habit. In preparation for quitting smoking, you can fortify your body by taking the following supplements daily: a high-potency multiple vitamin and mineral tablet; vitamin C, 1,000–3,000 mg; vitamin E, 400–1,000 IU (dry form); cysteine, 500–1,000 mg; and selenium, 50 mcg one to three times daily. In addition, take 10,000 IU of vitamin A daily for five days, then stop for two days.[6] A great book that explains how nicotine and other ingredients in cigarettes affect women's bodies is *How Women Can* Finally *Stop Smoking*, by Dr. Robert Klesges and Margaret DeBon.

Exercise

Exercise improves blood-sugar regulation and the receptivity of the cells to insulin. It works as a great hormone normalizer by slowly raising the level of those wonderful beta-endorphins and along with them your spirits and self-esteem. If you are faithful to an exercise program and start out slowly, exercise will increase your energy. Too many people set unrealistic goals. This can lead to feeling tired, achy, and drained after exercise, which all add up to a great temptation to quit. Do something fun, forget about setting any goals, and see how you feel.

Nutritional Supplements

Eating properly may not be enough for a person with a severe blood-sugar imbalance. Physicians who treat hypoglycemia find that additional nutrient supplements must be included. People whose diets have been deficient in vitamins and minerals, amino acids, and unsaturated fatty acids for years require greater than standard amounts of these nutrients to reverse the negative hypoglycemic cycle.[7]

B vitamins. Overconsumption of sugar and other white food products coupled with the inability to handle stress are major factors in the development of hypoglycemia. Both conditions quickly burn B vitamins, leaving the body devoid of energy. A B-complex vitamin supplement can compensate for this deficiency. I recommend a formula that contains 20–30 mg each of vitamins B-1, B-2, B-3 (niacin), and B-6, and 100–500 mg of pantothenic acid (B-5). Food sources rich in B vitamins include desiccated liver, wheat germ, peas, beans, and brewer's yeast. All the B vitamins generally occur in the same foods, so a deficiency of one usually indicates a deficiency of the others.

Vitamin A. A variety of nutrients participates directly and indirectly in maintaining blood-sugar balance. Without the complete array of these nutrients, glandular functions are diminished and hormonal output becomes erratic. For example, hormones from the adrenal cortex are very sensitive to a vitamin A deficiency. If an adequate supply of vitamin A is unavailable, cortisone, the adrenal hormone that balances the effects of insulin, will not be synthesized.

You may be eating foods containing vitamin A and still be deficient. While carotenes, which are food pigments that convert to vitamin A, occur in large amounts in green and yellow vegetables, many people have difficulty converting these into the usable nutrient through their bodily processes. Carotenes come in many forms; beta-carotene is the most important and most common. If you have difficulty converting carotene to vitamin A, you may need supplements. An appropriate range for most adults is 5,000 to 20,000 IU daily. Good sources of vitamin A (or of carotenes) include carrots, sweet potatoes, pumpkin, spinach, broccoli, and cantaloupe. (For the precise amount of this nutrient contained in certain foods, consult Appendix C.)

Vitamin C. Vitamin C is also important in the utilization of sugar. In 1977, Fred Dice of Stanford University reported that the dose of the hormone insulin required to control the sugar level in a diabetic who lacked the ability to produce the hormone was cut in half when the patient took high doses of vitamin C.[8]

The ability of vitamin C to produce energy and reduce fatigue has been noted by many scientists. It is thought that vitamin C cleanses the body of pollutants and blocks the metabolism of carcinogens found in foods and in the body. It also may prevent "tired blood" (blood that is low in oxygen, thereby slowing down its energy-producing functions) by increasing the production of leukocytes (white blood cells that fight infection) and hemoglobin (red blood cells that carry oxygen to all the cells). Without this important vitamin, energy-giving iron supplies in the body would be ineffective. In one study, over four hundred people were interviewed; those who took more than 400 mg of vitamin C per day clearly experienced less fatigue than people who were not supplementing.[9] Good sources of vitamin C include orange juice, broccoli, Brussels sprouts, grapefruit juice, strawberries, and raw tomato. (For the precise amount of this nutrient contained in certain foods, consult Appendix C.)

Minerals. The minerals magnesium, potassium, and chromium are all involved in the metabolism of carbohydrates and thus affect energy levels. Magnesium sparks more chemical reactions in the body than any other mineral, and an undersupply of this mineral can cause fatigue, weakness, and irritability. Most women fail to get enough of this mineral, which may partially explain pervasive complaints of fatigue.

Daily Supplements That Aid in Balancing Blood Sugar

- multiple vitamin and mineral supplement
- B-complex vitamins (20–30 mg), three times daily for extreme cases
- pantothenic acid (100–500 mg)
- vitamin A (5,000–10,000 IU)
- vitamin C (50–500 mg)
- magnesium (500 mg)
- potassium (2,000–3,000 mg)
- chromium (200 mcg)

Good sources of magnesium include peanuts, lentils, split peas, tofu, wild rice, bean sprouts, almonds, chicken, spinach, and beef.

Potassium deficiency can cause symptoms similar to those of low blood sugar. This was brought to public attention when American astronauts made one of their first lunar flights; they suffered heartbeat irregularities because the synthetic orange juice they drank lacked potassium. Excessive use of laxatives and diuretics, vomiting, diarrhea, or chronic low intake of water can lead to dehydration and possibly to potassium-deficiency symptoms. An adult typically ingests 1,875 to 5,625 mg daily. The recommended dosage for healthy people is 2,000 to 3,000 mg per day. Good sources of potassium include fish, potatoes, avocado, bananas, nonfat milk, fresh peas, and oranges. (For the precise amount of this nutrient contained in certain foods, consult Appendix C.)

Julian Whitaker, M.D., author of *Medical Secrets Your Doctor Won't Tell You*, routinely prescribes magnesium and potassium. He feels they are essential for good health and energy, and can be protective against heart disease, high blood pressure, and diabetes. He prefers a supplement of magnesium and potassium complexes with aspartate, an amino acid.[10]

Chromium is indispensable to the production of insulin and to the metabolism of glucose. Chromium is best taken in a brewer's yeast product that contains the chromium compound called *glucose tolerance factor* (GTF); this form is more easily absorbed and is better at stabilizing blood sugar than a standard chromium supplement. Studies show that a dosage of 200 mcg daily significantly improves glucose tolerance.[11]

Most Americans take in roughly 30 mcg of chromium daily, while the recommended range is 50 to 200 mcg. As with many minerals, absorption gradually deteriorates with age. Good sources of chromium include all-bran cereal, puffed rice, orange juice, and cheese.

Anemia

Anemia arises from a reduction of the amount of hemoglobin in the blood or a reduction in the number of red blood cells. In either case, the reduced amount of oxygen available to the cells causes decreased efficiency of body processes. The brain reacts to the lack of oxygen, causing headaches, dizziness, faintness, loss of memory, nervousness, irritability, and drowsiness. Other danger signs are rapid heartbeat, numbness and tingling in the fingers and toes, ringing in the ears, black spots in front of the eyes, and a craving for ice, dirt, clay, or laundry starch.

Anemia is never a disease in itself, but rather is always caused by other factors. The change in red blood cells may be due to the use of certain drugs, exposure to certain insecticides, infection or disease, endocrine disturbances, or bone marrow atrophy. Usually, however, anemia results from either chronic blood loss or a lack of adequate nutrients, most notably iron.

IRON

Since more than half the body's iron is present in the red blood cells as a component of hemoglobin, any blood loss results in iron depletion. Hemoglobin, the protein that transports oxygen from the lungs to the tissues and cells, not only houses the iron, but depends on it for its own production. Even hemorrhoids or ulcers can cause enough blood loss to deplete iron stores. Anyone who continually loses blood obviously requires more iron.

During her childbearing years, a woman's requirement for iron is greater than that of a man because she loses blood each month. If she has profuse or prolonged periods, or if she is using an intrauterine device (IUD), chances are she may be losing considerably more iron than is safe. IUD users are apt to develop iron deficiency because they lose up to five times the amount of blood that other women do during menstruation.[12]

Inadequate iron in the blood is a pervasive problem in both young and middle-age women. Many studies reveal that the vast majority of women take in only one-third to one-half their total daily requirement. The reasons for this are twofold: They are not consuming enough iron-rich foods, and the iron in the foods they are eating is not being utilized completely by the body.

It is difficult to eat adequate amounts of iron-rich foods. Unless you love liver and can handle several cups of beans a day, you are unlikely to get the 18 mg RDA (recommended dietary allowance) from diet alone. To combine foods high in iron is possible; unfortunately, not only would it require time and careful planning, but the amount of food needed would exceed three thousand calories daily. Even if you did make the effort to eat the required amount of iron-rich foods each day, you would still have to take into account the fact that iron is poorly absorbed by the body. Lack of adequate stomach acid makes it difficult for many postmenopausal women to absorb iron. According to most sources, only 10 percent of the iron ingested is used by the body.

Good sources of iron include liver, ground beef, dried apricots, blackstrap molasses, raisins, beans, cooked spinach, and chicken. (For the precise amount of this nutrient contained in certain foods, consult Appendix C.) For those who want to try to take care of their need for iron through diet alone, I offer some advice: When it comes to absorption, the best source of iron is liver. The other sources (spinach, peanut butter, legumes, nuts, wheat germ, molasses, apricots, and raisins) need nutritional assistance to do the job. James Cook, director of hematology at the University of Kansas Medical Center, suggests that if you combine grains, vegetables, and dried fruits with vitamin C, you can increase iron utilization as much as fourfold.[13]

Certain chemicals found in foods diminish the absorption of iron. Tannic acid (found in many teas), phytic acids (an ingredient in whole grains and cereals), and phosphates (a preservative added to most packaged bakery products, ice cream, and soft drinks) greatly decrease iron utilization.

Iron is also lost through body excretions, such as sweat. If you exercise frequently, you may lose significant amounts of iron and must therefore make sure your diet is generous in iron or take supplements.

A variety of iron supplements is available. Liver extracts provide the best meat source, called *heme iron*. Take this kind of tablet with meals. An absorbable form of nonheme, or nonmeat, iron includes iron bound to succinate, fumarate, ascorbate, glycinate, or apartate. These are better taken between meals, but if they cause abdominal discomfort, double the dose and take with meals.

Vitamin C aids in the absorption of iron and other minerals (especially calcium, copper, cobalt, and manganese). For optimum effect, take vitamin C with your iron-rich foods or as a supplement. If you eat a well-balanced diet or take a multiple vitamin and mineral tablet, you are already getting sufficient amounts of these "micronutrients."

FOLIC ACID AND B-12

Anemia and fatigue can be caused by a deficiency in nutrients other than iron. Lack of either folic acid (a B vitamin found in both vegetable and animal sources) or vitamin B-12 may produce fatigue, as well as symptoms such as apathy, withdrawal, and slowed mental ability. Like iron, folic acid is involved in creating normal red blood cells. A deficiency causes fewer cells to be produced, which means less hemoglobin and eventually less oxygen to all the cells. Folic acid deficiency is common in women, especially in women taking or making excess estrogen, pregnant women, alcoholics, and the elderly. Folic acid and vitamin B-12 interconnect biochemically and are best taken together. Again, a good multiple vitamin tablet will include the full range of B vitamins.

⪢ Underactive Thyroid ⪡

Unrelenting fatigue is a classic symptom of hypothyroidism before, during, or after menopause. Hypothyroidism, or an underactive thyroid, means that the gland is producing smaller than normal amounts of thyroid hormone. This condition is widespread, especially in women, yet frequently remains undetected. Researchers estimate that 17 to 20 percent of women will show subclinical signs of low thyroid output by their sixth decade.[14] *Subclinical* means that you know something's wrong because you don't feel right, yet the doctor can't detect anything from medical tests; blood hormone levels all fall within normal range.

The thyroid is a butterfly-shaped gland located in front of the neck, just below the Adam's apple. It controls every chemical reaction in each cell, tissue, and organ in the body. Therefore, obviously, when it fails to function at peak performance, other bodily functions are diminished to greater or lesser degrees. The first subtle complaints may be enough to signal that your body is at risk: fatigue, susceptibility to infection and disease, menstrual disorders, lowered metabolism, unexplained weight gain, sensitivity to cold, constipation, loss of hair, dry skin, puffy eyes, and cold hands and feet. Of course, these general indications could represent a number of problems. If you suspect they apply to you, follow up with self-help tests and, if indicated, check with your physician.

According to thyroid specialist Richard Shames, M.D., low thyroid output may masquerade as other illnesses. In his book, *Thyroid Power*, he explains that a patient's primary complaint may be any of the classic symptoms, but she may also exhibit a complex array of bizarre symptoms that don't seem to fit.[15] For example, an individual may suffer from extreme fatigue and inability to lose weight (a text-book case of hypothyroidism), but may also notice indigestion, gas, or constipation, indicative of a sluggish intestine. As lowered thyroid-hormone levels progress to the liver, the condition may result in abnormally high cholesterol and triglyceride levels. (Indeed, new evidence indicates that subclinical hypothyroidism, like overt hypothroidism, puts older women at risk for cardiovascular disease.)[16]

Other body parts are affected by inadequate thyroid-hormone levels, too. Sluggish skin can erupt in acne, eczema, or atypical rashes. For a menopausal woman, even if thyroid levels are borderline at the time of the change, her hot flashes, mood swings, and vaginal irritations can be made considerably worse. Younger women who are severely bothered by endometriosis or stricken by repeated miscarriages or infertility should consider the possibility that inadequate thyroid hormone may be partly responsible.

Recent research indicates that estrogen therapy decreases thyroid function. An article in the *New England Journal of Medicine* confirms that estrogen increases protein binding of thyroxine, creating symptoms of low thyroid hormone or increasing the severity of preexisting hypothyroidism.[17] John Lee, M.D., has also observed that women taking estrogen exhibited traditional symptoms of low thyroid hormone, yet fell within the normal range when tested. In a more recent newsletter he suggests that women can find relief from menopausal symptoms if they lower their estrogen dose and/or add progesterone, which balances the tendency of estrogen to decrease thyroid function.[18]

SUBSTANCES THAT DEPRESS THYROID FUNCTION

Everyday foods, additives, and drugs can compromise thyroid function. Cutting down or eliminating as many of these irritating substances from your diet can be an important step in relieving the effects created by an already sluggish thyroid.

Goitrogens, substances or chemicals that when taken in large enough quantities to result in an enlarged thyroid gland called a goiter, have a prominent effect. Foods that result in the release of goitrogens include soybeans, almonds, peanuts, pine nuts, sorghum, millet, sweet corn, and cassava (tapioca). Additionally, foods from the cruciferous vegetable family interfere with iodine uptake and are best to avoid; these include Brussels sprouts, cauliflower, cabbage, and broccoli. If you do eat these highly nutritious vegetables, cook them to neutralize some of the antithyroid properties.

I would like to single out one specific food mentioned above because many health authorities are advocating excessive use of it to relieve and/or treat menopausal symptoms, heart disease, cancer, and almost anything else that ails you. While soybeans and soy products can be healthful, in large quantities they also may prove deleterious to those with low thyroid function. My editor has a friend who followed a vegan diet and therefore ate four or five servings of soy per day. She suffered from subclinical hypothyroidism. After eliminating all soy from her diet, her hypothyroidism cleared up dramatically.

SELF-HELP TESTS FOR UNDERACTIVE THYROID AND LOW BLOOD SUGAR

The symptoms of hypothyroidism are similar to those of hypoglycemia. According to Broda Barnes, a well-respected doctor who published more than a hundred papers on the thyroid gland, there is a direct correlation between an underactive thyroid and blood-sugar imbalances; in fact, a drop in blood sugar is one of the symptoms of hypothyroidism.[19] As Barnes explains, when the thyroid is underactive, the liver is unable to release its stored glycogen and produce glucose, thereby

causing a low blood-sugar condition. This theory has been tested in the laboratory: When the livers of laboratory animals are removed, blood sugar declines rapidly, and death from hypoglycemia occurs unless glucose is injected intravenously.

Barnes suggests that both hypoglycemia and hypothyroidism can be diagnosed at home. For hypoglycemia, simple observation of symptoms is sufficient. To detect an underactive thyroid, take your basal body temperature (the temperature of the body at rest) before getting out of bed in the morning. If it reads below 97.8°F, there is reason to suspect a thyroid deficiency. Repeat for three or four days to be certain of your reading. (For accurate basal temperature measurement, place a thermometer at your bedside. As you are awakening, place the thermometer in your armpit and keep it secure for ten minutes. Menstruating women note: Take your temperature during the week of your period; body temperature is subject to greater fluctuation during the remainder of the month.)

IODINE

The manufacture of thyroid hormone is dependent on several nutrients, and the mineral iodine is at the top of the list. A deficiency of iodine or an inability to metabolize iodine results in an enlargement of the gland, a condition known as *goiter*. A sore neck sometimes indicates a possible glandular dysfunction.

The most important dietary source of iodine is iodized salt (containing 70 mcg of iodine per gram of salt). If you use salt in cooking or sprinkle it onto your food, there is little chance you need more iodine. Fast food, canned foods, and prepackaged foods contain significant amounts of iodized salt, so if these are part of your everyday diet there's no need to supplement further. (In fact, if you eat a diet high in processed foods, you may be getting too much iodine, which also harms the thyroid gland.)

Most salt is iodized, but if you use sea salt (which is not iodized), or if you are restricting your salt intake, and if you don't eat much fish, consider supplementing your diet with kelp tablets. One tablet, taken four times a day, will stimulate production of the thyroid hormone in most individuals. Susan Weed, authority on both herbs and menopause, is not fond of pills or capsules. She suggests that women use high-quality powdered kelp or dried pieces of kelp, totalling 3 to 5 grams per day.[20] Sea vegetables are an excellent way to obtain the trace minerals that help boost thyroid production, but they are not commonly consumed in the United States. If you're open to trying something new, kombu, another name for kelp, is a healthy addition to soup. Seaweed is found in several kinds of sushi as a wrapper for the fish and rice, and is also used in the Japanese diet as an ingredient itself.

TYROSINE

Along with iodine, the thyroid gland requires tyrosine, an amino acid found in specific proteins, to make thyroid hormone. While tyrosine is abundant in many common foods, thus making it rare for people to suffer from a deficiency of it, you may want to go over the list that follows and make certain these foods find a way into your meal plan: meat, aged cheese, yeast-containing breads and pastas, bananas, almonds, avocados, pumpkin, and sesame seeds. Another approach to increasing tyrosine levels in the diet—and certainly not my first choice, but rather an option—is to buy a mixture of amino acid powder at the health-food store, combine it with freeze-dried algae, kelp, or green vegetables, and stir it into your morning orange juice or shake.

SELENIUM AND ZINC

For the synthesis and metabolism of thyroid hormone, numerous nutrients and enzymes must work in concert. The importance of iodine is well established. The effects of selenium deficiency on thyroid-hormone concentration are less profound than those of iodine deficiency; however, a lack of both selenium and zinc leads to severe hypothyroidism and goiter in rats.[21] Check your daily multiple vitamin/mineral tablet to make sure it includes 25 mg of zinc and 10 mcg of selenium.

⇒ Tired Adrenal Glands ⇐

Fatigue generated by adrenal exhaustion is caused by unrelenting low-level stress. Whether the chronic stress is emotional or physical, good stress or bad, over time it takes a toll on the body, and our little adrenal glands pay. The crescent-shaped adrenal glands, which lie on top of each kidney, have the enormous and vital job of producing the important stress hormones adrenaline and cortisol, to name only two. These substances prepare us for action in the face of stress by increasing our heart rate and blood pressure and sending blood to the muscles and the brain. They enable the body's "fight-or-flight" response to kick in, and they also improve our ability to recover from the major and minor traumas of life. However, if living through many years of chronic stress means we come to menopause already "drained," otherwise normal symptoms might just push us over the edge into debilitating fatigue and depression. Interrupted sleep, one of the complaints of perimenopause, further exacerbates adrenal exhaustion. Rest and repair of the adrenal glands occurs somewhere between 11:00 P.M. and 1:00 A.M., and if you are awake during those hours, the repair process doesn't happen.

ARE YOUR ADRENAL GLANDS THE PROBLEM?

Adrenal fatigue is related to both hypoglycemia and hypothyroidism. When the adrenal glands fail to function properly, the blood-sugar response tends to become more sensitive and thyroid-hormone output tends to decline. Some of the symptoms of adrenal dysfunction are similar to hypoglycemia and hypothyroidism, but others help to distinguish it from these two conditions. Symptoms include dizziness (especially when getting up after sitting), headaches, inability to concentrate, heart irregularities, trouble getting out of the bed in the morning, tender spots in the muscles, throat irritation, and low blood pressure.

How do you tell if your fatigue and other symptoms are related to your adrenal glands rather than something else? Conventional blood tests may fail to indicate an abnormality, so you may want to consider ordering a saliva test to measure cortisol and DHEA levels (see Resources). James Kwako, M.D., finds that a salivary hormone level taken four times a day is particularly revealing, because cortisol has a very definite circadian (twenty-four-hour) rhythm. It's at its highest in the early mornings, between 3:00 A.M. and 9:00 A.M.; then it reaches a low at night, sometime between 11:00 P.M. and 2:00 A.M.[22]

PEPPING UP YOUR TIRED ADRENALS

Should the tests indicate elevated cortisol levels at the wrong time of day, you need to pay attention to rebuilding your adrenal strength. Start with dietary changes and stress-reduction techniques, but if they prove ineffective, supplementation may be necessary. An excellent book on the topic is *The Cortisol Connection: Why Stress Makes You Fat and Ruins Your Health—and What You Can Do about It*, by nutrition expert Shawn Talbott, Ph.D. It features a complete plan for counteracting the negative health effects of chronic stress, including several chapters devoted to designing a program of nutritional supplementation. If your salivary test also shows subnormal DHEA levels, it may be appropriate to supplement with this hormone, because DHEA protects against the overproduction of cortisol. Choose pharmaceutical-grade DHEA, and start with a daily dose of 10–25 mg. Retest in three months to see if your DHEA levels have increased adequately to put you in the normal range, and also to determine whether your cortisol level is more consistent with normal. If this is the case, you can taper off the DHEA. If not, your health practitioner may choose to keep you on the same dosage for three more months or to increase it.

If you have tired adrenals, finding ways to relax and minimize turmoil in your life is an obvious necessity. However, you need to be particularly careful to avoid dietary stressors *as well as* emotional stressors. You must devote time and effort to

discovering and practicing an eating plan that works for you. A hypoglycemic diet works well to keep blood-sugar levels balanced; consequently, it will give all your glands a chance to regroup. Avoid stringent weight-loss plans that eliminate any of the major food groups: fats, proteins, or carbohydrates. And consider taking the following adrenal-strengthening supplements: a B-complex vitamin with 50 mg/day each of B-1, B-2, and B-6, and 500 mg/day of B-12. Vitamin B-5 (pantothenic acid) should be taken twice daily with meals, in 200-mg doses. Vitamin C can be taken in doses up to 500 mg/day. Your health professional may advise larger doses of these vitamins in extreme cases.

⋙ Copper and Zinc Reversed ⋘

When all else fails in your search for unexplained fatigue, an imbalance in two trace minerals—copper and zinc—just may be the root of the problem. Nutritionist Ann Louise Gittleman presents an innovative theory in her book, *Why Am I Always So Tired?* Her premise is well researched, fascinating, and makes logical sense. Minerals often work in tandem with each other, and such is the case with copper and zinc. Ideally, they coexist best in a ratio of 1:8 copper to zinc. An overexposure to copper upsets the balance and the body's normal functioning. Gittleman cites many reasons why copper gains the upper hand, but stress and a weakened adrenal function lead the list. In a vicious cycle, the more stress we're under, the more likely we are to develop copper overload or zinc deficiency, either of which leads to adrenal insufficiency—and then the more likely we are to develop the adrenal insufficiency that leads to copper excess.[23] Furthermore, a skewed copper-to-zinc ratio suppresses both the thyroid and the liver, contributing to hypothyroidism and poor liver-enzyme function. Do you see how all these systems, glands, and hormones interreact and depend on each other for support and survival? Bolster one and you strengthen the others.

It's not a stretch to imagine how copper and zinc find themselves out of kilter when you consider all the potential factors that spike up the body's copper levels. Various environmental factors contribute greatly, because copper is found in everything from pipes to pesticides. Copper from the water pipes and the copper tubing installed in our homes leaches into the water supply and eventually gets into our bodies. Xenoestrogens (estrogen mimics) abound in our everyday world, in the pesticides blanketing our otherwise healthy fruits and vegetables, in the plastics we touch and handle regularly, and in the household products we clean our homes with. Because xenoestrogens resemble female estrogen molecules, they can build up

in our body, causing us to retain copper. Even certain healthy foods I've urged menopausal women to consume with regularity are particularly rich in copper: nuts, soy products, whole grains, and shellfish.

On the other side of this seesaw is zinc deficiency, which is rampant among American woman but could easily be reversed with a concerted effort. Zinc depleters are easy to spot and to control; they include coffee, alcohol, sugar, stress, and a high-carbohydrate diet. Common over-the-counter drugs impair zinc absorption, thus contributing to copper excess; these include Zantac, Tagamet, antacids, and many diuretics. Sadly, the diet that many women cling to—one that is low in fat, high in carbohydrate, and minimal in protein—is zinc deficient. This is particularly true when the carbohydrates we choose are the fat-free, sugar-filled nonfoods that hide in our cupboards. You can count white-floured pastas, breads, bagels, and muffins as part of the problem, too. Not only are they zinc-free; they lack such other nutrients as the B-vitamins and manganese needed for preventing copper toxicity. Due to special circumstances, such as surgery, injury, illness, weight loss, ERT, and pregnancy, some women need more zinc than the RDA of 12 mg/day.

Reversing the tendency of copper overload is simple. Avoid as many of the xenoestrogens as possible to limit excessive estrogen-like effects in the body. Check your home's pipes and water supply for copper plumbing. Wash your fruits and vegetables to lessen the amount of pesticide residue you ingest. Junk those sugary cookies, gooey deserts, and white pastry products, and replace them with whole grains and healthier goodies. Eat more fiber-rich foods, such as fruits, vegetables, grains, beans, and bran, because they help to carry the toxins out of the body. Add more foods that are high in zinc to your daily diet: eggs, red meat, and poultry. You don't have to force down large portions of these items; three ounces, or a serving the size of your fist, is adequate. Finally, consider supplementing with 15–30 mg of zinc/day.

☙ Herbs for Fighting Fatigue ❧

Once you've dealt with any underlying health issues that might be causing your fatigue, consider adding to your daily regimen one of the herbs that have traditionally been used to increase energy. But remember: Herbs are to be used as *supplements;* they are not a substitute for addressing chronic health troubles. If you're anemic or suffering from hypothyroidism, swallowing ginseng capsules isn't going to solve your problems. That's why I advocate using supplements only under the care of a qualified and knowledgeable health professional.

GINKGO BILOBA

Ginkgo biloba increases the flow of blood to the brain, improves memory, and has been successful in treating problems related to poor circulation. It has been shown to increase the uptake of glucose by brain cells and to improve the transmission of nerve signals.[24] An extract of the fresh leaves is marketed in the United States and Europe; the product should be standardized to contain 24 percent ginkgo flavonglycosides.

Ginkgo biloba is said to be the world's oldest surviving species and can be traced back 200 million years. It has been cultivated in China as a sacred tree, and now it is grown widely across the United States. Ginkgo leaves have been used in Chinese medicine for their beneficial effect on the brain. To increase your energy, take the standard dosage of 40 mg, three times a day. Pills are also available; take as recommended by the manufacturer.

GINSENG

For fatigue, take capsules of powdered Siberian ginseng in doses of 200 mg to 1,000 mg, three times a day, for one to three months. It is better to use lower doses for a longer time than higher doses for a shorter time. Herbs work at the cellular level, and their tonic effect is not dramatic. Expect to wait a few weeks before noticing results. If you are having difficulties sleeping, do not take ginseng close to bedtime.

≋ Setting Realistic Goals ≋

One last comment concerning fatigue: Don't overlook the obvious. You may be overtired because you are trying to do too much, trying to be everything to everybody, and running yourself ragged. Examine your daily routine and responsibilities; maybe your lack of energy is caused by an impossible schedule. A good source for more information about the so-called superwoman syndrome is Georgia Witkin-Lanoil's *The Female Stress Syndrome: How to Recognize and Live with It.*[25] Remember, workaholism is an addiction—and a disease.

CHAPTER 5

SEXUAL CHANGES

*With all the complexity, with all the difficulties, most midlife women
will say, "Sex? It's gotten better and better."*

— LILLIAN B. RUBIN, *Women of a Certain Age*

Menopause does not mean the end of sex. Quite the contrary; for many women, the midlife years are especially sexually satisfying and creative. Think about it: After nearly forty years, you are free from the fear of pregnancy and the bother of birth control devices, tampons, and pads. Better yet, opportunities that were few and far between when the kids were running in and out of the house are now available. An entire Saturday afternoon can be spent in a leisurely romantic interlude. You don't have to worry or hurry. Look forward to these days—they should be a time of celebration.

More good news: Some of the hormonal alterations women experience at menopause actually heighten their sexual response; for many women, sex is even more satisfying at fifty than at twenty. People who think that women change into asexual beings at menopause should consider these revealing statements from *The Hite Report:*[1]

"I believe sexual desire increases with age. Enjoyment certainly increases—I can vouch for that."

"I didn't know getting older would make sex better! I'm 51 now and just getting started."

"I thought that menopause was the leading factor in my dry and irritable vaginal tract. My doctors thought that it was lack of hormones...but with my new lover, I am reborn. Plenty of lubrication, no irritation."

Why do we expect the sexual charge to abandon us once we reach a certain age? I believe we are conditioned to expect this. All through life we are subtly—and not so subtly—indoctrinated by the media to believe that sex and beauty accompany youth. The ads in popular magazines and on TV confirm this. So it is not surprising that many older women, when they see a few lines on their faces and feel a few extra pounds on their figures, feel less desirable.

The emotional impact of these changes can be devastating for some women. Kaylan Pickford, a once-famous over-fifty model, observes that if a woman accepts the idea that only in youth is there beauty, sexuality, and therefore love, she falls into the trap of making unrealistic comparisons and becomes insecure. To compare the first spring bud with a late summer blossom is absurd. Pickford says that youth, middle age, and old age should never be compared. They are each as unique and beautiful as the changing seasons. Each offers a fresh perspective, a different experience.[2]

Sex: It's About More than Just Your Hormones

Although reaching—and passing—midlife in no way must mean a death sentence for sexual desire and fulfillment, real sexual issues can confront women in their menopausal years. Sexual health is an important factor in overall health and well-being. Diminished sexual capacity in "older women" deserves to be the focus of serious scientific research and media attention. While some women report little change in sexual activity during their midlife years, between 50 and 86 percent, depending on the study, do admit to some loss of sexual function. The most common complaints are a lack of interest in sex and painful intercourse due to vaginal dryness. Determining the cause of sexual disinterest and discomfort is difficult because so many factors influence sexuality—from physical to psychological, social to relational.

Factors Affecting Sexual Desire

- illness
- hormonal imbalances
- lack of sleep
- anxiety
- psychological issues
- lifestyle factors (nutrition, smoking, alcohol use)
- medications
- past experiences
- relationship issues
- current expectations
- social factors

It is beyond the scope of this book to delve into the myriad nuances of such a complicated issue as sexuality. But do note that if you no longer feel sexy, jumping on the estrogen bandwagon to solve all your problems may not be the right solution. Your situation could be more complicated and require a nondrug, nonhormonal approach. We tend to think that taking hormones dissolves all midlife symptoms, and this simply isn't true.

As Judith Reichman, medical correspondent for "The Today Show," advises in her book *I'm Not in the Mood: What Every Woman Should Know about Improving Her Libido*, before considering drugs or hormones, ask yourself if you may be depressed or overly anxious, or if you're concerned about your changing body or involved in a toxic relationship. Counseling to unravel such possibilities could be a positive step toward greater sexual enjoyment.

≫ Is It All in Your Head? ≪

"A woman's sex life after menopause is determined more by her psychological outlook than her physical changes," says John Moran, gynecologist and director of the Well Woman Centre in London. The fate of the libido seems to depend on a number of factors, such as genetic makeup, early childhood upbringing, and life experiences, all of which come into play long before menopause. Psychiatrists agree that the sex drive is predominantly psychological, though controlled to a degree by the amount of steroids circulating in the blood. It is possible that women who complain they do not "feel sexy" after the change also did not feel that way before menopause. An extensive Kinsey study found that some women use menopause as an excuse to curtail sexual relationships they were unenthusiastic about anyway.

To a large extent, however, how a woman responds sexually depends on the interest and response of her partner. Your husband or lover may be going through his or her own midlife crisis. While middle-age men do not experience the range of hormonal changes women do, they do undergo anatomical changes that can reduce their sexual responsiveness. Like the woman's ovaries, the man's testicles decrease in size. The vas deferens, the narrow tube that transports sperm, becomes narrower, and the sperm become thinner and less plentiful. It generally takes longer for the middle-age male to reach arousal and orgasm. If the man is unaware that this is normal, he may become overanxious, and he may transfer his insecurity to his partner. Researchers note that some women's psychological problems with sex during this time of life may be caused by men who, bewildered by their own changes in sexual performance, shift the blame to their partners.[3]

Around the half-century mark, both men and women confront new problems and must make adjustments. They sometimes switch jobs, realizing that if they intend to make a career change, it had better be soon. Children entering college may become a financial burden. Illnesses may result in physical adjustments, economic insecurity, and emotional stress. The uncertainty arising from all these changes may be more responsible for sexual and marital problems than either hormonal or physiological changes.

It is said that the most difficult part of aging sexually is accepting it. Men and women need to realize that our physical responses inevitably slow down as we age. This has nothing to do with our femininity or masculinity—it is normal. Allowing more time for sexual expression is important. The word *communication* may be overused, but maybe that is because talking honestly about your troubles is

a good, commonsense practice. Share with your partner what is happening in your body; together you can creatively pursue ways of finding mutual satisfaction.

Myths and misconceptions have defined sexual roles for too long. For modern adult women, it is time to differentiate between the facts and the fiction about aging, menopause, and sexual satisfaction. Correct information is the best ally we have in preparing for the change—or any change, for that matter.

Physical Changes

Now that we've taken a look at some of the most significant nonphysical factors affecting sexuality, let's examine the vital role played by our changing bodies—including our hormones. Women going through menopause experience physiological changes in their female organs and hormonal secretions, some of which may result in a temporary decline in their sexual responsiveness. As Dr. Moran explained to me, "The dramatic change in hormone levels during the menopause accounts for a variety of unpleasant symptoms: chiefly, tiredness, lack of energy, low self-esteem, and poor memory. If the common vasomotor symptoms—hot flashes, headaches, and night sweats—are present, these can also lead to a feeling of being unwell. With all these symptoms, it is not surprising that sexual pleasure is diminished."

In a study collecting data from a group of perimenopausal women, it was found that there was a close association between the number of hot flashes and the frequency of intercourse.[4] Women experiencing hot flashes had a lower level of sexual activity. This observation can be interpreted in two ways: Women who have hot flashes do not want sex more regularly, or regular sexual activity is protective against hot flashes. Both are possible.

Losing sleep and feeling overtired are reasons enough for anyone, at any age, to lose interest in sex. The cessation of menstrual periods and declining levels of female hormones, however, do not in themselves affect sexual desire. In fact, there is mounting evidence that in some women sexual interest and enjoyment do not decrease at midlife, but rather increase. This is because of the change in the ratio of male to female hormones. What few women realize is that the hormone most responsible for sexual arousal is the male hormone testosterone. Although testosterone is present in the female system prior to menopause, its effect is tempered by the larger proportions of estrogen and progesterone. As these female hormones decrease at menopause, the proportion of testosterone increases.

Declining female hormone levels may not directly affect sexual response, but they do subtly alter the reproductive tissues, often leading to uncomfortable and even painful intercourse. The changes are most evident in the vagina, which becomes smaller, shorter, thinner, smoother, drier, and less elastic. As estrogen levels decline, blood flow to the genitals diminishes and secretions of vaginal mucus dwindle. A woman generally is slower to lubricate in response to sexual arousal and often takes a little longer to achieve orgasm, although, according to Niels Lauersen, gynecologist and professor of obstetrics at Mt. Sinai Hospital in New York City, the difference is not great—between seconds and minutes.[5] In any case, women need not feel insecure if they take longer to lubricate; remember that it also takes longer for the mature man to achieve erection. Actually, for men and women close in age, this is probably the first time in the sexual relationship in which arousal time is almost equal.

Other parts of the female anatomy undergo minor changes. The cervix, ovaries, and uterus diminish in size; the labia majora (outer lips of the vulva) become thinner, paler, and smaller; the breasts lose some of their fat, firmness, and shape, and may even become slightly less sensitive; and clitoral stimulation may become irritating due to lack of lubrication. Some of these changes may be unnoticeable, while others may be annoying, but they are all normal.

Balancing Hormone Levels for Sexual Health

Maintaining adequate levels of sex hormones is key to a satisfying sex life—and this is true before, during, and after menopause. No hormone in the body acts independently, including the sex hormones: estrogen, progesterone, and testosterone. All are derived from the same original source, cholesterol, and their levels rise and fall depending on cues taken from each other. When one is inadequate, another will pick up the slack and cascade (be converted) into the other. A wonderful backup system exists among the sex hormones, so that when outside factors interfere with the balance, we are protected. To suggest that estrogen is responsible for all menopausal symptoms and that replacing estrogen alone will cure them is a myopic view of this complex system. All the sex hormones participate to keep our sexuality alive and healthy. Not only the female hormones, but also the male hormones, such as testosterone, must be present in specific amounts to insure sexual desire and satisfaction.

THE ROLE OF ESTROGEN

Researchers have concentrated on estrogen as the single most important hormone involved in menopausal symptoms, yet questions still exist as to how it contributes to sexual desire. Estrogen receptors are found all over the body, so it stands to reason that the hormone's systemic action—which means it stimulates everything, including brain, bones, skin, blood vessels, intestines, and genitourinary system—may exert at the very least an indirect role in sexual health. It is widely known that

dwindling levels of estrogen result in a thinning and drying of the vaginal tissue, causing uncomfortable and painful intercourse. Estrogen stimulates blood flow to sensitive areas; thus, an inadequate supply may make it more difficult to experience pleasurable stimulation and to reach orgasm. But does estrogen replacement therapy boost a flagging libido? Studies say no. HRT in the form of estrogen does improve vaginal dryness and pain from intercourse in women with vaginitis, but for women with sexual dysfunction and low libido, it has little or no effect at all.[6]

If lubrication is your main issue, natural remedies may be sufficient. Many women have shared with me that soy, vitamins, and herbs proved most helpful. Unfortunately, they didn't work for me—and I so badly wanted to boast about how soy cured all my symptoms! Instead, I had to try something stronger if I wanted any kind of a sex life. (Cringing during sex is not a turn-on for either party.) So I tried estriol—and let me just say *yeah!*

Estrogen replacement comes in many forms—some more gentle on the body than others. Estriol has a safer track record than its stronger counterpart, estradiol (a leading component of some conventional hormone therapies). Estriol effectively combats a dry vagina, making sex fun again. You can take it orally as part of a bi-est or tri-est formula, or use it as a vaginal cream. Christiane Northrup, M.D., also recommends estriol vaginal cream to relieve urinary symptoms. Since this method of delivery doesn't result in any appreciable absorption into the bloodstream, women worried about the risk for breast cancer can feel more comfortable using it.[7] Vaginal estriol must be prescribed by a physician and is available from compounding pharmacies. You apply the cream to the top surface of the vagina or insert it into the vagina with an applicator nightly for up to two weeks, and then as needed. Dosages vary from 0.5 mg/g to 1.0 mg/g. Consult with your doctor to determine the lowest amount that works for you. (See Chapter 2 for a detailed discussion of estriol therapy versus conventional HRT.)

PROGESTERONE IS A POSSIBILITY

The second female hormone, progesterone, has been studied less than estrogen as a libido enhancer, but women who use it swear that it works. In addition, ongoing research is finding links between progesterone insufficiency and lowered sexual energy. Progesterone is a precursor of both estrogen and testosterone, which means that if they are in short supply, progesterone comes to the rescue and produces more. On the other hand, if progesterone recognizes too much estrogen and testosterone present in the blood, it can dampen the effects of oversupply, leveling out the imbalance. Progesterone has been labeled the "feel-good" hormone because it enhances mood, improves sleep, and normalizes other hormones.

In a clinical setting, Dr. John Lee noticed that his female patients who complained of losing interest in sex also had an array of other symptoms: water retention, fibrocystic breasts, depression, dry, wrinkling skin, and irregular and sometimes heavy periods.[8] He came to understand that these signs were indicative of a progesterone deficiency and possibly also of an estrogen dominance. To balance an estrogen excess, you can take progesterone orally in doses of 25 to 100 mg or use a cream of equivalent dose. Talk to your health-care professional regarding specific instructions for your symptoms.

TESTOSTERONE AND WOMEN

Many women are surprised to learn that their bodies make male hormones, called *androgens*, and that production of these hormones declines with age. Testosterone, one of the most well-known of the androgens, is gaining popularity as "the hormone of desire" because it has been shown to successfully treat women with low libido. Although most of the studies using testosterone replacement have included only women who have undergone a complete hysterectomy, more recently women going through natural menopause have found testosterone supplementation to heighten sexual satisfaction for them as well. Psychiatrist Susan Rako knows from both her own experience and her extensive research on the subject that if the body isn't producing enough testosterone, the deficiency may lead to a complete inability to experience sexual desire, sexual fantasy, arousal, and/or orgasm. She explains, "No matter how hard a woman might try to assemble the building blocks of healthy sexual functioning—the required amounts of other hormones, a loving partner, adequate stimulation, possibly a good sexual fantasy—it cannot work if she does not have the basic foundation of enough testosterone."[9]

Symptoms of Testosterone Deficiency

- overall decreased sexual desire
- diminished vital energy and sense of well-being
- decreased sensitivity to sexual stimulation in the clitoris
- decreased sensitivity to sexual stimulation in the nipples
- overall decreased arousability and capacity for orgasm
- thinning and loss of pubic hair (in some women)

Symptoms of androgen deficiency frequently go unidentified and untreated because the medical community has been slow to address, recognize, and research sexual dysfunction in women. Dr. Rako lists the most obvious signs of testosterone deficiency in her book, *The Hormone of Desire*.

Dozens of articles have been published in medical journals demonstrating that women who had undergone surgical menopause (bilateral oophorectomy, or removal of both ovaries) and were treated with both estrogen and testosterone reported higher rates of sexual desire and arousal and a greater number of fantasies than those who were given either estrogen alone or left untreated.[10] One study found that in some women, supplemental estrogen alone at menopause may be counterproductive, because it can decrease testosterone levels in the blood and worsen sex drive as well as other recalcitrant menopausal symptoms.[11] The authors of this study concluded that ERT ultimately may represent an incomplete preventive hormonal treatment. Continuing studies suggest that testosterone replacement can markedly improve sexuality in postmenopausal women.

A major concern of women and health-care providers unfamiliar with supplemental testosterone is its potential unattractive masculinizing effects. Not to fear. Clinical evidence indicates that such changes (facial and body hair, lowered voice, acne, male-pattern baldness, and larger muscles) are infrequent and readily reversible once the supplement is stopped.[12] Studies of women who ended up with these unwanted symptoms found that they had taken the full dose of the commercial product Estratest. This commonly prescribed oral estrogen-testosterone combination comes in two strengths, and many physicians who have used it with their patients contend that both doses are set too high.

Many physicians prefer the oral synthetic form of testosterone, called *methyltestosterone*, because natural testosterone converts too quickly to estrogen. Compounding pharmacies can special order either natural or synthetic versions of testosterone and can help to regulate the dosage, keeping it at the lowest dose necessary to reduce symptoms. Compounders can formulate products into capsules, creams, gels, ointments, and lozenges. A prudent goal is to keep blood levels of the hormone within a normal physiological range. Blood tests and saliva tests can be taken periodically to maintain and monitor appropriate levels.

Natural Remedies for Vaginal Dryness

In a few women, decreased elasticity of the vagina, along with the reduced ability to lubricate, may cause vaginal dryness so severe that intercourse becomes uncomfortable or painful. In severe cases, it may even cause bleeding. The usual medical treatment for vaginal dryness and irritation is estrogen replacement therapy. However, if estrogen is contraindicated for you, or if you would rather not take hormones, internal as well as external lubricants are available.

DIETARY AIDS

Phytoestrogens may provide natural internal lubrication by improving blood flow to uterine tissue. Plants such as soybeans and herbs such as ginseng that work within the enzyme system as adaptogens can stimulate a woman's body to produce additional estrogen—but they only have this effect if she needs it.[13]

Of all foods, tofu, or soybean curd, contains the greatest amounts of isoflavones, which are phytohormones with estrogen-like properties.[14] (See Chapters 3 and 15 for more discussion of phytohormones and soy.) Soy is now widely available in the United States in many forms. You can experiment with recipes by substituting soybeans for beans in soups, stews, and casseroles. Soy flour can replace wheat flour in breads, rolls, pancakes, and muffins. Vegetarians are familiar with soy-based alternatives to meat. If you have not sampled veggie burgers, frozen soy desserts, or soy cheese, I highly recommend them. And even your favorite latte or cappuccino (decaf, of course) can be made with soy milk.

Daily Nutritional Support for Female Tissues	
Vitamin A (beta-carotene)	5,000–30,000 IU
Vitamin C	500–5,000 mg
Bioflavonoids	500–2,000 mg
Vitamin E	400–1,200 IU

(For the precise amount of these nutrients contained in certain foods, consult Appendix C.)

Essential fatty acids (EFAs) help keep all the tissues of the body, including the skin, hair, and genital tissues, well lubricated internally. In our concern to limit the fats in our diets, we may go overboard and eliminate necessary essential fatty acids. Two oils are classified as "essential" because the body cannot manufacture them; they must come from the diet. Linoleic acid, an omega-6 fatty acid, is primarily found in nuts and in seeds such as flax, pumpkin, sesame, and sunflower seeds. The oils derived from these sources are good choices for use on salads and for taking as a supplement (about 1 to 2 tablespoons per day). Linolenic acid, of the omega-3 family, is primarily found in oils of fish such as salmon, trout, and mackerel. If you would rather not rely on your diet for EFAs, there are many capsule supplements of essential oils that will help to internally moisturize your tissues. Try evening primrose oil, flaxseed oil, black currant seed oil, and borage oil. The typical dosage is two to eight capsules per day. Diabetics should not take supplemental fish oils, but can eat cold-water fish such as salmon, tuna, trout, herring, and sardines.

Women bothered by vaginal dryness need to avoid substances that will further sap moisture from the membranes, including alcohol, caffeine, diuretics, and antihistamines. They should also keep the body well hydrated by drinking one to two quarts of water each day.

Specific vitamins and vitamin-like substances support and maintain the health of the vaginal and urinary tissues. Without them, these organs atrophy and dry out. See the table "Daily Nutritional Support for Female Tissues" above for recommended amounts of these nutrients.

Note: If you have high blood pressure, diabetes, or a rheumatic heart condition, do not take more than 30 IU of vitamin E without first consulting your physician.

HERBS

The herb chaste tree (vitex) contains flavonoids, glycosides, and micronutrients that enhance hormonal production and revitalize vaginal tissues. Dosage is generally one capsule up to three times a day, taken on an empty stomach, or twenty drops of tincture one or two times a day. Motherwort and dong quai may also stimulate vaginal lubrication and your sex life.

EXTERNAL LUBRICANTS

Vegetable oils can help moisturize the vagina, increasing sexual enjoyment. The most popular choice is vitamin E oil in liquid or suppository form, though most unscented massage oils will also work. Mineral-based products such as petroleum jelly and baby oil should not be used since they tend to coat the vaginal lining and inhibit one's own natural secretions. In this age of AIDS, it is important to know that petroleum-based products weaken and break down latex condoms—another reason to avoid them. Water-based products plump up the vaginal tissue by providing additional moisture. Everyone is familiar with the old standby, K-Y Jelly, but there are new names on the market, such as Astroglide, Sensell, Probe, and calendula cream.

For women who do not want to bother with lubricating just prior to intercourse, there is a moisturizer gel called Replens that lasts up to three days. It is inserted as a suppository and has the additional benefit of protecting against vaginal infection.

Natural progesterone creams, discussed in Chapter 2, are also recommended. John Lee started using natural progesterone for menopausal women who could not take estrogen and found that, in many cases, it not only reversed osteoporosis but reduced vaginal atrophy.[15]

Natural Remedies for Bladder and Vaginal Infections

Fifteen percent of menopausal women experience recurrent bladder and vaginal infections. Typical symptoms are frequent and painful urination, increased nighttime urination, feeling a need to urinate even when the bladder is empty, pain in the lower abdomen, and a strong or unpleasant smell to the urine. Infections sometimes get out of control and require medical attention. If this is the case, see a doctor. Frequent urination itself could indicate a diabetic condition. It is important to determine when it is appropriate to use natural methods and when professional services are necessary.

Vaginal tissue, like tissue in the bladder and urethra, depends on a constant supply of estrogen to maintain its thickness, strength, and general health. When estrogen levels drop, many women experience symptoms of itchiness, discomfort, and painful sex. Vaginal acid balance changes with lowered estrogen levels. When estrogen drops, the pH or acid measurement goes up, meaning the vaginal tissue becomes less acidic and less resistant to harmful bacteria. Maintaining a normal pH in the vagina is especially important for women prone to infections. The primary goals in treating bladder infections naturally are (1) to enhance the normal environmental condition within the bladder and vagina (i.e., to encourage friendly bacterial growth), and (2) to prevent harmful bacteria from invading and propagating within the urinary tract.

A woman's urethra is considerably shorter than a man's, and a woman is more susceptible to bacterial infections throughout her life. The following commonsense precautions can ward off a pesky problem:

- Do not delay emptying your bladder, and always empty it completely. Retaining urine for any length of time will increase your risk of infection.

- Always empty your bladder immediately after sexual contact to keep unfriendly microbes from entering the urethra.

- Avoid tight clothes—jeans, underwear, or pantyhose—and wear cotton-crotch underwear or underwear made from the new "wicking" fabrics (created for active- and athletic-wear to pull moisture away from the skin) to keep the vaginal area as dry as possible; bacteria multiply in a warm, moist environment.

- Hygiene sprays, bubble baths, and soaps may cause further irritation; if you suspect an infection, discontinue their use.

- Take hot baths to relieve the pain associated with infection. Add one cup of vinegar to a shallow bath, and sit in it with your knees up so that water can enter the vagina. Vinegar discourages microbial growth and restores acid balance.

- Frequent use of chlorinated swimming pools and hot tubs can lower the acidity of the vagina.

After menopause, the internal environment of the vagina changes from slightly acidic to alkaline. If you are taking estrogen or antibiotics, or overindulging in sugar and processed foods, this change may be more pronounced. This change coupled with the fact that the outer vulval lips are now smaller and provide less protection for the vagina, urethra, and bladder, make it so that infections can begin more easily and spread quickly.

ACIDOPHILUS

Several natural solutions exist for maintaining and restoring vaginal pH balance. Douching with a plain lactobacillus acidophilus yogurt or powdered acidophilus is quite successful. Add a few tablespoons of plain yogurt or powder to warm douche water, or, if you prefer, insert several teaspoons of plain yogurt into the vagina with a tampon and then lie down for five to ten minutes. Yogurt is even more effective when taken internally; add it to your diet to create a beneficial environment in the intestine.

Acidophilus is also available in supplemental form and helps to reestablish friendly bacteria in the colon and to detoxify harmful substances. Because it is sensitive to heat, store it in a cool, dry place. Take one to two capsules on an empty stomach in the morning and one hour before meals. Many types and brands of acidophilus are on the market, such as Maxidophilus and Megadophilus. You can even get a milk-free variety, such as Kyo-Dophilus. A nondairy yogurt with live acidophilus is available in most health-food stores and some general markets. Milks and other dairy products are now often fortified with acidophilus. If you are on antibiotics, wait until you have finished the series before taking acidophilus orally.

CRANBERRY JUICE

The urinary tract contains built-in defenses against bacterial growth. The lining of the bladder has antimicrobial properties that prevent bacteria from adhering to its surface cells. This is the reason why cranberry juice can relieve bladder infections—once again, an example of folk remedies gaining scientific authenticity. Studies show that substances in cranberry juice reduce the ability of *E. coli* (a resident bacteria in the body that can get out of control) to adhere to the walls of the bladder and urethra.[16] The juice of the blueberry also possesses the antiadhesive agents that prevent bladder infections.

At the first indication of infection, start drinking pure, unsweetened cranberry or blueberry juice, or juice sweetened with apple or other sweet juices. Stay away from juices with added sugar or high-fructose corn syrup. Ten to sixteen ounces a day will probably be enough without irritating your stomach. If the juice is too strong, dilute it with water. Some women find it easier to take three capsules of concentrated cranberry juice three times a day.

OTHER REMEDIES

Drinking plenty of water helps dilute the urine and flush bacteria from the bladder. Cleansing the system with natural diuretics such as celery, parsley, and watermelon also helps to relieve discomfort.

When fighting an infection, stay away from foods and drinks that drain the system rather than build it up: Caffeine, carbonated beverages, chocolate, alcohol, and sugar should be eliminated, or at least kept to a minimum. Eating foods and taking supplements that fight infection may help lessen the severity of an infection or prevent frequent recurring symptoms. Vitamin C is known to fight infection. It helps create an acidic environment in the bladder and urinary tract, which discourages bacterial growth. The recommended dosage once infection is well underway is 500 mg every two hours or until you notice loose stools; then decrease the dosage until your bowels return to normal. If you have not yet added a multivitamin and mineral supplement to your diet, now would be a good time to rebuild your defenses by doing so.

Garlic, long reported to ward off vampires and witches, also fights infection. With the emergence of more and more new strains of bacteria that are resistant to modern drugs, scientists are once again looking at garlic's infection-fighting capabilities. Scientific studies show that garlic helps to prevent and to treat infections of all kinds. Take it whole, raw, baked, or cooked with vegetables. If you prefer, garlic is available in capsule form; take three to four a day.

One of the more effective botanical antimicrobial agents for the treatment of bacterial infections is goldenseal. Take one teaspoon in a cup of hot water as a tea or tincture, three times a day. You also might try dandelion tea or extract, or bearberry (uva ursi).

Exercises for Enhancing Your Sex Life

Exercising the vaginal, stomach, and back muscles will greatly extend your years of sexual pleasure. Keeping the muscles surrounding the internal organs toned and tight will prevent many common complaints, such as backache, fallen organs, involuntary urination, and excessive dryness. The most commonly recommended exercises are the Kegel exercises. Developed more than forty years ago, they strengthen the pubococcygeus (PC) muscle, the band of muscle that extends from the pubic bone in front to the coccyx (tailbone) in back. Since the PC muscle supports the vaginal tissues as well as the internal pelvic organs, it requires continual strengthening.

Kegel exercises can be started when a woman is in her teens, although better-late-than-never works just fine in this case, too. They can improve sexual satisfaction, make childbirth easier, and are useful for women of any age who suffer from poor bladder control and leaking urine.

If you are unsure where the PC muscles are, the next time you go to the bathroom, try to stop the flow of urine. The muscles you contract are the PC muscles. If you try it without urinating, you will be able to exert even more pressure. You don't have to strain to gain benefit, however, so take it easy and breathe naturally when doing the exercises described below. Kegel exercises can be done anytime, anywhere, and there are variations if you tend to get bored doing only one kind of exercise.

Kegel Exercises

1. Contract the PC muscle tightly. Hold for three seconds, relax for three seconds, and repeat. Gradually build to ten-second contractions.

2. Contract and release the PC muscle as rapidly as you can, starting with ten repetitions and working up to one hundred.

3. Doing the exercises in a lying-down position works both the PC muscle and the internal organs. Lie on your back, with your knees bent and your feet on the floor. Raise your pelvis until you feel the stretch, and then begin squeezing.

Kegel exercises are the most popular exercises for strengthening and toning the vaginal muscles. However, other muscles in and around the reproductive organs also require strengthening and toning. All of the muscles in front of, behind, and surrounding the female organs work best at protecting the lower body if they are tight and firm.

As with any other muscle, disuse of the vaginal muscle results in diminished tone and decreased flexibility and eventually atrophy. Many sex therapists recommend regular and frequent intercourse to ensure adequate lubrication, muscle tone, and continued sexual health. Ralph W. Gause, a doctor and sex therapist, observes that the decrease in estrogen and the lack of sexual activity work together: "The estrogen level may fall, but if the vagina is sexually active, it remains fully functional."[17]

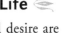 Maintaining a Healthy Body for a Healthy Sex Life

A satisfying sex life depends on a healthy body. Sexual function and desire are closely linked to hormone production and the condition of the endocrine glands. To function optimally, all the hormone-producing glands—including the thyroid, pituitary, adrenals, and sex glands—require nutritional support.

LOW THYROID FUNCTION

An underactive thyroid (hypothyroidism) may be a cause of low sexual desire. A low metabolic rate caused by a sluggish thyroid not only produces fatigue, lethargy, and weight gain, but may be responsible for decreased sexual interest, less sexual fantasy, and poor response to sexual stimulation. Conversely, an overactive thyroid (hyperthyroidism), a condition that speeds up the body's basal metabolism, can result in rampant sexuality. People who take supplemental thyroid hormones often report an unusually strong interest in sex.

HRT is commonly recommended for menopausal women when what is actually lacking is thyroid hormone. This is because physicians too often assume that any fifty-year-old woman with medical complaints needs female hormones. However, if the thyroid is the culprit and is corrected, HRT may prove unnecessary. Additionally, too much estrogen opposes thyroid function, and taking natural progesterone can augment thyroid therapy. Moreover, women who are taking thyroxine for hypothyroidism should be aware that estrogen therapy may increase their need for thyroid medication, requiring them to adjust their dosage of thyroxine.[18]

Certain menopausal symptoms seemingly unrelated to the thyroid respond well to thyroid treatment; these include thinning of the vaginal walls as a result of dropping estrogen levels, as well as the resulting itching, discharge, and painful intercourse. Women who have endured unremitting vaginal dryness that is unresolved with vaginal creams or HRT are often found to be low in thyroid hormone.[19]

A number of nutrients, such as iodine, copper, zinc, and the amino acid tyrosine, are important in activating the thyroid gland in individuals with diminished thyroid activity.[20] On the flip side, certain foods may inhibit thyroid glandular secretion and thus sexual interest; turnips, kale, cabbage, and soybeans contain an antithyroid substance and should be avoided by individuals with decreased thyroid activity. Fasting, although sometimes a healthful practice, may inhibit thyroid function. When the body does not get enough calories, it slows down to conserve energy. Regular fasting may induce a slowed metabolic state and inhibit sexual urges. If you want to increase or maintain your sexual activity, eat regularly.

If you suspect a thyroid problem, check it out with your doctor. (For a more complete discussion of hypothyroidism, including a home method for detecting an underactive thyroid, see Chapter 4.)

EXHAUSTED ADRENALS

The adrenal glands are critical to sexual development and drive. If you suffer from adrenal exhaustion, which can be caused by continued external stress (death, divorce, moving, family problems), internal stress (overuse of sugar, fat, coffee, or alcohol), or both, you may not feel very romantic. Finding ways of handling stress is vital for a more enjoyable sex life.

Keeping your adrenal glands healthy is important throughout life because they assume a starring role at menopause, when they become the primary producers of estrogen. Many symptoms we attribute to menopause—fatigue, lethargy, dizziness, headaches, forgetfulness, food cravings, allergies, and blood-sugar disorders—may actually be more related to reduced adrenal function.

If you suspect that your adrenals are exhausted, you can revitalize them by providing a respite from both external and internal stress. Start by changing something over which you have control: your food selections. Avoid foods and substances that aggravate and overstimulate the system: concentrated sugars, fried foods, alcohol, caffeine, tobacco, processed foods, and salt. Or at least reduce your use of them (sometimes denying yourself completely can be much more stressful than reducing your intake). Emphasize fresh, whole, raw fruits and vegetables (foods that are easy to digest), whole grains, and low-fat chicken and fish. Supplementing with a multiple vitamin and mineral tablet will help replace nutrients that have been in short supply and will thus enable your adrenals to rebuild and repair. Exercise also helps to relieve stress and to stimulate healthy adrenal function. (See Chapter 4 for more discussion of healthy adrenal glands.)

MEDICATIONS AND OTHER STRESSORS

Sexual desire and performance can be adversely affected by many things: certain drugs (tranquilizers, muscle relaxants, antidepressants, amphetamines, diuretics, antihypertensives, and hormones, to name a few), alcohol, marijuana, cigarettes, coffee, overwork, tension, frustration, and depression. The general effects on the body include stress on the adrenal glands and depletion of a wide variety of nutrients.

VITAMIN E

Vitamin E is concentrated in the pituitary gland and is essential for the production of sex hormones and adrenal hormones. It is also required for normal brain functioning and muscular reflexes, which are involved in sexual arousal. Acting as an antioxidant, it protects body organs and glands from destruction by oxygen. Vitamin E directly and indirectly touches all the cells of the body, protecting them from aging.

It is difficult to obtain even the minimum RDA of vitamin E exclusively from food because processing and refining destroy so much of the vitamin. Still, it is good to get what you can from food sources; wheat germ, nuts, seeds, eggs, leafy vegetables, and vegetable oils provide the richest supply. In addition, most people can supplement with up to 400 IU of vitamin E daily; however, if you have rheumatic heart disease, diabetes, or high blood pressure, consult with your doctor first.

ZINC

Zinc, like vitamin E, is found in high concentrations in the pituitary gland. Its role as a nutrient involved in sexual enjoyment has to do with its close association with blood histamine levels. Studies have shown that women with low histamine levels are often unable to reach orgasm, whereas women with high blood histamine levels achieve orgasm easily. Likewise, the higher the histamine level in men, the quicker the ejaculation; and the lower the count, the slower the response. Men and women who take antihistamines regularly need to be aware of the possibility of decreased sexual desire, delayed orgasm, and ejaculation difficulties.

Zinc deficiency is common in women because they lose significant amounts during menstruation, and diet often reinforces this loss. Refining grains and cereals removes 80 percent of the zinc found therein, rendering these foods useless as viable sources of the mineral. The recommended dosage for a healthy sex life is 15 to 30 mg per day, usually supplied in a multivitamin and mineral tablet. Good sources include oysters, beef, turkey, crab, sunflower seeds, almonds, and beans. (For the precise amount of this nutrient contained in certain foods, consult Appendix C.)

VITAMIN B-3 (NIACIN)

Niacin is another nutrient that may be associated with histamine production. Life-extension researchers Durk Pearson and Sandy Shaw report that niacin not only causes the release of histamines, but also stimulates the formation of mucus in response to sexual activity.[21] Take niacin as part of a multivitamin tablet or B-complex unit, making sure that the major B vitamins range between 25 mg and 50 mg. Good food sources include the following: tuna, liver, turkey, salmon, beef, brown rice, and enriched bread. (For the precise amount of this nutrient contained in certain foods, consult Appendix C.)

A good diet is the foundation of a good hormone balance. It not only increases your libido, but it often minimizes the problems of menopause—such as hot flashes, insomnia, and vaginal dryness—that put a damper on your sex life. With those hindrances out of the way, you can begin to enjoy the sexual freedom of your later years.

Also, remember that the enjoyment of sex may have as much to do with attitude and continued sexual practice as with any of the age-related changes. If you have enjoyed a rewarding love life before menopause, you have every reason to believe it will continue. Should temporary symptoms arise, they can, for the most part, be treated with natural methods. A combination of a sound knowledge of the aging process, acceptance of yourself, and an understanding attitude toward your partner will enable you to learn new, creative ways of finding sexual pleasure.

CHAPTER 6

DEPRESSION, MOOD SWINGS, AND MEMORY LOSS

Sometimes I feel like a figment of my own imagination.

— LILY TOMLIN

Historically, menopause has been associated with irritability, nervousness, emotional instability, and depression. If a woman of fifty cries or is cranky or melancholy, her feelings are blamed on shifting hormones. This is a harmful attitude. First, it makes a woman feel she has no choice but to give in to her chemical "controls." Second, if she is clinically depressed or if other conditions are responsible, she may postpone seeking appropriate professional help. When emotions cannot be explained, all possibilities need to be examined—family situations, fear of the change or of aging, and health status.

≶ Internally or Externally Induced? ≷

Whether depression and mood swings during menopause are psychological or biological in origin is still hotly debated by scientists and clinical practitioners. Opinions are divided into two main schools of thought, each with profoundly different implications for research and clinical treatment. One viewpoint holds that depression and mood swings are associated with or triggered by endocrine changes at midlife. A second and more recent view holds that these experiences are related to social issues encountered by women in their forties and fifties.

Studies from different countries, encompassing a broad age range and spanning various socioeconomic strata, reveal that, while depression is common among women, there is no indication that menopausal women are more susceptible than

other women. An extensive research project, involving approximately twenty-five hundred randomly selected pre- and postmenopausal women, came to the following striking conclusions:[1]

1. Depression was not associated with the natural changes of menopause or with the hormonal changes accompanying the event.

2. The only midlife women who reported depression were those who recently had experienced a surgical menopause. The rate of depression in this atypical group of women was twice as high as in the pre- to postmenopause group.

3. The most marked increase in depression was related primarily to events and situations likely to occur in midlife but unrelated to menopause itself.

4. The factor associated most strongly with depression was ill health, as measured by the number of physical symptoms reported. An even stronger association was noted in those people who had recently been diagnosed with chronic conditions.

Other studies show that depression is associated significantly with marital status and education. Widowed, divorced, and separated women with fewer than twelve years of education are the most depressed group. Never-married women have low rates of depression, while married women fall in the middle.

In other words, clinical depression as well as less-debilitating mood swings are associated with factors other than female hormonal fluctuation. These factors include physical disorders (underactive thyroid, endometriosis, stomach upset, headaches), nutritional deficiencies, poor lifestyle habits, stress, deprivation of light, lack of sleep, and unresolved psychological issues.

It is important to remember that not all women entering menopause become depressed or sing the blues all day. Some women sail through the change happy, rewarded, and secure—cultural conditioning, hormonal imbalances, and all. Sadja Greenwood, assistant clinical professor at the University of California Medical Center at San Francisco, claims that women who value themselves in their work (as homemakers or in a career), and women who have interesting jobs, steady incomes, a sense of purpose, and things to do usually report fewer problems with menopause.[2] Feeling secure and worthwhile contributes to our physical, as well as emotional, health.

⟆ The Impact of Hormones on Brain Function ⟅

In some cases our state of mind is indeed related to hormone levels. Researchers at Harvard Medical School report that there is a difference in blood hormone levels between depressed and nondepressed people. A sharp drop in hormone levels may lead to significant changes in behavior. Certain women experience greater hormonal highs and lows throughout their lives. Women who have suffered from premenstrual syndrome can testify to the reality of the physical and emotional symptoms they experience when their hormones fluctuate. But just as all women don't have PMS, not all women experience a large drop in hormones at menopause. By maintaining a healthy body in the years prior to menopause, a woman is less prone to the biochemical extremes that can alter behavior.

Biochemical and hormonal factors may induce depression in an otherwise healthy individual. The endocrine and nervous systems are closely linked, and when any hormone—sex-related or otherwise—is out of balance, emotions can be affected. For example, during the first several days and even weeks following the birth of a baby, the mother experiences an abrupt decline in circulating estrogen, progesterone, and cortisol. This, coupled with the physiological drain of labor, causes many women to experience a significant emotional low known as *postpartum depression*. Even women who have had an uneventful pregnancy and an easy delivery may experience it. I did, and my pregnancy was textbook normal. If some wise woman had told me that uncontrollable crying was to be expected, I probably would have experienced less guilt. Just knowing in advance about the possibility of postpartum depression can relieve anxiety.

Estrogen and progesterone can affect mood and memory in complicated and interrelated ways. The brain and other parts of the nervous system are filled with countless receptor sites for these sex hormones and are highly sensitive to any imbalance. Estrogen orders the release of chemical messengers such as beta-endorphins and serotonin, which promote clear thinking, good feelings, normal memory, and reduced anxiety. When estrogen levels fall, the feel-good hormones follow. If the drop is abrupt, as with a hysterectomy or ovariectomy, chances of extreme mood disturbances increase. This rapid drop in hormones happens in about 15 to 20 percent of women who have had hysterectomies.[3]

Many menopausal women have praised their hormone regimen because of the enhanced sense of well-being they felt while on it. Doctors have postulated that the reason estrogen in particular has been so popular is because it quelled women's hot flashes and night sweats and allowed them a good night's rest, which enhances

anyone's mood. We're all cranky when we don't get our rest. Now there is preliminary scientific evidence that estrogen itself may be responsible for alleviating mild perimenopausal depression. In a double-blind study, researchers found that 80 percent of the women who received estradiol were less sad, less irritable, and enjoyed life more compared to those who took a placebo. Moreover, the presence or absence of hot flashes did not influence the outcome of either group.[4] It needs to be noted that not all studies have found similar results, and researchers remind us that low-dose estrogen is inappropriate for treating serious depression. Furthermore, crabby moods, low energy, and inability to concentrate that have failed to respond to estrogen alone may improve with the addition of testosterone.[5]

It is generally accepted that women who still have their uterus and who take estrogen replacement should balance it with progesterone, the hormone produced in the second half of the menstrual cycle and which helps guard against endometrial cancer. However, too much or the wrong kind of progesterone decreases estrogen receptors in the brain; this may be one of the reasons women complain of irritability and depression when this component is added to HRT, especially in a synthetic form. Progestin (the synthetic form of progesterone) is widely known to cause depression in women, whereas bioidentical, or natural, progesterone seems to be better tolerated. (See Chapter 2 for a detailed discussion of bioidentical versus synthetic hormones.)

The decline of the body's estrogen levels has been implicated in the increased incidence of Alzheimer's disease in aging women. However, as the studies unfold, it appears that estrogen replacement is not a primary factor in slowing the progression of Alzheimer's. According to a double-blind, nationwide study conducted by the University of California at Irvine, there is no evidence that estrogen therapy helps at all to treat Alzheimer's.[6] Good news from research reported in 2002 says that a high intake of vitamin E from food seems to cut the risk of this debilitating disease.[7] (Check Appendix C for food sources of this vital nutrient.)

Clinical Depression Versus the Blues

Whatever your life stage—whether premenopausal, perimenopausal, or postmenopausal—if you're feeling persistently beset by a serious case of the blues, it may be worth determining if you are suffering from clinical depression. Clinical depression is distinguishable from feelings of depression arising out of life transitions and losses. Most of us struggle at some point in our lives with periods of feeling unhappy or out of focus. We may cry for weeks after losing a loving pet, or fall into a dark funk when our son leaves home for college in a distant country.

Nagging work conflicts may erode our otherwise healthy attitudes and positive feelings about life in general. Many situational life experiences, especially when they descend in bunches, wear us down physically and emotionally. But usually, with the help of time, wise friends, trusted counselors, and our individual coping skills, we work through these experiences and move on. These feelings of sadness, grief, and lack of purpose associated with life changes and loss are different from clinical depression.

Major depression is more than having a series of bad days. According to psychiatrist Deborah Sichel, M.D., clinical depression is a continuing downward spiral associated with changes in other bodily functions such as appetite, concentration, sleep-wake cycles, and energy levels.[8] You don't get over real depression by distraction or avoidance, getting busy, helping others, putting on a false smile, taking drugs, or even praying. These were some of the remedies suggested to me before I sought professional counseling for my clinical depression. Like others suffering from depression, nothing I tried worked. Intense sadness followed me like a black cloud even during the happiest moments of my life.

To help you determine if you are "down" or "depressed," Dr. Sichel, in her book *Women's Moods*, provides specific criteria for diagnosing clinical depression. Symptoms of major depression, including persistent sadness and melancholy coupled with the loss of interest in all or most of your usual activities, must be present continually for at least two weeks or more, and must be associated with at least five of the following additional symptoms:

- increased or decreased appetite

- weight gain or loss

- agitation and restlessness, or lethargy

- onset of panic attacks or pervasive anxiety

- difficulty with sleep, sleeping either too much or not enough

- feelings of hopelessness, worthlessness, or inappropriate guilt and shame

- difficulty thinking, concentrating, or making decisions

- recurrent thoughts of death or suicide

We can probably all claim some experience with these feelings. The difference is that the clinically depressed individual experiences most of these feelings most of the time—and usually to a high degree.

DEPRESSION FROM UNRESOLVED ISSUES

Whether or not depression manifests itself more often at midlife than at other times in a woman's life, we should avoid dismissing its significance by masking symptoms with hormones and tranquilizers. Traditional psychology teaches that emotional symptoms reflect an underlying conflict the individual is attempting to resolve. If a woman has not come to terms with a particular issue, such as early childhood hurts or her own identity, her depression could be symptomatic of a continuing problem that has flared up at midlife. Some psychiatrists believe that menopause, like any other major life event, can stimulate the resurgence of unresolved psychosocial conflicts from earlier stages.[9] If this information had been presented to me when I started researching menopause nearly twenty years ago, it would have remained merely theory to me. However, the events of the past several years have shaken my reality—not just in relation to menopause, but regarding underlying family issues I had never reconciled. When I was forty-eight years old, my husband was transferred. Though I wasn't overjoyed at the idea of leaving my children, extended family, friends, church, nutritional-consulting practice, and social network, I tried to think of it as "God's calling." Anyone might expect that a major move would take major adjustment, so at first I wasn't too concerned about my daily crying jags and bouts of staring into space for hours. After a year without much improvement despite genuine attempts to get over it by trying all the self-help strategies that had worked so well in the past—exercise, fresh air and sun, long baths, vitamins, and prayer—I knew I needed professional help.

At first, I strongly rejected any suggestion that the experiences of my early years were related to my present sadness. It took the skill and sensitivity of a wonderful therapist to show me how the abrupt loss of my life as I knew it had triggered other, earlier memories of losses that I had ignored and suppressed—childhood wounds that were still festering and needed healing. I never would have dreamed that, at almost fifty years old, I needed to grieve a situation I would rather not even have remembered. Allen Chinen, author of *Once upon a Midlife: Classic Stories and Mythic Tales to Illuminate the Middle Years*, believes that confronting and dealing with past traumas is a major midlife task for women and men.[10] When depression is real, there is no substitute for counseling. Hormones, tranquilizers, even exercise and the best diet in the world will not work—at least not for long.

I know that many doctors are quick to prescribe Prozac and other types of antidepressants and tranquilizers to their depressed patients, but I must agree with internationally known psychotherapist Alice Miller that drug therapy for depression is not always beneficial. In a book that was particularly helpful to me, *The*

Truth Will Set You Free, she says that most such medications interfere with clients' interest in their childhoods or leave them even more in the dark about their own past reality than they were before, thus undermining the potential success of psychotherapy.[11] Understanding what happened in our early years is key to liberating ourselves from the depression that's absorbing our daily lives. I discovered that Dr. Miller was right when she wrote that the past *does* catch up with us, especially in our relationships with other people. But we can change our feelings and behavior by becoming aware of what we ourselves suffered, uncovering the beliefs we adopted in childhood as gospel truth, and then confronting those beliefs with what we know today.[12] To deny wounds inflicted on us is to perpetuate the cycle to the next generation. And don't we all want not only to heal ourselves but also to help insure that our children will be free of our own unresolved garbage?

Midlife is a monumental transition for some individuals, and it may be a time when we are forced to confront repressed emotional issues. According to William Bridges in his book *Transitions*, "The transitions of life's afternoon are more mysterious than those of its mornings and so we have tended to pass them off as the effects of physical aging."[13] You might consider the possibility that early issues were passed over as you cared for your family and made a living. Even if you think you came to terms with deep-seated hurts, you might examine them again to make sure they are not still eating away at your happiness.

THE ROLE OF SELF-ESTEEM

Judging from the higher rates of depression in women compared to men, in both the United States and Europe, it seems women in our culture struggle more than men with role perception and self-identity. In *Revolution from Within: A Book of Self-Esteem*, Gloria Steinem writes about the pervasiveness of women's poor self-opinion: "Wherever I traveled, I saw women who were smart, courageous, or valuable, who didn't think they were smart, courageous, or valuable—and this was true not only for women who were poor or otherwise doubly discriminated against, but for supposedly privileged and powerful women, too."[14] At some time in our lives, we all need to deal with the question of what we are really worth.

Studies reveal that most women see themselves in terms of either their bodies or their various roles. Psychologist Lillian Rubin found that, when asked to describe themselves, most women started with their physical attributes: "I'm short, tall, blond, fat, pretty, not so pretty anymore, average."[15] One should not find these responses surprising in a culture in which youth and beauty are women's most valued attributes; however, they don't say much about who we really are.

Women who are overconcerned with their physical appearance or who have defined their role in terms of husband and children seem to have the most difficulty accepting the change of life. Certain female roles increase the incidence of emotional loss. For example, women who are overprotective of their children are more likely than other women to suffer depression after their children leave home.[16] Mothers who have sacrificed their own dreams to live vicariously through their children are more likely to experience the "empty-nest syndrome" when their children move away.

A woman's emotional life prior to menopause will determine, at least in part, how she will react to physiological changes. If she has not defined her identity as a woman in the years prior to menopause, there is strong evidence that menopause may be a difficult emotional transition. If she has unfinished emotional business, it may bubble up and flood her life.

In light of the many facets of depression presented in this chapter, how do you know if your feelings are hormonal or psychological? My experience is this: Keep your mind open to all the facts and information, and then go with your gut intuition.

⇒ Food and Mood ⇐

Food—or the lack of it—has a potent effect on mood, thinking, and behavior. Many women are undernourished due to excessive dieting or poor food selection. Government surveys show that women on average barely take in half the RDAs (recommended dietary allowances), a minimum requirement for health.

My editor Kelley Blewster told me about her personal epiphany regarding the amount of food that her body requires and what occurred when she tried to diet below her optimum needs. It's a story that I have heard often and one that we midlife women must pay attention to as we try to maintain our girlish figures:

> Five and a half years ago, I weighed ten pounds less than I do now. Then I met and started dating my (now) husband. Within a few months of beginning to date him, I had put on eight to ten pounds—simply because I was eating more at meal times and eating less often and on the run. At first, of course, I panicked and grew discouraged, and swore to lose the weight (I hated no longer fitting in most of my size-6 clothes). But before long, I realized something: Whereas before, I'd consistently suffered from frequent, nagging headaches, crankiness, and feelings of hopelessness that seemed to come out of the blue, now I hadn't had a headache in three months! Another thing: Whereas I'd always craved a

high-sugar snack once or twice a day, I simply wasn't craving sugar any longer. It came as a revelation to me that I just needed to eat more than I had been eating in the past. At 130 pounds, my body simply wasn't being nourished adequately! So I decided that about 140 is the right weight for my body—screw the Hollywood ideal! (Oddly, making the link between food and mood was helped by the fact that my husband is a type-1 diabetic, diagnosed at age four. For his entire life, he's known that if he's beset by feelings of hopelessness or spaciness, he needs to eat something. Now I follow the same practice. And it works!)

Proper functioning of the brain, more than any other organ, depends on what we eat. In the early 1970s, Richard Wurtman, a neuroendocrinologist from MIT, found that mood is related to concentrations of certain chemicals in the brain called *neurotransmitters*, and that by eating certain foods or taking specific nutrients, an individual can raise the level of these brain chemicals and thus feel better.[17] The three neurotransmitters that most influence behavior are serotonin, dopamine, and norepinephrine.

SEROTONIN

Serotonin is the neurotransmitter known to ease anxiety and promote a sense of well-being. Generally speaking, we can raise serotonin levels in the brain by simply eating carbohydrates. Other nutrients that aid this chemical conversion are the amino acid tryptophan and vitamin B-6. Tryptophan is abundant in proteins such as chicken, seeds, and nuts, and is normally available in the body from previous meals. When carbohydrates are consumed, the increase in insulin removes from circulation other amino acids that compete with tryptophan; therefore, tryptophan easily enters the brain to make serotonin.

Factors That Can Lower Serotonin Levels and Your Mood

- lowered estrogen levels
- higher than normal progesterone levels
- congenital hormonal abnormalities
- low-carbohydrate diet
- excessive carbohydrates
- weight fluctuations
- consuming 80 percent or less of daily RDAs
- alcohol and drug abuse
- light deprivation

Serotonin is produced quickly when we eat starchy foods such as breads, pastas, and cereals. That is why if you are feeling down, as few as one or two crackers or half a bagel may raise your spirits. Sugar in small amounts also works, but remember that blood-sugar imbalances caused by too much sugar can induce depression. As with most recommendations, there are exceptions. Some women—particularly those who are 20 percent or more over their ideal weight or are premenstrual—may

need more carbohydrates to trigger serotonin production.[18] Carbohydrate-sensitive women may fail to respond at all to these guidelines. They instead feel more than relaxed after a carbohydrate meal; in fact, they may just go to the couch and fall asleep. Finding out how carbohydrates react in your body is an easy and fun experiment. (See Chapter 4 for more on the topic.)

Several lifestyle conditions may lower serotonin production and bring you down emotionally. These include stress, overwork, and trauma. Balance and moderation are probably most conducive to feeling good.

DOPAMINE AND NOREPINEPHRINE

Dopamine and norepinephrine are called *psychic energizers* because they produce chemicals that stimulate the mind. When the brain produces these substances, people report thinking more quickly and feeling more alert and motivated—that experience where everything just clicks into place. Eating protein is the prescription for energizing the mind. Whenever you eat protein by itself (such as a piece of chicken or a hard-boiled egg), or in combination with a small amount of carbohydrate (as in a sandwich), you allow more of the amino acid tyrosine to reach your brain. Tyrosine, with the help of B vitamins, produces dopamine and norepinephrine. All you need is three to four ounces of protein to stimulate this conversion.

ENDORPHINS

Endorphins are another class of brain chemical that, when produced in adequate amounts, will make you feel content and happy. The endocrine system and nervous system are closely linked; any sudden drop in hormones is likely to create feelings of anxiety. During menopause, if estrogen drops abruptly, there is a concomitant decrease in endorphins in the central nervous system.

The good news is that there are natural methods to elevate endorphin levels. The most accessible one is exercise. An exercise program that includes both aerobic and resistance training has been shown to increase the concentration of several brain chemicals in menopausal women, including endorphins and serotonin.[19]

Exercise is considered by some to be more effective in relieving depression than the most commonly used tranquilizers. In 1978, John Greist, of the University of Wisconsin, found running to be as useful as psychotherapy for depression. Even when the study was over, the once-depressed subjects continued to run, finding that when they quit, their depression returned.[20] Running may not be the answer for you, but walking is a good alternative, and there are any number of other forms of exercise you can do. If you feel down, get out and start your heart pumping four times a week for at least twenty minutes. Doing so will undoubtedly raise your spirits.

You may try other approaches to boost your endorphins. Have you ever wondered why menopausal women go ballistic over candy bars and truffles? It's because chocolate elevates endorphin levels. But don't think this gives you license to devour an entire box of Godiva chocolates; all it takes to trigger the endorphin surge is one small ounce. Before you decide to trade in your running shoes for bakeware, however, remember that exercise is twenty times more effective than chocolate in raising endorphins.

Other practices that may help raise your spirits are laughing, crying, water submersion (in hot baths or tubs), relaxation techniques, acupuncture, sex, coffee, and cigarettes. Obviously, some choices are better—that is, healthier—than others.

MAINTAINING BLOOD-SUGAR LEVELS

As discussed in detail in Chapter 4, maintaining a constant level of glucose in the blood is important to well-being. The brain and nervous system are especially sensitive to disturbances in blood-glucose levels. The central nervous system does not store glucose, and it needs more of it than any other part of the body. The primary component of that system, the brain, is the first to feel the deficiency when the glucose level is low. The brain and nervous system are so hypersensitive to disturbances of body chemistry that a defect in the utilization of sugar can result in an erratic mental state, with a list of symptoms and complaints that reads like the label on a bottle of snake oil: dizziness, fainting, headaches, fatigue, muscle pains, cold hands and feet, insomnia, irritability, crying spells, nervous breakdown, excessive worry, depression, illogical fears, suicidal thoughts, crawling sensation, loss of sexual drive—and the list goes on.[21]

The brain is more dependent for proper functioning on what we eat than any other organ. Diets high in sugar, caffeine, and alcohol can cause a roller-coaster ride of emotions, especially in the middle years. Tolerance to sugar declines with age, so strong reactions may be noticed after eating foods you once enjoyed. Maybe you have already noticed that desserts, espressos, or other combinations of food and drink set you off both physically and emotionally, or that going all day without eating no longer serves you well. Be careful about eating on the run or forgetting a meal; doing so may trigger mood swings.

We all experience sporadic blood-sugar fluctuations at various times in our lives. If you are feeling low and can't explain why, examine your eating habits. Do they include drinking a lot of coffee or alcohol or eating large amounts of sugar and processed foods? All of these can contribute to unnatural highs and lows. To stabilize your blood-sugar level, eliminate these stresses from your diet and eat foods high in protein and complex carbohydrates.

The number of meals you eat each day can affect your mood as well. Six small meals a day are much more conducive to a slow release of insulin from the pancreas, which allows for the gradual release of glucose, than three large meals.

Emotional Effects of Certain Nutrients

Psychological disturbances are some of the earliest symptoms of nutritional inadequacies. The normal production and function of neurotransmitters demands a full range of amino acids and supporting nutrients. For example, vitamin B-6 is needed in both the conversion of the amino acid tryptophan to serotonin and the conversion of the amino acid tyrosine to dopamine. The B vitamin niacin is likewise instrumental in converting the amino acid tryptophan into the neurotransmitter serotonin.

What follows is a discussion of certain amino acids and other supplemental nutrients that can have a beneficial effect on mild depression. A note of caution: Do not take amino acids or herbs with MAO inhibitors or other antidepressants unless you are under the care of a knowledgeable doctor. Mixing therapeutic levels of nutrients with other meds is just as dangerous as combining certain drugs.

AMINO ACIDS: BUILDING BLOCKS FOR THE BRAIN

Tryptophan

For years the amino acid tryptophan was used in supplemental form almost exclusively by nutritionally minded health professionals to treat depression and insomnia. It effectively raised serotonin levels in the brain and had minimal side effects. Research confirmed that in double-blind studies it compared similarly to other, more powerful antidepressants such as Prozac. Tryptophan was sold over the counter in health-food stores and supermarkets until 1989, when the FDA ripped it off the market after one contaminated batch from Japan killed thirty-seven people and seriously hurt hundreds of others. It is difficult for me to comprehend why this safe, effective, natural antidepressant was withdrawn when it was the contaminant and not the product that caused harm. How many other products, from Tylenol to Evian, have had similar bouts with bad batches and yet are still publically available?

At this time, the only way to obtain therapeutic doses of tryptophan is to find a doctor to prescribe it and then to have a compounding pharmacist fill the prescription. It is more expensive—not to mention less convenient—than it was when we bought it at the local drugstore.

Recommended doses of tryptophan start at 500 mg per day and in special cases can go as high as 9 grams per day. It is best to work with your doctor when you use tryptophan, to avoid the risk of overmedication. As a starting place, if you suffer from mild depression, consider raising your serotonin levels naturally by getting regular exercise and eating foods rich in tryptophan.

5-HTP

Closely related to tryptophan is another substance that occurs naturally in the body called *5-hydroxytryptophan*, or 5-HTP. It is made from L-tryptophan and is similarly converted into serotonin, thus elevating the brain-hormone levels in the body. Moreover, 5-HTP also triggers an increase in mood-elevating endorphins and other neurotransmitters that result in depression when blood levels are low. A multitude of studies have shown that 5-HTP is as effective as drugs such as Prozac, Zoloft, Paxil, and tricyclic antidepressants, and its side effects are fewer and less severe.

Vitamin B-6 and magnesium are needed for the first step of the conversion from tryptophan into 5-HTP, demonstrating again the interrelationship between nutrients, amino acids, and brain hormones. Dr. Susan Lark suggests starting with 50–100 mg of 5-HTP twice a day, and taking it together with 50–100 mg of vitamin B-6 and a small carbohydrate snack (cracker, fruit) to facilitate uptake into the brain.[22] *Note:* Taking too much 5-HTP could potentially cause anxiety and high blood pressure.

Tyrosine

Tyrosine is a precursor to vital hormones and neurotransmitters that direct brain behavior and regulate moods, including adrenaline, noradrenaline, dopamine, and cortisol. Shortage of this amino acid can lead to inadequate production of any one of these substances, resulting in lack of energy and focus, anxiety, and depression. Not necessarily every depressed woman will respond to tyrosine supplementation, but it appears to be particularly helpful to people with low thyroid-hormone levels.

Dr. Michael Lesser, founder of the orthomolecular psychiatry movement, which focuses on nutritional and vitamin therapy to regulate moods, recommends 1.3 to 3 grams daily of supplemental tyrosine.[23] When using the upper doses for depression, it is advisable to be supervised by a physician.

Phenylalanine

Phenylalanine is an amino acid that the body converts into another amino acid, tyrosine. Tyrosine is then made into the brain hormones listed above. Phenylalanine is also converted into the stimulant and mood enhancer PEA, a substance that is

found in chocolate. Phenylalanine is a relatively fast-acting antidepressant; it can help a person feel better within twenty minutes. Those of us who dash for the chocolate when faced with anxiety and stress know the powerful tranquilizing effects it can have. Like the other amino acids and nutrients, phenylalanine is only effective for treating mild depression.

In his book *The Brain Chemistry Diet*, Dr. Lesser recommends beginning with 500 mg a day of phenylalanine and increasing gradually until you feel the effect; do not exceed 3 to 4 grams a day.[24] Two types of this protein product are available at health-food stores: L-phenylalanine is best for stabilizing moods; and D, L-phenylalanine is useful for chronic pain associated with PMS, arthritis, or migraines. Don't take either form with MAO inhibitors. You should also avoid this supplement if you are pregnant or nursing, or have anxiety attacks, diabetes, high blood pressure, phenylketonuria, Wilson's disease, or skin cancer.

SAMe

S-adenosylmethionine (SAMe) has been used predominantly in Europe for the treatment of major depression and arthritis. While it is not technically an amino acid, it is created from another amino acid, methionine, which is prevalent in many protein foods. SAMe is involved in the formation of key brain hormones; decreased levels have been discovered in the brain of individuals with Alzheimer's disease and depression.

Even though it is said to equal other antidepressants in activity, many women have not experienced relief from using SAMe. Dr. Christiane Northrup believes it doesn't work unless taken in the proper form and dosage, because it is very unstable and quickly loses its potency when exposed to air. Dr. Northrup has learned from her own experience that to protect SAMe from being deactivated by stomach acid and to maximize absorption, consumers should purchase an enteric-coated tablet in a form called *butanedisulfonate*.[25] Brand names to look for are Nature Made and GNC. Start with 400 mg per day and slowly add 200 mg every three to seven days until you reach a therapeutic dose. Those with severe depression may require as much as 1,600 mg a day, but unless you are under a physician's care, you should not experiment with this higher range.

NUTRIENT IMBALANCES AND MENTAL SYMPTOMS

Even one deficient nutrient can play havoc with a person's nervous systems. Roger Williams, the biochemist who discovered pantothenic acid, has done extensive work in the field of vitamin research. He discusses the importance of nutrients in the control of mental problems and says the most important way to improve the environ-

ment of the brain cells in a threatened individual is to supply her or him with the full nutritional requirements.[26]

If you suffer emotional distress, what are the chances that your diet is missing a crucial vitamin or mineral? Check whether any of the following symptoms are familiar to you:

- vitamin B-1 (thiamine): loss of appetite, depression, irritability, memory loss, sensitivity to noise, inability to concentrate, fatigue, reduced attention span

- vitamin B-3 (niacin): insomnia, nervousness, irritability, confusion, depression, hallucination, loss of memory

- vitamin B-5 (pantothenic acid): depression, inability to tolerate stress

- vitamin B-6: anxiety, depression, irritability, insomnia

- vitamin B-12 (cobalamin): difficulty concentrating and remembering, stuporous depression, severe agitation, hallucinations, manic behavior

- folic acid: irritability, weakness, apathy, hostility, anemia

- vitamin C: increased stress and fatigue

- vitamin E: depression, lethargy, poor memory

- potassium: nervousness, irritability, mental disorientation

- magnesium: paranoid psychosis

- calcium: anxiety, neurosis, fatigue, insomnia, tension

- zinc: anemia, poor mental function

- iron: depression, lethargy, poor concentration, irritability, decreased attention span, personality changes, anemia

- essential fatty acids: anxiety, irritability, insomnia

(Besides these deficiencies, an excess of copper in the system can cause racing mind, insomnia, and chronic depression.)

The chemical makeup of the brain requires an ample and constant supply of essential nutrients. Vitamins, amino acids, fatty acids, and enzymes are all interrelated, each dependent on the others for absorption and utilization; moreover, a shortage of one vital element can render all the others less effective. That is why nutritionists urge people to eat a variety of nutrient-dense foods.

⇒ **Diet and Exercise Stimulate Memory** ⇐

I've never really had a quick and sharp memory, so I can't tell if it's getting worse with my advancing calendar years. But I seem to misplace my jewelry with regularity. Since I divide my time between two homes, it's very disconcerting to wonder if I really lost my pearl dinner ring or an earring, or if it's just tucked away in my sock drawer at the second house. Mostly, I've noticed difficulty finishing sentences. I will start out with a subject and verb, but before I reach the object, my brain pauses. It's usually only a few seconds until the word comes to mind, but my children often complete the missing thought before I manage to spit it out. Is this normal? I hear my friends complain of forgetting where they placed their keys, or not remembering to pick up bread at the grocery store. I guess the way our memory changes is just as individual as other symptoms of menopause or aging.

There is good research indicating that one's general health and nutritional state may enhance—or diminish—memory and cognitive ability. A study reported in the *American Journal of Epidemiology* showed that poor dietary habits—specifically, inadequate food intake, skipping meals, and low levels of vitamin E—led to memory loss in the elderly. Only 7 percent of participants who ate consistent meals suffered memory problems, compared with about 20 percent of those with an inadequate diet. Blood levels of vitamin E were the kicker: Researchers found that memory skills declined as levels of vitamin E dropped. Vitamin E, an antioxidant, may protect against free-radical damage to brain cells.[27] (For more explanation of antioxidants, see Chapters 9 and 10.)

A second study shows another way in which diet can affect cognitive functioning. You've probably encountered all the press touting the benefits of the Mediterranean diet (which is really a complete lifestyle, as discussed more fully in Chapter 14). There may be another benefit to such a diet besides protection from heart disease: prevention of cognitive problems associated with advancing age. In an Italian study reported in the journal *Neurology*, a diet rich in monounsaturated fats appeared to enhance global cognitive functioning and attention to detail in men and women ages sixty-five to eighty-four. (The diet didn't seem to affect story recall, the third function measured.) The more olive oil, canola oil, walnuts, and avocados the participants ate (foods in plentiful supply in the so-called Mediterranean diet), the better the respondents scored on the tests, after the researchers controlled for education and other variables. Why? Researchers speculate that it may be because unsaturated fatty acids, an important component of cell membranes, help keep brain-cell membranes healthy. Additional research is called for to confirm and expand these findings.[28]

In case you needed one more reason to take up regular aerobic exercise—or to stick with your program if you already exercise—new research suggests that sedentary older people who begin walking regularly can improve mental agility, even if they've never exercised before. The University of Illinois recruited more than one hundred couch potatoes ages sixty to seventy-five. Members of one group walked briskly three times per week (increasing over time from fifteen to forty-five minutes per session). The others performed toning and stretching exercises. After six months, those who walked showed better scores on computer tasks, while the calisthenics group showed no improvement.[29] Aerobic exercise increases oxygen to the brain and probably slows the decline of the part of the brain associated with mental agility. Remember, it's never too late to start healthy new habits!

Exercising the brain as well as the body may help to prevent memory loss and increase mental fitness. Lawrence C. Katz, Ph.D., professor of neurobiology at Duke University Medical Center, has developed eighty-three so-called neurobic exercises; they are described in his book *Keep Your Brain Alive*.[30] Neurobic exercises are designed to stimulate the production of nutrients that grow brain cells, thereby helping to keep the brain stronger and potentially younger. According to Dr. Katz, a neurobic exercise must meet a series of conditions. For instance, the activity needs to involve one or more of a person's senses in a novel context. An example of this would be to get dressed for the day with your eyes closed. A second condition is for the exercise to engage the person's attention by changing something in his or her daily routine—for example, turning the pictures on your wall upside down, or taking your child to work with you. Breaking a routine activity in an unexpected way is a skill I often practice by taking a new route when I walk, or reversing the order of cleaning the house. The object is to change your everyday life, learn new ways to do old things, and stimulate your mind and senses. By doing so, Dr. Katz asserts, you will keep your brain alive and active.

Natural Ways to Improve Mood

- First rule out physical illness and psychological issues, including clinical depression.
- Maintain even blood-sugar levels.
- Practice moderation in the use of sugar, alcohol, drugs, and caffeine (highly sensitive people may have to eliminate one or all).
- Do not overindulge in food.
- Eat small carbohydrate meals and snacks for relaxation.
- Eat proteins for mental alertness.
- Do not try to lose more than one to two pounds per week if you are dieting.
- Exercise a minimum of twenty minutes four times per week.
- Expose yourself to the sun or to bright, full-spectrum light every day.
- Take hot baths, or lounge in a hot tub for twenty minutes.
- Learn relaxation techniques.
- Laugh.
- Cry.
- Try acupuncture.
- Take a multiple vitamin and mineral supplement daily.
- Use natural herbs.

⋙ Herbal Remedies ⋘

A number of herbs and nutrients have been proven to calm anxiety, reduce tension, and stimulate the brain and memory. It is advantageous to use herbs and supplements in conjunction with positive changes in nutrition and lifestyle.

Ginkgo biloba has been widely prescribed in France, Germany, and other European countries to improve blood flow to the brain. Hundreds of studies have substantiated the ability of ginkgo biloba to improve mental health. A 1993 study indicated it actually improves transmission of nerve signals and is capable of relieving symptoms such as depressive moods, anxiety, tiredness, confusion, poor memory, and absentmindedness.[31] The recommended dose is 40 mg three times a day; take it four to six weeks before expecting results. Precautions: Ginkgo biloba prolongs bleeding, so don't take it with vitamin E or aspirin, if you're on anticoagulants, or if you have high blood pressure or a history of bleeding.

St. John's wort has become well known as a natural antidepressant (for situational rather than clinical depression). Several studies in the 1990s validated this fact, something natural practitioners already knew. A meta-analysis of twenty-three randomized trials of St. John's wort extract in 1,757 patients with depressive disorders concluded that the herb was significantly superior to placebo, and that its effectiveness compared with standard antidepressant drugs.[32] It also is used clinically for alleviating anxiety, sleep disturbances, and insomnia. Recent research has indicated that the herb's antidepressive effect may be largely due to its ability to inhibit the reuptake of serotonin, a process mimicked by such synthetic antidepressants as Prozac.[33] Dose: Using a standardized extract of 3 percent hypericin, take 300 mg three times per day. St. John's wort may cause stomach upset if taken on an empty stomach, so take it with food. Do not use it long term or with other antidepressants.

Kava kava, a member of the pepper family, is used in traditional Polynesian cultures as a calming beverage, for celebration, and in religious ceremonies. Certain European countries have approved its use as a relaxant or mild sedative for anxiety. An antispasmodic, it also helps with menstrual cramps. Aim for 45 to 70 mg of standardized kavalactones (30 percent kavalactone), three times per day. Do not take it with alcohol or use it with other antidepressants or if you're pregnant or nursing.

Other helpful herbs to make you feel better include chaste tree (vitex), oat straw, Siberian ginseng, dandelion root, garden sage, passionflower, skullcap, and chamomile.

CHAPTER 7

OSTEOPOROSIS

Scientists agree that adequate nutrition can reduce the impact of osteoporosis by as much as one half or more.

— *Journal of the American Dietetic Association,* JUNE 1994

Osteoporosis, a bone-thinning disease that leads to fractures and disability, affects 25 million Americans. Along with heart disease and breast cancer, it is one of the three most serious diseases affecting women. Half of all women between the ages of forty-five and seventy-five show beginning signs of osteoporosis; one in three of these women has full-blown osteoporosis, and by age seventy-five, the number jumps to nine in ten for extreme bone deterioration.[1] Despite these grim statistics, osteoporosis is for the most part preventable. Scientists now agree that adequate nutrition can cut these figures in half and possibly even more.

The word *osteoporosis* literally means "porous bones," or bones filled with tiny holes. It is not clinically considered a disease, but rather the progressive and severe loss of bone mass. Because of the loss in density, osteoporotic bones fracture more easily and heal more slowly. While some softening of the bones is normal in both men and women who are of middle age and older, weakness to the degree that prohibits one from functioning properly is not normal. In women, the loss of bone begins sooner and proceeds six times more rapidly than in men (primarily because women's bones are smaller and therefore have less mass to spare to begin with).

Our bones are made of living tissue that is continuously recycled. While the inner bone is breaking down, the outer surface is reforming. A delicate balance of the two processes is maintained in response to the demands of the body. If the body needs calcium, bone is broken down; if it doesn't, bone is rebuilt. When more calcium is withdrawn from the bones than is deposited, bones become soft and weak. Reversing this process is the primary step in preventing and treating osteoporosis. There is confusion and conflict about specific recommendations for how

to do so, however, because of the numerous factors that contribute to bone health: genetic predisposition, hormonal output, nutritional status, age, physical activity, and lifestyle habits. It is necessary to examine all the factors involved in this complex problem.

Osteoporosis is expensive. The average cost for two weeks of hospitalization after a hip fracture is roughly ten thousand dollars, not including home care and rehabilitation expenses. In the United States alone, more than a billion dollars is spent each year for the general care and treatment of women with osteoporosis.[2]

The severity of the problem cannot be overemphasized. Osteoporosis is painful and crippling. After menopause, a woman's chances of fracturing a bone increase dramatically; even a minor fall or vigorous hug may lead to a break. Bone fractures often result in immobilization, hospitalization, and dependence—and, in extreme cases, even death. Although fractures of the spine are the most common outcome of osteoporosis, hip fractures are more debilitating. They often lead to long-term disability, depression, and accelerated death. Between 15 and 20 percent of women die within three months of a serious hip fracture, either from the injury or from secondary complications; about 30 percent die within six months; and those remaining are at risk for recurring fractures or permanent disability.[3]

The physical deformities caused by this condition cannot be concealed: An older woman with advanced osteoporosis loses height, is hunched over, has a protruding abdomen, and often walks with a shuffling, unsteady gait. As the bones of the spine lose density, the vertebrae collapse, forcing the rib cage to tilt downward toward the hip. A curvature in the upper spine creates a second curve in the lower spine, pushing the internal organs outward. The stomach protrudes so prominently that the woman may look pregnant.

Because of the compression in the spinal column, up to eight inches in height can be lost. The resulting "dowager's hump" is one of the classic stereotypes of the aging woman—and unfortunately it is not a myth.

As the compressed organs shift positions and put pressure on other organs and systems, internal functions may be impaired. Constipation becomes a problem, and breathing may become labored. Aches and pains throughout the body, particularly in the lower back, may arise from pressure on the nerves emanating from the collapsed vertebrae. Life evolves into a series of problems.

A woman's appearance and self-esteem may change drastically when osteoporosis reaches an advanced stage. Along with being uncomfortable and, to varying degrees, incapacitated, she tends to feel awkward, unattractive, and old. Clothes don't fit properly, and a fashionable look is next to impossible. Realizing that the body can never fully return to its premenopausal shape, many women with osteo-

porosis experience stress, anxiety, feelings of helplessness, and dread of the future. Psychologically, the loss of self-esteem and the emotional adjustments may weigh heavier than the physical inconveniences.

⇒ Diagnosing Osteoporosis ⇐

Osteoporosis is difficult to detect early because it sneaks up on a person gradually. Often, the first sign is a broken bone. The standard X-ray technology used to identify other bone fractures is not sensitive enough to detect osteoporosis until the disease has taken up to 40 percent of bone mass. More sophisticated tests are available, however, to evaluate potential risks at an earlier stage. Several of these are discussed below.

The following early physical warning signs might alert you to a potential problem:

- chronic low back pain
- loss of height
- nocturnal leg cramps
- joint pain
- transparent skin
- rheumatoid arthritis
- hypothyroid disease
- restless behavior (foot jiggling, hair twisting)
- insomnia
- tooth loss
- periodontal (gum) disease

A combination of these symptoms may be a reason for taking the next step for further diagnosis.

⇒ Testing Your Bones ⇐

Screening for bone health is an important part of preventive care for the midlife woman. Several types of tests are available, some more accessible and less expensive than others. It is a good idea to have a baseline test to determine your bone status and consider your options. If you do show considerable bone loss, you might

undergo a follow-up test six months to a year later to make sure that your program is working and you are no longer losing bone mass.

Osteoporosis is now defined in terms of standard deviation (SD) from the norm. The results are expressed as a "T-score," referring to the trabecular, or spongy, part of the bone, which turns over faster than the cortical, or rigid, type of bone. The T-score actually compares your bone status to that of the average thirty-five-year-old woman with peak bone mineral density. The World Health Organization has suggested classifications based on the following T-scores:

- Greater than –1 (meaning no more than one SD below the mean peak value in young adults) indicates normal bone mineral density, or a low risk for fractures.

- Between –1 and –2.5 indicates low bone mineral density.

- –2.5 or lower indicates osteoporosis.

Several bone mineral density (BMD) tests exist; four are described in this section. You might consider asking your doctor to test you if you are a candidate for osteoporosis (see the section "Who Is at Risk?" on page 130), or if you want to establish a benchmark for evaluating your rate of bone loss as you develop a plan of preventive action.

DEXA

Because of its precision, DEXA (sometimes called *DXA*, short for dual-energy X-ray absorptiometry) is considered the gold standard of bone densitometry, or bone-density measurement. Typically used to measure bone mineral density in the hip and the spine, DEXA offers a lower dose of radiation and a shorter exam time than other X-ray methods.

DEXA has a few drawbacks. It is an expensive procedure, and usually insurance will not cover it for purely preventive reasons (that is, an existing condition of osteoporosis must warrant the test). Furthermore, it provides only a static measurement of bone mineral density, which means a second test is necessary to indicate whether the patient is losing or building bone. Finally, DEXA may not be the best analysis for small-boned women, because it may indicate that their bones are brittle when in fact they are not.

URINE PYRILINKS-D TEST

A bone-screening test that indicates what's happening in your bones right now, and not just what has happened already, is the best, especially when used in conjunction with a test such as DEXA.

Osteoporosis is not just a bone disease; it's also a collagen disease. Collagen keeps your skin looking plump and keeps it from sagging. The same is true for collagen in your bones. As physician and women's-health writer Christiane Northrup, M.D., puts it, the bones are like a string of pearls. The pearls are the calcium, and the string that holds them together is the collagen.

Just as your skin begins to sag with age, your bones are affected by the same collagen-breakdown process. It's important to know the rate at which this is happening in the bones. A urine test, which looks for excess breakdown of collagen in the urine, can tell you this and, thus, whether you're building bone or losing it.

The pyrilinks-D analysis tests for deoxypyridinoline (Dpd), a specific urinary marker for bone resorption (loss). A Dpd level higher than 6.5 means the rate of bone loss is greater than that for healthy women.

Aeron Labs offers a home urine test for measuring bone loss, as well as saliva tests for determining hormone levels. The tests are mailed to you; you administer them yourself in the privacy of your home and return the materials to the lab. The results are then mailed to you or to your health-care provider, who can read the results and offer a possible protocol. All in all, it's a very easy way to determine what is happening in your body before deciding to undergo any hormone or drug therapy. I have taken both the bone-density and the hormone tests to monitor my status and will continue to use them as a tool to reevaluate and revise my personal program. The tests are not inexpensive; together the two cost me about two hundred dollars, not reimbursed by my insurance. I feel it is worth the price to know the status of my bone health and to gain the advantage offered by monitoring my own individualized program.

Aeron is not the only lab that offers this service, but it is one of the oldest and enjoys an excellent reputation. It also sends easy-to-understand consumer information. (See Resources for Aeron's address and website.)

PDXA

Peripheral DXA (pDXA) is a newer, less expensive modification of the DEXA test. It measures bone density in the arm. The procedure is performed in about five minutes with a scanner the size of a desktop computer. Thus, although pDXA isn't considered as reliable as DEXA, it is portable and therefore handy for use in clinicians' offices, workplaces, and shopping centers. Its convenience makes it a good option for initial screening.

SONOMETER

The sonometer, a portable device introduced in 1998, employs ultrasound to measure bone density at the heel. The procedure takes less than a minute and provides

a computer printout with a T-score as well as an estimate of bone density in grams per square centimeter.

With these lower-cost bone-measurement options, variation exists among the equipment used from center to center. Therefore, to monitor your bone density, you should use the same type of device every time you get tested. You should also test at the same place on your body every time.

Who Is at Risk?

ARE YOU AT RISK FOR OSTEOPOROSIS?

If you answer yes to two or more of the following questions, consider undergoing one of the tests described and continue reading to see what you can do to prevent further bone loss.

- Has any member of your family had bone disease?

- Are you short, thin, and small-boned?

- Are you fair-skinned or freckled?

- Were your ovaries removed before age forty-five?

- Did you have an early, natural menopause?

- Have you ever given birth?

- Are you a diabetic or hypoglycemic?

- Are you lactose intolerant or do you avoid dairy products?

- Do you have an underactive thyroid gland?

- Do you have celiac disease, kidney disease, or liver disease?

- Are you sedentary?

- Do you drink more than two cups of caffeinated beverages per day?

- Do you have more than two alcoholic drinks per day?

- Do you smoke cigarettes?

- Have you been involved in prolonged dieting or fasting?

- Is your diet high in salt?

- Do you take in less than adequate calcium, magnesium, and vitamin D?

There are enough indicators to allow us to guess, with a fair degree of accuracy, who will or will not develop osteoporosis. They include the following:

GENETIC PREDISPOSITION

Let's start with genetic inheritance. If a woman's mother, aunt, or sister incurred fractures because of weak bones, the woman probably will too. I do not agree, however, that we have no control in such a situation. A family tendency toward osteoporosis does not mean that a woman must suffer fractures. Her relatives may have unknowingly aggravated their conditions. Were their diets poorly balanced? Did they take medications or have preexisting medical conditions? Were they active or sedentary? As I discuss in this chapter, lifestyle is key to both preparing for and coping with osteoporosis.

BODY SIZE

Body size is a valuable clue in evaluating risk. Small-boned, thin women—women who wear petite sizes—are at dramatically greater risk than larger women, simply because they have less bone to lose. This is the same reason why men are less susceptible to breakage. Bones respond to a higher weight load by forming new bone tissue to meet the demand: The heavier you are, the greater the stress on your body, and the more bone is formed. Research suggests that those who weigh less than 140 pounds have increased chances of developing osteoporosis. However, this should not be interpreted as a case for being overweight, which carries far greater health risks than this one benefit. Exercise can provide the same weight-bearing advantages as a larger body.

The inadequate nutrition that is often the cause of thinness, and the lack of estrogen resulting from inadequate body fat, predisposes young women to osteoporosis. Studies show that women and girls suffering from anorexia, bulimia, and other eating disorders already have decreased bone mass.[4] Amenorrhea, the lack of menstrual periods due to inadequate body fat, causes estrogen production to stop and increases the risk of bone loss. Young athletes often fall into both these situations. The numbers are staggering: Eating disorders and their consequences involve 50 percent of all competitive runners, 44 percent of ballet dancers, 35 percent of noncompetitive runners, and 12 percent of swimmers and cyclists.[5] These shocking statistics help explain why researchers refer to osteoporosis as a childhood disease with a midlife outcome.

SKIN PIGMENTATION

The fairer your complexion, the greater your risk of bone loss. Studies of different ethnic groups have shown that women with northern European ancestry, such as English, Dutch, or German, are at greater risk for osteoporosis, and women with African-American ancestry are at the least. Women of Hispanic and Jewish origin appear to fall somewhere in between.

PREMATURE GRAYING OF THE HAIR

A puzzling risk factor for osteoporosis is premature gray hair (meaning that half the hair has turned color by the age of forty). Scientists at the Maine Center for Osteoporosis Research found that subjects with no identifiable risk factors but with graying hair were 4.4 times as likely to have osteopenia (lower than normal bone mass) than those who maintained their natural color.[6] The researchers suspect that the genes controlling early color change are the same as, or close to, those that control bone density. Other possible conditions associated with premature graying are thyroid disease and premature menopause, both contributors to bone loss.

PREMATURE MENOPAUSE

Women who undergo premature menopause (before age forty-five) endure a more rapid decline in bone tissue than women who experience menopause naturally. The relationship between osteoporosis and estrogen became clearer during those years when hysterectomies routinely included removal of the ovaries. Surgeons now try to avoid removing the ovaries of premenopausal women to help prevent premature bone deterioration. If you have undergone a surgical menopause, or are experiencing natural menopause at an early age, read *Sudden Menopause*, by Debbie De Angelo, RNC, for further insights into risk factors, HRT, and uniquely related issues (see Resources).

MEDICAL CONDITIONS

Medical conditions may make women vulnerable to bone deterioration. Diabetes, kidney or liver abnormalities, celiac disease, Crohn's disease, hypothyroidism, and stomach surgery are some of the common medical conditions that, for different reasons, impede absorption and utilization of calcium and other important nutrients necessary for the building of bone.

Bone recycling is a complex process involving interactions of organs, hormones, and minerals. Any defect or disease that affects the nutrient-transport system, endocrine system, liver or kidney functioning, or any illness that requires extended bed rest, causes calcium loss and consequent bone loss.

MEDICATIONS

Several medications interfere with calcium absorption. Some can easily be avoided; others cannot. Ask your doctor how your prescription drugs affect calcium balance. If you must take any of the following drugs, ask about the advisability of calcium supplementation.

Corticosteroids (cortisone, hydrocortisone, prednisone, dexamethasone). Used extensively, these can cause severe bone porosity, leading to osteoporosis. They not only create a negative calcium imbalance, but suppress the formation of new bone.

Anticonvulsants (phenytoin, phenobarbital, primidone, phensuximide). These stimulate the production of enzymes that break down vitamin D, leading to deficiencies of both vitamin D and calcium and, in turn, severe bone loss.

Antacids containing aluminum. These cause an increase in calcium excretion. Aluminum-containing antacids do not cause osteoporosis per se, but they can be a contributor if taken on a regular basis. Check the label when buying antacids—or any product for that matter. A few antacids that do not contain aluminum are Alka-Seltzer, Bisodol, Eno, Titralac, and Tums.

Diuretics. Women often take diuretics to reduce blood pressure and body fluid. Some are thought to have an adverse effect on bone mass. Long-term usage may cause the blood-calcium level to rise and the excretion of calcium to fall. Morris Notelovitz, director of the Center for Climacteric Studies in Gainesville, Florida, writes that Furosenide increases urinary calcium excretion, while Thiazide reduces the amount of calcium lost in urine and thus is more appropriate for osteoporosis-prone women.[7]

LIFESTYLE FACTORS

The speed with which our bones break down depends on the way we treat our bodies: what we regularly put into them and how much we use them. Virtually everything we do is, in one way or another, related to bone health.

ANIMAL PROTEIN

Many studies of societies around the world have proven a correlation between diet and advanced bone disease. For instance, a vegetarian diet helps prevent osteoporosis. Especially after the age of fifty, heavy meat eaters lose almost twice as much calcium as do vegetarians. The latest study to date suggests that the important issue is not so much total intake of animal protein; rather it's the ratio of animal to vegetable protein in the diet. The women in the study whose diets favored animal

sources of protein (average ratio of 4.2:1 animal to vegetable protein) suffered significantly higher rates of bone loss than women who relied more on vegetable protein (average ratio of 1.2:1).[8] The results were the same even after all other risk factors, such as calcium intake, estrogen levels, exercise, and body weight, were taken into account. According to the authors of this study, the point isn't that we all have to adopt a vegetarian lifestyle and avoid all animal protein, but rather that we should integrate more vegetable protein into the diet, add more fruits and vegetables, and focus on balance.

It is well accepted that protein intake beyond what our body needs creates acidity in the stomach, a condition that leaches calcium from the skeleton. With age, our kidneys are less able to neutralize stomach acid, so when stressed with acid excess, the body withdraws alkaline minerals from the bones. There are two ways to deal with this situation: We can cut down on animal protein if it is overburdening our diet, or we can supply a base in the form of fruits and vegetables, which will neutralize the acid. Once again, these findings build the case for greater amounts of fresh fruit and vegetables in the diet every day.

Animal-based protein has a second downside. Meat is high in phosphorus, a mineral that when taken in amounts over our bodily needs has a similar effect of creating acid and thus depleting calcium from the bones. The body's acid/alkaline balance is critical to bone health specifically and to total health in general. To maintain equilibrium within your body, curtail acid-producing foods; these include red meat, carbonated drinks, alcohol, salt, and refined sugar and flour. In their place, beef up the amount of vegetables in your diet. (For a discussion of the benefits of plant-based proteins, see the section "Nutrients Beneficial to Bones," starting on page 145.)

FATS

Both the amount and the kind of fat you eat affect calcium absorption. If fat consumption is too high or too low, calcium absorption is depressed. This has been a major criticism of weight-loss diets that call for nonfat milk and other fat-free products. Calcium requires the presence of some fat for its absorption, so for the sake of your bones, don't eliminate all fat from your diet, even when you want to lose weight.

A certain amount of fat is needed every day for functions that cannot be performed by any other nutrient. Essential fatty acids (EFAs) are necessary for the metabolism of calcium and must be obtained from food. The preferred forms of fat are those found in whole natural foods, such as raw seeds and nuts, vegetable oils,

and fish. Butterfat in fermented products such as yogurt and acidophilus milk encourages calcium absorption. Even people who are sensitive to milk can usually tolerate these foods because they are partially predigested.

Many women shun fat in their diet at all costs. If you have eliminated most fats from your life, I encourage you to find ways to integrate the essential fats into your food plan or to supplement with capsules. Essential fats can normalize your hormones, protect your arteries, decrease tumor growth, and, strangely, even help you maintain your weight. The most significant food source of EFAs comes from cold-water fish, such as tuna and salmon. Because eating these foods on a daily basis isn't practical, I recommend the vegetarian source, flaxseed, as an easier way to assure yourself of obtaining adequate essential fats. There's a bonus to your bones with flaxseed. Due to its antioxidant properties and its ability to minimize calcium loss in the urine, it exerts a positive effect on bone metabolism. A study examining the effects of flaxseed intake on postmenopausal women not on HRT found that when 38 grams (four tablespoons) of ground flaxseed was integrated into their daily diet, it reduced the rate of bone resorption.[9] Flaxseed comes in a variety of forms: as seeds to grind, as prepackaged ground flaxseed, and as oil.

The fats to avoid—those that alter digestibility and utilization of nutrients—are saturated fats, such as those found in meat, dairy products, shortening, and processed foods, and certain vegetable oils, such as coconut and palm oil. And keeping fat-calorie intake to no more than 25 percent of total calorie intake is generally healthy.

SUGAR

Those of us with a penchant for sweets run a greater risk of developing osteoporosis. A high sugar intake encourages acidity, which, as discussed above, causes calcium to be excreted from the bones. Imagine the effects on your body of being both a voracious meat eater and a sugar fanatic!

SALT

Most people know that excess sodium can raise blood pressure and increase the risk of hypertension and heart disease. Few people realize that too much salt brings another risk: the loss of large amounts of calcium from the bone. The more salt you eat, the more calcium you excrete. It is recommended that daily sodium intake not exceed 2,000 mg (the amount contained in approximately one teaspoon of table salt). Watch out for hidden offenders: condiments and dressings, processed and canned foods, cheese, hot dogs, cured meats, and pizza.

CAFFEINE

Coffee, cigarettes, and alcohol all react in the body to produce bone porosity. Young women who drink the equivalent of two cups of coffee a day are putting themselves at risk for osteoporosis in later life, according to a study of 980 postmenopausal women.[10] Caffeine acts as a diuretic, speeding up the loss of calcium and magnesium from the body. This study also showed that it is possible to balance the harmful effects of caffeine by adding eight ounces of milk a day, or the equivalent of 300 mg calcium.

ALCOHOL

Heavy alcohol intake has been linked to inadequate absorption of calcium, so most nutritionists counsel high-risk individuals against drinking. This is probably because alcohol has diuretic effects, but it also damages the liver, interfering with vitamin D metabolism. A British study rather surprisingly has suggested that alcohol might increase bone mass, since it causes the conversion of androgens to estrogen.[11] I think the rule of moderation applies to alcohol as it does with other substances that can harm us when we overindulge.

CIGARETTES

Female smokers lose bone faster than female nonsmokers. Smokers generally experience menopause several years earlier than nonsmokers, and the premature drop in estrogen may be responsible for diminished absorption of calcium into the bones. Cigarette smoking may also interfere with the body's metabolism of estrogen, although the mechanism by which this happens is unclear. Smoking frequently accompanies consuming caffeine or alcohol—a combination that may be worse than the sum of the individual parts.

The Exercise Connection

There is no controversy concerning the benefits of exercise in building and maintaining strong bones. Like muscle, bone grows stronger with use. Bone density depends directly on how much the bone is stressed: As stress on the bone increases, the amount of calcium deposited in the bone increases. Bones of athletes and physically active individuals are considerably denser than the bones of those who do not exercise.

You don't have to be a marathon runner to get results from regular physical activity. Muscle-strengthening exercises, like the ones pictured at the end of this book, help reverse the decline in muscle mass and muscle strength that comes with aging and may increase bone density. Research at the Center for Climacteric Studies in Florida showed that postmenopausal women on hormone therapy experienced an 8 percent increase in bone mass when they performed muscle-strengthening exercises.[12] A comparison group of women who were on estrogen replacement therapy (ERT) but didn't exercise neither gained nor lost bone mass. Even in a group of ninety-year-old women, high-intensity resistance training was found to increase muscle strength and reduce the risk of osteoporotic-related falls.[13]

It doesn't require an unreasonable time commitment to realize results with exercise. In a research project at Nassau County Medical Center in New York, post-menopausal women who exercised for one hour three times a week not only stopped losing calcium, but also they actually added some to their bones.[14] The amount of exercise one gets does relate to the amount of bone mass she will gain. Women who exercise four times a week will have denser bones than those who exercise two times a week.

Osteoporosis is a multidimensional problem, and the many factors that contribute to bone loss must be evaluated as part of a preventive or recovery program. In a study of older women, it was found that exercise alone was not as effective as exercise plus calcium. In the women who exercised and took calcium, bone loss nearly stopped. Among the women who took estrogen while exercising, bone density increased about 3 percent a year, but estrogen therapy may not be an option for all women.[15]

It is never too late to improve your body. If you are not physically active, start a program as soon as possible, if for no other reason than to protect your bones from deteriorating. The best exercises for bone strengthening are those that put a load on your bones: jogging, aerobic dance, skipping rope, brisk walking, stair climbing, dancing, and strength training. I've said it before but it bears repeating: Don't underestimate walking for exercise. If, like me, you used to run and now can't, you can still get a good workout by walking fast, walking hills or mountains, or wearing weights on your body when you walk. (*Caution*: Wearing ankle weights while walking does more harm than good by placing unwanted stress on the knees and ankles.) My dear thin friend Karan came up with a plan to further load her bones: She carries ten-pound weights in a backpack when we're out for our early morning trek up and down the hills of Sausalito.

To reap the fullest benefits, as you've probably heard before, exercise for twenty to thirty minutes at a pace fast enough to accelerate your pulse moderately. Frequently, women concentrate on aerobic exercises or exercises for the lower body and ignore the upper body. This is why so many women have relatively weak arms and shoulders. For a thorough workout, put all your bones and muscles through

137

their full range of movement. Walk or dance for the lower extremities, then add arm and shoulder exercises or work out with weights. Strength training can even be practiced sitting down or in a wheelchair. Charlene Torkelson's *Get Fit While You Sit* provides some interesting ideas about how to exercise if you are mobility impaired or require low-impact exercises (see Resources).

Some great exercise videos are designed specifically for women—some even for menopausal women. I recommend Kathy Smith's *Moving Through Menopause*. She includes it all: a low-impact cardio routine, a strength-training workout, plus a stress-reducing yoga session. Actually, all of Kathy's tapes are fantastic. I also like Denise Austin. Besides her videos, she leads a regular early-morning workout on TV that you can follow for free. My preference for exercise instructors are people who have studied exercise physiology and who keep current with the latest scientific information—not "celebrities" who just look good in shorts.

There comes a time in our lives when we are forced to change our exercise programs. I hated having to discontinue running and am grateful that my younger friend Linda, who still runs up to five miles a day, will hold back and walk hills with me. I also find that some of the low-impact aerobic workouts hurt my knees and the balls of my feet. I'm not recovering from exercise pain as quickly as I once did. It's difficult giving up something that has been enjoyable and so much a part of one's life. Believe me, I fought changing as long as I could, but my body told me loud and clear that I had to find gentler alternatives. Now that I've adjusted to my new routine, I love speed walking, hiking mountains, and my dance aerobics class. I plan to experiment further with new classes, maybe yoga or ballet. What is true for me may also be reality for you. Not everyone should engage in high-impact aerobic activities. Orthopedic consultant to the Pennsylvania ballet company, Nicholas DiNublie, M.D., warns that people with musculoskeletal ailments should refrain from high-impact exercise. Additionally, people with foot and ankle problems and those with arthritis or osteoporosis would be better served by sticking to low-impact activities.[16] Elderly people, as well as those who have neurologic conditions that affect balance, run the risk of falling and should be careful with the exercise they choose.

Remember that domestic activities, such as gardening and housework, also help to maintain physical fitness. The more you move your body, the healthier you will be—and the fewer physical complaints you will suffer.

Prevention is the best—and for some the only—way to avoid the skeletal fractures, severe discomfort, and permanent disfiguration of osteoporosis. Once detected, osteoporosis can be controlled and reversed only to a limited extent, so the safest course is to begin preventive measures now. Exercise will add mass to your bones and possibly years to your life.

⇒ The Hormone Connection ⇐

The research clearly indicates that hormones are directly involved in bone metabolism. It remains less clear as to which hormone plays the predominant role, what sources are best, and what amounts are adequate and safe for postmenopausal women. Estrogen, progesterone, and testosterone all contribute to bone health prior to menopause, but is taking these hormones necessary for all postmenopausal women, or only for those at risk for osteoporosis or those who already suffer signs of bone deterioration?

The important role of estrogen in bone health has been recognized for decades. Estrogen preserves bone mass by slowing down the loss of bone. Note, however, that it doesn't build any new bone cells; it only slows down the process of bone loss. Thus, any loss that has already occurred cannot be reversed by taking estrogen alone. A woman's estrogen levels throughout life greatly determine her chances of developing osteoporosis after menopause. Because you need a certain amount of estrogen per month to lay down bone, anything that interferes with your hormonal cycle and with estrogen production prior to menopause will also interfere with bone production. Some of these conditions include the age at which you begin your period (starting later means less estrogen production), the age at which you reach menopause (reaching it earlier means less estrogen production), and the skipping of menstrual cycles (which means less estrogen production). On the other hand, exercise, especially in the earlier years, helps to build bone. Furthermore, carrying a little extra body weight doesn't hurt, especially after menopause. This is because fat converts to estrogen, which translates to less bone deterioration.

Estrogen improves calcium and magnesium absorption and reduces the amount of these minerals excreted in the urine. Because the early literature on menopause focused exclusively on the role of estrogen and bone, the conventional wisdom has suggested supplementing estrogen at midlife when hormonal levels begin to wane. To derive optimal bone benefit from ERT, one must start it early in the perimenopausal years, when the rate of bone loss is at its peak, and then continue for up to nine years.[17] Other research indicates that estrogen must be taken for life, since discontinuation results in immediate bone loss, possibly at an accelerated rate. This is discouraging news to women who are aware that an increased risk for breast cancer exists when usage exceeds five years.[18]

What to do when one is faced with this dilemma is not an easy question, nor can anyone offer a blanket recommendation that will apply to all women. The condition of your bones and the total count of all your risk factors combined will help lead you to the decision that is right for you. For starters, not all women are candidates for ERT; this includes women with cancer of the uterus, estrogen-related cancers, endometriosis, uterine fibroid tumors, high blood pressure, liver or gallbladder disease, diabetes, migraines, or a tendency toward blood clotting. Other women find hormonal therapy intolerable because of such side effects as anxiety, mood swings, fluid retention, weight gain, abdominal bloating, withdrawal bleeding, nausea, and headaches.

A growing number of women just don't feel comfortable with the idea of trying to control a natural life process by taking conventional hormones that have proven harmful or drugs with dangerous side effects. Even if a chance exists that the therapy is protecting them against bone loss, the unknowns concerning its long-term effects disturb many women enough to make them hold off. Fortunately, many natural, less invasive practices exist that offer bone protection. A friendlier estrogen, estriol, has been effective in reducing many of the common menopausal symptoms; however, it hasn't yet been studied adequately enough for us to know with certainty if it will prevent bone loss as effectively as the stronger estradiol (a common component of many conventional forms of HRT). That said, several Japanese studies find encouraging results; it appears that estriol may prevent bone deterioration in postmenopausal women.[19] (See Chapter 2 for a detailed discussion of natural, or bioidentical, hormones such as estriol.) In addition, a host of nutrients protects bone from further loss, as discussed in the section "Nutrients Beneficial to Bones," below. Foods such as soy offer an estrogen-like effect that can strengthen bones; soy tablets and other supplements are now being marketed for the woman who struggles to find ways to integrate enough soy into her diet. If foods, nutrients, and friendly hormones fail to work for you, then consult with your doctor for a medical treatment.

A hormone that makes bones stronger by actually working to restore bone tissue is progesterone. Research from the United States is scant when it comes to the role of this other female hormone in treating menopause, because the researchers thought they had the answer to menopause—estrogen. Progesterone was only added to the ERT mix as a protection against endometrial cancer. The most significant studies on progesterone at this time come from the University of British Columbia. Testing both animals and humans in a variety of scientific settings, Dr. Jerilynn Prior found that progesterone not only put a stop to bone loss; it actually formed new bone and/or increased bone turnover.[20]

John Lee, M.D., is one of the pioneers who has tested natural progesterone in a clinical setting. He, too, finds that progesterone is the key to building bone. Since 1982, Dr. Lee has treated postmenopausal women with a natural progesterone cream plus a dietary program that includes vitamin and mineral supplements and moderate exercise. He found true reversal of osteoporosis even in patients who did not use estrogen supplements.[21] Read more about Dr. Lee's work in his books *What Your Doctor May Not Tell You about Menopause* (with Virginia Hopkins) and *What Your Doctor May Not Tell You about Premenopause* (with Jesse Hanley, M.D., and Virginia Hopkins).

Natural progesterone cream is available over the counter in some pharmacies and health-food stores. *Note:* The number of creams on the market now is growing rapidly, and the names can tend to sound similar, but not all of them contain real progesterone, so buyer beware. Aeron LifeCycles Clinical Laboratory has evaluated a number of commercial cream products with potential hormonal activity for progesterone content (a list of these products can be found in Chapter 2).

Synthetic progesterones, called *progestins*, such as those found in Provera and other traditional HRT treatments, may offer some of the bone-building benefits of progesterone; however, the serious side effects make them intolerable to many women. (See Chapter 2 for more about natural versus synthetic progesterone.)

Recent advances in the study of androgens show that testosterone also stimulates new bone growth and contributes substantially to bone density. A two-year investigation of an oral combination of estrogen and methyltestosterone confirmed that the duo not only prevented bone loss (as did estrogen singly), but also produced significant increases in spinal bone mineral density (not an effect of estrogen alone).[22] Furthermore, men who have lower testosterone levels have a higher incidence of osteoporosis.

Even though the research on women is minimal at this time, it is probable that some postmenopausal women may benefit from testosterone replacement. Checking hormone levels, testing for osteoporosis, and following symptoms are advisable before starting any hormone treatment.

Nonhormonal Drugs

Now that HRT has been discredited, drug companies are standing in the wings waiting to promote their bone-building products to concerned women. I have no numbers to support this theory, but it's not a stretch of the imagination to expect sales of Fosamax, Evista, and newer look-alikes to soar within a very short time. From what I've read (outside of the mainstream media), both Evista and Fosamax need careful consideration before a woman embarks on treatment using them. The

benefits of Fosamax (generic name: alendronate) remain questionable because of the type of bone it creates. Part of the problem with this drug is that we lack any long-term studies. Still, several researchers are highly suspicious that over the years alendronate may actually cause bones to fracture more easily. Its side effects are frightening as well; these include permanent damage to the stomach and esophagus. Nor do the advertisements play up the fact that the drug causes deficiencies of calcium, magnesium, and vitamin D—minerals that are definitely crucial to strong bones.

Evista (raloxifene) is gaining in popularity as a nonhormonal bone builder. Before you try it, however, know that it can worsen menopausal symptoms, especially hot flashes, and can increase the risk for fatal blood clots. As the drug companies introduce the latest bone-building wonders, read about all potential side effects before making your decision.

The Marketing of Fear?

I'd like to offer one final word about how profitable osteoporosis promises to be for drug companies out to corner the market of aging consumers. I do not want to underplay the devastation, inconvenience, and financial drain a broken hip can cause, but a handful of medical writers are reporting that as a health problem, osteoporosis has been blown out of proportion. Gill Sanson, a women's health educator from New Zealand, has extensively reviewed the literature on osteoporosis and finds that the information contained in patient brochures, advertising, and the media is misleading, often inaccurate, and has been allowed to proliferate without public policy and objective analysis.[23] She points out that low bone mineral density doesn't necessarily lead to fractures, and that to label low BMD as osteoporosis is like labeling high blood pressure as a stroke, or high cholesterol as heart disease. On the other hand, to hype reduced BMD, a condition that millions of elderly people have lived with for thousands of years, as a global epidemic provides potentially unlimited commercial return for the bone-testing, pharmaceutical, dairy, and calcium-supplement industries. Before you decide on drug treatment, you may want to take a look at Sanson's book, *The Osteoporosis "Epidemic": Well Women and the Marketing of Fear*. Check out her website at www.bonestory.com.

The Calcium Connection

The process that ends in osteoporosis begins thirty to forty years before the first fracture. The early years are when you build bone health; the longer you wait, the harder it is to catch up. Prevention is the best way—and the only certain way—to maintain bone health. And the story begins with calcium. Getting the calcium into the bones and keeping it there is the trick, and it is not as easy as drinking a glass of milk before bedtime.

To say that calcium is important to the body is an understatement. Because calcium is instrumental in brain function, blood clotting, and muscle contraction, the body is equipped with an elaborate system of hormonal checks and balances to ensure that an adequate amount is circulating in the bloodstream at all times. When blood-calcium levels fall, special hormones and glands respond immediately by withdrawing whatever is needed from the faithful storehouse: the bones.

An adequate amount of calcium in the blood is essential for ensuring that a continual withdrawal does not leave the body, decades later, with weakened bones. The RDAs for calcium have recently been increased to the following:

Calcium Sources

Food	Portion	Calcium Content (mg)
Nonfat or low-fat (2%) milk	1 cup	300
Sardines (with bones)	1/4 lb	300
Frozen yogurt	1 cup	200
Yogurt	1 cup	290
Cheddar cheese	1 oz	205
Ice cream	1/2 cup	190
American cheese	1 oz	175
Spinach, cooked	1 cup	150
Tofu	4 oz	145
Broccoli, cooked	1 cup	130
Almonds	1/4 cup	80

Women ages 19 to 50: 1,000 mg (including women who are pregnant or lactating)

Women age 50 and above: 1,200 mg

In preventing and treating osteoporosis, we need to consider three issues: (1) Are we getting enough calcium in our diets? (2) If we are, what may be preventing us from absorbing the calcium for building bone strength? (3) Is supplementation necessary?

Taking calcium into the body in the form of food should be a top priority, but there are factors that mitigate against doing so. Some women simply do not drink cow's milk or eat cheese; dairy products don't agree with them. It is possible that they can no longer digest cow's milk; this is true for the majority of African Americans and Asians, who are lactose intolerant. If this describes you, and yet you would like to get more of your calcium from dairy products, you can try Lactaid milk or add enzyme drops to your milk. Alternatively, I have found rice and soy milks to be good with cereal and in cooking, and both are now fortified with calcium.

Dairy products, however, may not be the answer to the calcium question and to bone health. The hip fracture rate is the highest in Western countries, where dairy foods are consumed in large quantities.[24] Incorporating more of the other food sources of calcium may be a better solution, but consider some of the top contenders: sardines (with the bones), boiled turnip greens, and almonds. Be honest—how many times a week would you really eat these foods? My favorite calcium-rich food is broccoli, but I would have a difficult time forcing down twelve cups to get my daily recommended requirement. (Check the list on page 143 and add up your approximate daily calcium score.)

Consuming calcium-rich foods is only the beginning of the process that takes calcium through the digestive system, into the blood, and to the bones. Since calcium is poorly absorbed by the body, you may need even greater amounts to compensate for the inefficiency. While absorption of any nutrient varies with the individual, at best only 20 to 40 percent of the calcium you ingest is usable, and even that percentage decreases with age. Consider some of the complex aspects of calcium absorption:

- Your genetic makeup determines whether or not you are an efficient absorber.

- Disease and illness decrease the amount retained.

- Estrogen enhances calcium absorption, which helps explain the rapid loss of bone after menopause.

- Calcium absorption declines with increasing age in both men and women, but the decline begins earlier for women.

- Exercise increases absorption; inactivity decreases it.

- Medications, drugs, cigarettes, caffeine, and certain foods impede absorption, increase excretion of nutrients, and decrease utilization.

- Stress depletes your immediate supply as well as your storehouse of calcium.

- Lack of other specific nutrients will deter absorption, especially vitamins D, C, and K, and the minerals magnesium, phosphorous, and boron.

Supplementation, then, is absolutely necessary for most women and is proven to be effective in reducing bone loss in postmenopausal women.[25] Choosing which supplement to buy can be frustrating. Calcium carbonate is clearly the most popular and widely available source, largely because it contains the most elemental, or actual, calcium; however, it is not the best choice for the mature woman. Calcium citrate is the preferred form, since it is better tolerated by individuals with low stomach acid, a condition common among older adults.[26]

The safety of certain calcium supplements has also been questioned. For several years, health educators have warned the public about dolomite and bone meal, because they contain the toxic metals lead and cadmium. Recently, significant amounts of lead and aluminum have been found in one of the more popular sources of calcium, the calcium carbonate labeled "oyster shell" or "natural source."[27] Calcium citrate does not contain these metals.

Absorption of calcium is enhanced when calcium intake is spread out over the day. Dole out your portions and take them with each meal. If you forget to take calcium during the day, be sure to remember at night, when bone loss is greatest.

Many women ask about the superiority of name brands over generic products when choosing supplements. In the case of calcium, the National Osteoporosis Foundation does recommend that you stick to brand-name supplements. There is a way to test for quality and dissolution time. Drop one tablet into a small container of vinegar. If it takes more than 30 minutes to dissolve, shop elsewhere.

Nutrients Beneficial to Bones

Our information about the interrelationships among nutrients constantly expands. Bone health involves not just calcium, but also an array of cofactors and other substances.

PLANT-BASED ALTERNATIVES: SOY AND HERBS

A soy-based diet appears to be advantageous for preserving bone, and the fact remains that women from cultures that consume large amounts of soy-based foods do not experience many of our common menopausal symptoms, including bone loss. Japanese women, for example, who traditionally ingest about five servings of soy daily, experience much lower rates of breast and endometrial cancer, heart disease, and osteoporosis. Japanese people who begin following a traditional Western diet, on the other hand, have disease rates the same as ours.

Soy protein does not cause calcium excretion, as animal protein does. In one study, subjects who ate protein from soy sources excreted about 50 mg less urinary calcium than those eating protein from animal sources.[28] Soy foods, such as tofu and tempeh, are rich sources of calcium and phytoestrogens. A 1992 study suggests that the isoflavones in soybeans also bear a direct benefit on bone health, possibly by inhibiting bone resorption.[29] Furthermore, it is known that the isoflavones genistein and daidzein, both contained in soy, are similar to the synthetic estrogens used in HRT, which are effective in preventing or retarding bone loss.

Whereas early research found that isoflavones bore only a modest effect on bone tissue, more recent studies appear quite encouraging. A University of North Carolina study showed that soy protein prevented bone deterioration in rats whose ovaries had been removed (which would normally result in a diminished estrogen supply and attendant bone loss). The results were compared with those from another group of rats, which were on Premarin (the most common ERT medication, made from the urine of pregnant mares). They showed that soy could prevent bone loss almost as well as this synthetic hormone preparation.[30]

In a University of Illinois study, women who took soy protein containing 90 mg of isoflavones every day for six months were found to have higher bone mineral density in their spines than women who drank milk. Doses of isoflavones below 90 mg did not work. (Researchers pointed out that the studies need to be extended to three years.)[31]

An analysis of published reports from several types of studies—including population studies, lab cultures on cells and tissues, and experimental studies on animals—concluded that taking isoflavones (especially genistein and daidzein) at optimal doses resulted in improved bone mass.[32]

How much isoflavone does it take to treat and prevent bone loss? While some experts have speculatively recommended daily intakes of between 16 and 20 grams of soy protein (which would provide 16 to 60 mg of isoflavone) for prevention, remember the study that demonstrated success with a minimum of 90 mg of isoflavones. This translates into three or four servings of soy per day. Other experts recommend 150 to 200 mg of isoflavones per day, or five to six servings of soy foods. (If this seems daunting, see Chapter 3 for a discussion of soy supplements. Also review Chapter 15 for practical tips for including soy in your diet.)

I want to mention a specific synthetic derivative of isoflavone, ipriflavone, which originally showed promise as an alternative to estrogen replacement for reducing bone loss. In the fourth edition of this book I cited studies suggesting that ipriflavone had increased bone mass in rats and menopausal women, and based on that information I chose it over HRT to keep my osteoporosis under control. After eight months on ipriflavone, I assessed my progress by getting a urine bone density test, and much to my surprise I found I was losing rather than gaining bone mass. Forced to rethink my plan, I noted that my options were to take either drugs that were unnatural to my body or hormones that were. (I'm following all the dietary and exercise practices recommended, yet with my risk factors I still need additional support.) As mentioned earlier, I opted for taking a natural hormone preparation, and worked with my doctor and a compounding pharmacist to establish a formula that was right for me. It was after deciding to discontinue ipriflavone

that I read about a large, randomized, double-blind study involving 474 post-menopausal women which found that ipriflavone neither prevented bone loss nor reduced fracture risk.[33] Sometimes it is very frustrating to lack a definitive answer to these difficult postmenopausal questions. Still, my approach remains the same as it always has been: Start with the least harmful remedy that is effective based on the best science to date, and use it until proven otherwise.

Speaking of safer and often effective remedies, the wisdom of the ages has always encouraged the use of herbs in caring for one's health. Whereas modern medicine and its reliance on synthetic drugs is only a few generations old, herbal remedies have been used for millennia. As discussed in earlier chapters, many herbs encourage hormone production. Black cohosh, hops, sage, sweetbriar, alfalfa, buckwheat, horsetail, roses, and shepherd's purse promote estrogen production; chaste tree (vitex), sarsparilla, wild yam, and yarrow promote progesterone production. These natural sources of both estrogen and progesterone can be incorporated into your regimen for building bone. Plant phytosterols are safer than synthetic hormones. They encourage your own body to produce small amounts of hormones—but no more than what you need. Unlike with estrogen replacement therapy or hormone replacement therapy, excess dosages are not a worry. In fact, researchers have found that the phytoestrogens, such as those found in soy, have a protective effect on breast tissue.

VITAMIN D

Vitamin D is vital to calcium absorption. Without it, the small intestine cannot absorb calcium adequately no matter how much is available. A lack of vitamin D has been found in 30 percent of postmenopausal women with bone deterioration.[34] Vitamin D and calcium taken together can inhibit hip fractures even after eighty years of age. This is the finding of a research project directed by a team of French scientists who set out to see if they could prevent bone fractures in a group of more than three thousand ambulatory women living in nursing homes. For eighteen months, half of the women were given daily supplements of 1.2 grams of calcium and 800 IU of vitamin D; the other half received inactive tablets (placebo). At the end of the study, the women receiving the supplements had a 40 percent lower rate of hip fractures and a 32 percent lower incidence of wrist, arm, and pelvic fractures. The scientists noted few side effects and concluded that calcium plus vitamin D was a safe and effective way to prevent fractures.[35]

Getting sunlight is the most effortless way to promote the manufacture of natural vitamin D in the body. Just thirty minutes a day of direct sun exposure is all that is necessary for the skin to convert a type of cholesterol into vitamin D. If

this is not possible for you because you live where there is little sun, you usually stay indoors or cover yourself outdoors, or you are exposed to sunlight primarily through a window or screen, then supplementation as part of a multivitamin and mineral program is probably called for.

In fact, most of us don't get enough sun or eat enough fish, eggs, dairy foods, and fortified cereals to obtain adequate amounts of vitamin D. A number of studies published in the late 1990s suggest that vitamin D deficiency is much more common than previously thought. In 1997, the Food and Nutrition Board (part of the National Academy of Sciences) began a program to revise the RDAs in line with the growing understanding of the importance of nutrition in the role of preventing disease and optimizing health. Under the new system, when evidence supports a recommendation higher than the RDA, an adequate intake (AI) is suggested. The new AIs recommended for vitamin D are 400 IU for those over age fifty, and 600 IU for those over age seventy. Some experts recommend that everyone take 800 IU of vitamin D, regardless of age.

Good dietary sources of vitamin D include salmon, tuna, shrimp, fortified milk, and egg yolks. For the precise amount of this nutrient contained in certain foods, consult Appendix C.

VITAMIN C

Vitamin C is necessary for the manufacture of collagen, a fibrous protein that is found in connective tissue and cartilage and is essential for proper bone formation. Since the need for collagen regeneration increases with age, vitamin C is required in greater amounts as one gets older. With age, the stomach tends to produce less acid. Vitamin C also facilitates the absorption of calcium by creating the weak acidity level necessary for proper digestion. Good sources include kiwi fruit, raw green peppers, oranges/orange juice, broccoli, grapefruit (including grapefruit juice), watermelon, and grapes. (For the precise amount of this nutrient contained in certain foods, consult Appendix C.)

VITAMIN K

Low blood levels of vitamin K—the form that is found in green leafy plants (kale, collard greens, lettuce, and parsley)—were found in patients with fractures due to bone loss. The more severe the fracture, the lower the level of circulating vitamin K.[36] The good news is that the ongoing Nurses' Health Study reported in 1999 that vitamin K may offer powerful protection against hip fractures. Of more than seventy-two thousand women middle-aged and older, those with the highest intake of vitamin K suffered the lowest risk of sustaining a hip fracture over a ten-year period.

Women who ate lettuce (even iceberg) at least once a day had about half the risk as women who ate lettuce once a week or less. Other bone-health issues were factored in, such as calcium and vitamin D intake.[37]

The newly updated AI for vitamin K is 90 micrograms (mcg) for women, but the Nurses' Study indicated that the protective effect on bone health was achieved at lev-

Daily Nutritional Support for the Prevention and Treatment of Osteoporosis	
Nutrient	**Amount**
Calcium	1,000 mg before menopause; 1,200 mg after
Vitamin D	400–800 IU
Magnesium	500 mg before menopause; 600 mg after
Vitamin C	75–1,000 mg
Vitamin K	100–500 mcg
Boron	3 mg

els of 100 to 150 mcg per day, an amount relatively easy to include in your diet. Besides lettuce, good sources include spinach, broccoli, Brussels sprouts, cabbage, kale, and asparagus. (For the precise amount of this nutrient contained in certain foods, consult Appendix C.)

MAGNESIUM

The mineral magnesium is instrumental in converting vitamin D to its usable form and in keeping calcium soluble in the bloodstream. A magnesium deficiency disturbs the calcification of bone, impairs bone growth, and reduces calcium. Tests have shown that diets deficient in magnesium can lead to skeletal abnormalities, including osteoporosis.

Increasing your intake of calcium, vitamin D, or phosphorus increases your body's magnesium requirements, thus emphasizing the importance of nutrient interrelationships. Evidence suggests that the balance between calcium and magnesium is especially important. If the calcium level is increased, magnesium intake must be increased as well. The optimum calcium/magnesium ratio is two to one; thus, if you are taking 1,000 mg of calcium, you need 500 mg of magnesium. Calcium and magnesium are available in the correct proportion in single tablets. Good sources of magnesium include peanuts, Bran Buds, lentils, tofu, wild rice, bean sprouts, and chicken. (For the precise amount of this nutrient contained in certain foods, consult Appendix C.)

PHOSPHORUS

Phosphorus is necessary to metabolize calcium, but deficiency of the mineral is uncommon. Anybody who eats a typical modern-day diet of red meat, white bread, processed cheeses, soft drinks, and packaged pastries gets more than his or her quota of phosphorus.

149

The ratio of calcium to phosphorus affects the amount of calcium absorbed by the bones. Ideally, the balance should be two to one in favor of calcium. With the abundance of phosphorus found in today's foods, the balance has tipped four to one in favor of phosphorus. Not only is this change detrimental to calcium retention; it accelerates bone demineralization by stimulating the parathyroid glands, which secrete a bone-dissolving hormone called *parathyroid hormone.*

To reestablish the correct mineral ratio, you should drastically reduce your intake of high-phosphorus foods. Concentrate on eliminating processed foods, which often offer little nutrition anyway. These include almost all processed or canned meats (hot dogs, luncheon meats, bacon, ham, sausage), processed cheeses, instant soups, puddings, packaged pastries, soft drinks, breads, and cereals. Check the labels of packaged goods for ingredients such as sodium phosphate, potassium phosphate, phosphoric acid, pyrophosphate, or polyphosphate; if you find them, put the products back on the shelf.

BORON

Boron, a mineral needed in very small amounts in our bodies, has gained attention as another protective factor against osteoporosis. Supplementing the diets of postmenopausal women with 3 mg of boron a day reduced urinary calcium excretion by 44 percent and dramatically increased the levels of the most usable form of estrogen. In its active form, boron also appears to activate vitamin D conversion. Fruits and vegetables are the main dietary sources of boron, and, typically, American diets are deficient. Only 10 percent of diets meet the minimum requirement of these foods.[38]

Other nutrients that may be instrumental in building bone include zinc, copper, manganese, and silicon.

CHAPTER 8

BLEEDING, CRAMPS, PMS, BREAST DISEASE, INSOMNIA, ARTHRITIS

— AND THE GOOD LIFE

From month to month, from birth to the giving of life to the change of life, women face a unique challenge to keep their body chemistry in balance.

— RICHARD KUNIN, *Mega-Nutrition for Women*

The majority of women do not experience a major disruption in their lives due to menopause, although many are temporarily bothered by a number of physical concerns. Getting appropriate treatment during midlife years appears to be more challenging than at any other time in a woman's life. Depending on a physician's attitude and clinical experience with women going through the change, a woman's symptoms may be overtreated, undertreated, or misdiagnosed. If the doctor views menopause as a hormonal deficiency disease, unnecessary medications may be prescribed. On the other hand, some physicians regard all complaints as hormonal and may overlook something more serious.

In defense of the medical community, when real symptoms surface at menopause, diagnosing whether the problem is due to hormonal changes, an undetected physical abnormality, or the natural aging process can be challenging. When questions arise over a symptom, inform yourself about natural signs of menopause, consult medical professionals to rule out any functional cause, and then make an educated decision about the best course of action for you.

⋙ Heavy Bleeding (Menorrhagia) ⋘

Erratic periods with heavy bleeding are a common perimenopausal symptom. If an egg is not released for a month or more and progesterone is not produced, estrogen continues to build up the uterine lining. Finally, the sheer bulk of the blood-rich tissue causes an especially heavy flow, which may also be accompanied by large clots. Long, profuse periods can be uncomfortable and a bit frightening. Some women report periods of up to ten days with flow so continuous that the combination of a tampon and a super-absorbent pad cannot contain it. The amount of blood lost over a week can be draining and may cause extreme fatigue.

Heavy or continuous bleeding is occasionally a symptom of something more serious, such as uterine fibroids, polyps, and, in rare cases, uterine or cervical cancer. Should your heavy bleeding last for more than a few months, check with your physician.

Many doctors prescribe progestins (synthetic progesterone) to compensate for the body's reduced production of natural progesterone. By preventing the buildup of the endometrial lining, progestins create a more regular monthly period and relieve excess bleeding. They do not, however, alleviate bleeding in all women, and some women find the side effects of depression, fatigue, bloating, and breast tenderness too unpleasant to continue with the treatment. Not all physicians are aware that there are natural progesterone creams on the market that help to control bleeding in many women, without the side effects of the synthetics. If, however, progesterone cream proves unsuccessful for you, your doctor can prescribe a stronger natural, oral progesterone, which can be formulated by a compounding pharmacist. Also available is a commercial oral micronized progesterone tablet, which your doctor may be more inclined to prescribe. It is called Prometrium. (For more specific information about natural hormones, read Chapter 2.)

Unexpected bleeding can be scary, but if it is temporary, it is usually a sign of hormonal changes. Nutritionally, several important remedies exist that will help you feel better and build up your body during periods of excessive blood loss.

IRON

Blood loss is well known as a major cause of iron-deficiency anemia. It is less well known that chronic iron deficiency can itself cause menorrhagia (severe menstrual bleeding). Iron deficiency may be the most prevalent nutritional deficiency in the United States, and women, throughout their lives, are at risk because of their increased need.

Iron comes in two dietary forms. Heme iron, the most efficiently absorbed, is found in red meats, egg yolks, and fish. Nonheme iron, the plant variety, comes from grains, beans, and dried fruits. It must be ionized by stomach acid and then transported by a complex mechanism before it can be used by the body; thus, absorption is trickier. Lack of stomach acid makes absorption even more of a challenge for menopausal women, and blocking agents such as fiber, phosphates, and preservatives prevent absorption. If you shy away from meat, you can enhance absorption of your vegetarian sources by taking in a vitamin C source at the same time you eat your iron-rich food. Good sources of iron include liver, clams, oysters, beef, shrimp, poultry, prune juice, almonds, raisins, spinach, and split peas. (For the precise amount of this nutrient contained in certain foods, consult Appendix C.)

Because it is difficult for women to eat enough iron-rich foods, supplemental iron may be required to replenish low iron stores. A daily dose of 100 mg elemental iron has been used therapeutically to treat excessive bleeding.[1] Liver extracts provide an excellent source of heme iron; take two 500 mg capsules with meals. Several nonheme iron supplements on the market are also very good; those containing iron bound to ascorbate, succinate, fumarate, glycinate, or aspartate are better absorbed and tolerated. Take these forms on an empty stomach unless they cause you discomfort, in which case take them with meals. The recommended iron intake for women who are still menstruating is 18 mg per day; however, if you suffer iron deficiency approaching anemia, you may need two or three times this amount to restore iron levels. Have your doctor monitor your levels until they fall within the normal range.

VITAMIN C AND BIOFLAVONOIDS

Vitamin C not only aids in iron absorption; it, along with bioflavonoids, has also been tested as a treatment for heavy menstrual bleeding. Both nutrients effectively decrease menstrual flow by strengthening capillary walls. Increase your fruit and vegetable intake, especially emphasizing blueberries, grapes, cherries, and blackberries. It requires a considerable effort to eat enough of these foods to reach suggested dosages, so supplement with vitamin C (1,000–4,000 mg) and bioflavonoids (500–2,000 mg) per day as needed.

VITAMIN A

Vitamin A is important for the support and restoration of the skin and mucous membranes, including the vaginal and urinary tissues. Deficiencies often result in alterations in both skin and mucous membranes that resemble precancerous conditions. This finding has promoted more research into vitamin A as a possible anticancer agent or cancer preventive. Studies show that women who bleed excessively have significantly lower levels of vitamin A than women with more moderate periods and that treatment with vitamin A normalizes blood flow.

The best sources of vitamin A are a wide variety of fruits and vegetables that contain beta-carotene, which is converted in the body to the vitamin's active form. While vitamin A from animal sources can produce toxicity in large amounts, beta-carotene is completely safe even in high doses. Recommended dosage is between 25,000 IU and 50,000 IU per day. Good sources include liver, carrots, sweet potatoes, pumpkin, spinach, cantaloupe, papaya, and watermelon. (For the precise amount of this nutrient contained in certain foods, consult Appendix C.)

B VITAMINS

As far back as the early 1940s, medical literature recorded that B vitamins were instrumental in regulating estrogen levels in the liver.[2] When B vitamins are insufficient, estrogen levels escalate. Furthermore, excess estrogen creates B-vitamin deficiency, and a vicious cycle ensues. Since heavy menstrual flow can be caused by excess buildup of estrogen in the body, it is imperative to keep adequate amounts of B vitamins circulating in the system. Dietary sources of many B vitamins include whole-grain products, desiccated liver, brewer's yeast, wheat germ, beans, and peas. For women with heavy periods, the amounts needed to create a therapeutic benefit cannot be met by food alone. Supplement with a multivitamin and mineral tablet or a B-complex tablet containing at least 50 mg each of B-1, B-2, and B-6.

ESSENTIAL FATTY ACIDS

Essential fatty acids (EFAs), fats that our bodies require but cannot manufacture, can normalize heavy periods. Sprinkle one to two tablespoons of the following onto salads or vegetables, or take two to eight capsules per day: borage oil, black currant seed oil, flaxseed oil, evening primrose oil. Store these sources of EFA in the refrigerator, and do cook with them.

HERBS

Several herbs can be useful in relieving profuse menstrual flow. Dandelion leaves contain an absorbable source of iron and are used to prevent iron-deficiency anemia. They are also a natural diuretic and digestive aid and enhance liver and gallbladder function. Take one capsule up to three times a day, or mix ten to thirty drops of liquid extract in juice or water.

Vitex (chaste tree) and wild yam root both can stimulate progesterone precursors to stabilize hormones and remedy excessive bleeding. Take either herb in capsules (one to three taken throughout the day) or in tincture form (twenty to twenty-five drops several times a day) for several months.

⇒ Menstrual Cramps ⇐

Monthly cramping during perimenopause intensifies in some women and subsides in others. The culprit is a substance called *prostaglandin*. When menstrual cramps are accompanied by nausea, vomiting, diarrhea, fatigue, tension, and headaches, the sufferer is probably producing greater than normal amounts of this hormone-like chemical. The reason for this overproduction has not yet been determined; my own bias leads me to suspect that nutrition is involved.

DIET

Several researchers have found a strong correlation between hormonal imbalances and vitamin and mineral deficiencies, and most menstrual problems seem to be caused by hormonal imbalances. When the nutritional deficiency is corrected by diet or supplements, hormone levels often return to normal.[3] This suggests that a lack of proper nutrients can result in a wide array of symptoms.

A diet primarily consisting of complex carbohydrates, calcium-rich leafy green vegetables, and fatty fish, especially during the week before the period, seems to help many women. Holding off on sugar, caffeine, dairy products, and red meats generally works well too. If this is not enough to relieve your cramps, supplement with a multivitamin and mineral complex that includes a B-complex (10–30 mg of each B vitamin), vitamin C (100–1,000 mg), vitamin E (400 IU), calcium (1,000–1,500 mg), magnesium (500 mg), and zinc (30–60 mg). Additional magnesium relaxes smooth muscle; you may want to try an extra 300–500 mg a day, not to exceed 1,000 mg total. For some women, four tablespoons per day of fresh ground flaxseed has proven helpful for cramps.

EXERCISE

If you are bothered by cramps, remember that vigorous exercise four or five times a week will help prevent them. Exercise forces deep breathing, which brings more oxygen to the blood, relaxing the uterus and raising endorphin levels to relieve pain naturally. Yoga, stretching, and long, hot baths also relax the body, allowing tension and pain to recede.

CRAMP BARK

Cramp bark, as its name implies, is one of the best herbal remedies for menstrual cramps. It acts to reduce muscular tension and spasms and has also been used for threatened miscarriages. Some of its properties are aspirin-like and help to reduce general pain. Make a tea of cramp bark using two teaspoons of the dried bark or

herb in one quart of boiling water, and simmer for fifteen minutes. Drink up to three cups a day. If you prefer powdered capsules, take $1/2$ gram to 1 gram three times a day. **Caution:** Do not take cramp bark if you are on blood-thinning drugs because it also works as a blood thinner.

Other herbs that ease menstrual cramps include vitex, ginger, and garden sage. Make a tea or down a capsule for convenience.

Premenstrual Syndrome

For years I refused to admit, even to myself, that my minor recurring irritability and outbursts were in any way related to my menstrual cycle. Eventually I discovered, first through research and then through experience, that my premenstrual syndrome (PMS) symptoms were brought on or exacerbated by the foods I chose. For me, the amounts of sugar and coffee I was consuming were more reflective of my symptoms than was the time of month; I was being controlled by my eating habits, not my hormones. PMS has generated widespread interest among medical researchers and practitioners around the world. Clinics have cropped up, books are increasingly available, and new products are being formulated. Doctors are experimenting with a variety of theories about the causes of PMS, from the hormonal, biochemical, and neuroendocrinologic to the psychological and psychosocial. Possible causes being explored include an excessive amount of estrogen, a deficiency of progesterone, an imbalance of prolactin, excessive amounts of prostaglandins, hormone allergies, decreased endorphins, hypoglycemia, various vitamin and mineral deficiencies, abnormal metabolism of essential fatty acids, stress, and psychological factors. There is not enough scientific data to establish one theory above all others. What clouds the issue is that no single treatment works for all women: Some women respond to progesterone therapy, some to dietary changes, and others to placebos.

This suggests that PMS is a condition involving a host of interacting factors. The treatment you require will depend on your circumstances. (The treatment you get will probably also depend on your doctor's prejudices.) Before undergoing hormonal therapy, you may want to try the safest and least invasive methods: diet, nutritional supplements, and exercise. Diet and exercise alone will not work for every woman, but they may be the only remedy for some and will at least help to minimize symptoms in most.

The connection between nutrient deficiencies and hormonal imbalances works something like this: Without adequate nourishment our endocrine glands cannot manufacture hormones in normal quantities. Nutritional deficiencies also lower the threshold for stress, increasing the hormonal imbalance.

HOW CAN YOU BE SURE YOU HAVE PMS?

Even this point arouses controversy. The classic definition says that if you have one or more regular, recurring physical and psychological symptoms one or two weeks prior to menstruation that improve after the onset, you are a likely candidate. Katharina Dalton, a physician who has written extensively on the subject, emphasizes, "It is the absence of symptoms and the change of mood after menstruation back to being a happy, energetic, vivacious woman once more, which clinches the diagnosis."[4]

There are currently no definitive medical, hormonal, or psychological tests available for PMS. The diagnosis remains a subjective one, most likely made by the woman herself. Symptoms include irritability, mood swings, depression, hostility, confusion, coordination difficulties, fatigue, food binges, headaches, fainting, bloating, weight gain, constipation, acne, joint pain, and breast tenderness, to name a few. In fact, more than 150 symptoms have been associated with premenstrual syndrome.

Most experts agree that the best method for determining whether or not you have PMS is to keep a daily record of your symptoms for three months. You may use a calendar you already have, design your own, or use one of the professional charts put out by various authors and groups. If you are using a home calendar, mark down the date your symptoms occur and when you menstruate. I suggest you also chart your food intake; this information will be a significant help in establishing necessary dietary changes.

DIET

Certain foods provoke and aggravate premenstrual symptoms. The following red-light foods should be eliminated a week or two before menstruation and minimized the rest of the month:

- Sugar, alcohol, caffeine (in coffee and tea), and cigarettes: Women who suffer from PMS are often hypoglycemic, so maintaining a consistent blood-sugar level is important.

- Red meats: These are high in fat (which decreases the liver's efficiency in metabolizing hormones) and in phosphates (which use the body's calcium).

- Salt and high-sodium foods: These increase water retention and cause breast tenderness.

- Dairy products: These interfere with magnesium absorption and are high in sodium and fat.

157

⊙ Cold foods and drinks: These can contribute to cramping by reducing abdominal circulation.

In addition to reducing your intake of foods that aggravate PMS, increase your consumption of foods that encourage relief of symptoms. Beneficial foods include complex carbohydrates, such as whole grains, vegetables, beans, rice, and fruits. Since fluid retention is widespread among women with menstrual problems, drinking at least two quarts of water each day will help. Natural diuretics such as watermelon, strawberries, artichokes, asparagus, watercress, and parsley will also help.

ESSENTIAL FATTY ACIDS

Essential fatty acids are important for women during all stages of life and can specifically reduce cramps and other monthly symptoms. Evening primrose oil (EPO), which is richly supplied with an essential fatty acid, has been tested in both the United States and England. British studies have found that EPO relieved PMS in two-thirds of women who were not helped by any other means; another 20 percent were greatly improved.[5] EPO has also been found useful in treating women with heavy and prolonged menstrual bleeding and women suffering from fibrocystic breast disease.

EPO is by far the richest source of gamma-linolenic acid (GLA), one of the building blocks from which the body creates a prostaglandin called PGE1. A deficiency of PGE1 allows the hormone prolactin to become excessive in the body. Prolactin is another hormone found in greater than normal amounts in the PMS woman.

To be effective, EPO must be taken daily. Take six to eight capsules, along with 50–200 mg of vitamin B-6 (pyridoxine), divided into two or three doses during the day. Vitamin E (100–600 IU) plus the other nutrients involved in the biochemical conversion process are generally helpful and can be found in a multivitamin and mineral tablet. Start slowly, with smaller doses, and increase as necessary. Remember, too, how slowly the bodily environment changes. Two to three months is not an unreasonable length of time to wait before noticing results.

EPO is expensive, so I was pleased to read that Richard Kunin has found that the EFAs in fish oils are just as effective in treating PMS. As little as 10 grams or two teaspoons of salmon oil a day can be effective.[6] Other good sources of the necessary EFAs include flaxseed oil, wheat germ oil, borage oil, and omega-3 fish oils. Diabetics should not take supplemental fish oils but can eat more cold-water fish, such as salmon, tuna, trout, herring, and sardines.

Daily Nutritional Supplements and Their Potential Effects on PMS

Nutrient	Effect
B complex (10–30 mg)	Regulates estrogen activity
Vitamin B-6 (50–300 mg)	Reduces water retention; calms nervous tension; preserves higher levels of magnesium
Magnesium (500–1,000 mg)	Normalizes glucose metabolization; produces calming effect
Calcium (1,000–2,000 mg)	Reduces pelvic pain, insomnia, bloating, nervousness
Vitamin E (200–600 IU)	Reduces breast pain and tenderness; normalizes production of sex hormones; acts as a mild prostaglandin inhibitor
Vitamin C (500–1,000 mg)	Reduces allergic response; relieves pain
Lecithin (1 teaspoon)	Helps prevent excessive fatty deposits in liver; deactivates estrogen
Zinc (30–50 mg)	Improves glucose tolerance; helps regulate prostaglandins

OTHER SUPPLEMENTS

Many supplements designed specifically for PMS can be found in retail and health-food stores. If you are taking a multiple vitamin, check to see that you are getting at least the minimum therapeutic doses of the nutrients listed in the chart above.

Dong quai is an all-purpose herb for PMS, painful periods, cramps, hot flashes, and other symptoms related to hormonal fluctuations. Rich in vitamins and minerals, it is also taken to treat insomnia, anemia, and high blood pressure. Take one to three capsules a day, or drink one to two teaspoons in eight ounces of hot water.

The herb vitex agnus castus, or chaste tree, commonly found under the product name vitex, is effective in treating many common PMS symptoms. In a double-blind study from Germany, researchers observed 178 PMS sufferers, 86 of whom were given a 20 mg tablet daily of chaste-tree berry while the others received an inert pill. After three cycles, over half the women taking vitex reported major improvement in their symptoms: less irritability, anger, mood swings, headache, and breast fullness.[7] Vitex has been used widely in Europe with effective results and minimal side effects. It is available as a tablet, capsule, or tincture. Remember that herbs act more slowly than drugs; it may take two or three months of consistent usage before noticing results.

⮞ Fibrocystic Breast Disease ⮜

Fibrocystic breast disease (FBD), also called *cystic mastitis,* is the most common non-cancerous breast condition among women. It is not a disease per se, but a growth of fibrous tissues that most frequently appears when a woman is in her late thirties or forties and disappears with menopause. Fibrocystic breasts are uncomfortable, but the condition is not serious. Some 20 percent of the female population may, at some time in their lives, develop breast tenderness, swelling, discomfort, or noticeable lumps.

Breast cysts are influenced by the menstrual cycle and hormonal fluctuations, enlarging and becoming more painful just prior to the onset of the period. An imbalance in the estrogen/progesterone ratio seems to be responsible for both the cysts and the enlargement, but whether the important factor is the overproduction of estrogen or the underproduction of progesterone is not yet agreed upon by scientists.

Certain situations that result in a shifting hormonal balance may bring on FBD; it has been found in teenagers who have not achieved regular menstrual periods, women who have children late in life, women who have gained weight, women on estrogen treatment, and women under stress. Pregnancy and breast-feeding tend to improve the condition, as does menopause—unless, of course, estrogen hormone is taken.

Breast lumps are common and are usually a problem only because they are difficult to distinguish from cancerous lumps. A lump that fluctuates with your period usually indicates a harmless cyst. If you are past menopause, check the lump at the same time each month. (If you have FBD, you will continue to have cystic changes in your breasts even though your periods have stopped.) If the lump stays the same or increases in size, have a gynecologist examine your breast.

There is no sure way to reduce breast lumps, but dietary intervention has been found to help. John Minton, professor of clinical oncology at the Ohio State University College of Medicine, found a connection between chemicals called *methylxanthines* and FBD. When a group of women with FBD abstained from coffee, tea, chocolate, soft drinks, and various drugs, all of which contain methylxanthines, 65 percent became free of breast lumps in one to six months.[8] This should be good news for drinkers of coffee, black tea, or caffeinated sodas who are suffering from breast tenderness: You can reduce your intake of xanthine compounds by reducing—or giving up entirely—your consumption of these liquids.

CAFFEINE

Since Minton's study, other researchers and clinicians have had similar success. Penny Budoff conducted a test on herself and some of her patients who had premenstrual breast tenderness. Abstaining from coffee, they all felt they had better months—less pain, less irritability, and milder cramps.[9]

VITAMIN E

Supplemental vitamin E, at levels of 400–800 IU per day, has been found effective in the treatment of breast tenderness. In a study in which vitamin E was combined with reduced consumption of the xanthine compounds, improvement was found in 85 percent of subjects.[10]

B-COMPLEX VITAMINS

The B-complex vitamins regulate estrogen activity by promoting healthy liver function. Early studies showed that when women supplemented their diets with the B vitamins, they found relief from symptoms related to excess estrogen, including heavy menstrual flow, PMS, and fibrocystic breasts.[11] B vitamins can easily be taken as part of a multivitamin and mineral tablet.

Other dietary remedies for FBD that help some women include cutting down on fat, salt, and cigarettes.

≥ Insomnia ≤

Sleep patterns are commonly interrupted during the transition years. Hot flashes and night sweats may wake us from a sound rest; frequent trips to the bathroom disturb us and keep us from going back to sleep. Many women report that bad dreams and unsettled feelings prevent them from getting adequate rest even when they do sleep. One night, maybe even a few nights, like this may not be noticeable, but repeated episodes leave us drained and unable to think and act clearly, and often lead to depression and mood swings.

Evaluating one's lifestyle, activities, and food intake is the first step in combating sleeplessness. The kinds, amounts, and timing of foods and drinks you consume may prevent you from falling asleep or wake you during the night. Eating a large, heavy, fatty meal after 9:00 P.M. is a sure ticket to catching the late-night movie. It is hardly news that the caffeine in coffee, chocolate, sodas, and tea can keep one alert until dawn, but you may be unaware that alcohol fails to stimulate restful sleep. Although you may fall asleep quickly after several glasses of wine, its diuretic action will awaken you several times during the night.

BLOOD-SUGAR LEVELS

Erratic blood-sugar levels interrupt sleep. The brain is highly dependent on glucose (sugar) as an energy source, so a drop in blood sugar may trigger a wake-up call. Some people can handle moderate amounts of sugar with relative ease; others cannot. With age and overworked adrenal glands, our ability to tolerate extremes may

be impaired. Many factors other than overindulgence in sugar can contribute to blood-sugar fluctuations, and remember, the higher the high, the lower the low.

Maintaining an even blood-sugar level throughout the day and night is necessary if you want a good night's sleep. The diet recommended is no different from what is healthful for most situations: high in complex carbohydrates, high in fiber-rich foods, low in fat, and moderate in protein. As many as 50 percent of individuals must reduce starches in favor of more protein, but most individuals only need to adjust amounts and timing of meals. It is important to eat small meals or snacks often (about every four hours) and to avoid overindulging in concentrated sugars (even fruit juices for the highly sensitive), caffeine, alcohol, and refined, processed foods. Exercise will help stabilize hormonal levels, and a good multivitamin and mineral supplement will ensure that nutritional errors will not aggravate the condition. A chromium supplement of 200 mcg improves glucose tolerance, helping to regulate blood-sugar levels.[12] (For more discussion of the effects of blood-sugar levels on health and well-being, see Chapter 4.)

SEROTONIN

Serotonin, a brain neurotransmitter, regulates mood, pain, eating habits, and sleep. The synthesis of serotonin within the brain is dependent on the availability of tryptophan (an amino acid), the ingestion of a starchy food, and the cofactors vitamin B-6 and magnesium. Short-term insomnia might be helped by eating a nighttime snack of foods rich in tryptophan, such as milk, yogurt, tuna, turkey, almonds, bananas, or peanut butter. Accompany this snack with a piece of bread or a few crackers, and crawl under the covers.

Vitamin B-6 levels are often under par in women, especially those who are on the Pill or who take ERT. All the B vitamins are involved in maintaining a healthy nervous system, so when even one is lacking, symptoms of anxiety, nervous tension, and insomnia result. Although the recommended dietary allowance (RDA) of vitamin B-6 for women is 1.3 to 1.5 mg per day (higher for those pregnant or lactating), many health professionals recommend doses between 50 mg and 200 mg. Do not exceed 300 mg a day of vitamin B-6, as studies have found that in some people higher levels may result in damage to nerve tissues. Good sources of B-6 include bananas, avocado, hamburger, chicken, enriched cereals, cheese, fish, potatoes, and spinach. (For the precise amount of this nutrient contained in certain foods, consult Appendix C.)

Another B vitamin, B-3 (niacin), may be useful for women who fall asleep but later wake up. Like the other B vitamins, niacin functions in more than fifty body processes, but it also has a specialized effect for calming the nerves. Niacin can be

produced in the body from the amino acid tryptophan. Again, the interrelationship of the vitamins, amino acids, and brain chemicals points out the importance of optimum diet to good health. Studies indicate that one type of niacin, niacinamide, has an action similar to that of a low-dose tranquilizer; supplemental doses of between 50 and 100 mg may help you to get to sleep and stay asleep.

The other form of niacin, nicotinic acid, is regarded as one of the substances of choice for lowering blood-cholesterol levels. Those who take therapeutic doses over 100 mg experience a burning sensation in the face and neck and other side effects including nausea, headaches, cramps, and altered heart rate. Larger doses of nicotinic acid (over 2,000 mg) may result in liver toxicity. At these levels, it must be prescribed and monitored by a physician. Good sources of this vitamin include chicken, salmon, beef, peanut butter, and peas. (For the precise amount of B vitamins contained in certain foods, consult Appendix C.)

Causes of Blood-Sugar Fluctuations	
Increases Blood Sugar	**Decreases Blood Sugar**
Overeating	Skipping meals
Concentrated sugars	Endurance exercise
Alcohol	Alcohol
Stress	Stress
Infection, surgery	Large doses of aspirin
Estrogen	Anabolic steroids
Cortisone	Barbiturates
Lithium	Beta-blockers
Thiazide	Blood-thinning drugs
Nicotine	
Caffeine	

The full complex of B vitamins is vital for maximum benefit to the nervous system. Because they are water soluble, they readily pass through the system and constantly need replenishment. Take the full complex in a multivitamin tablet; for specific purposes, take the individual B vitamin. Many people find that taking B vitamins too close to bedtime is too energizing, so try to work them in at breakfast or lunch.

Magnesium, the second cofactor needed for the transformation of tryptophan to serotonin, also functions in muscle relaxation, contraction of nerve transmission, and conversion of food to usable energy. Menopausal women need 400 to 750 mg a day to ensure these jobs get done. Magnesium is best taken together with calcium in a two-to-one ratio of calcium to magnesium; the pair of minerals is available in supplements in the correct ratio. Even if you're supplementing, it's still a good idea to add more magnesium-rich foods to your diet. Good sources of magnesium include peanuts, split peas, tofu, cashews, fortified breakfast cereal, spinach, beef, and milk. (For the precise amount of this nutrient contained in certain foods, consult Appendix C.)

MEDICATIONS

Medications frequently contribute to sleeping problems. Check the labels on your prescriptions and over-the-counter drugs. A few common drugs that interfere with restful nights are appetite suppressants, decongestants, high-blood-pressure medications, and pain relievers and cold remedies that contain caffeine. Strangely, even drugs that help you sleep and calm you can eventually reach a point in your body where they not only are ineffective but trigger the opposite reaction.

HERBS

Many plants cause sedative actions in the body. Consult an herbalist for ones that might work best for you. They might include the following:

Passionflower. Hailed as one of nature's best tranquilizers, passionflower relieves anxiety, muscle tension, restlessness, and headaches. Since tryptophan was taken off the market because of one contaminated batch, passionflower has become its replacement for promoting sleep. You can steep the dried herb for tea, or mix fifteen to fifty drops of extract in liquid as needed. Do not take before driving or operating heavy machinery.

Valerian. Tagged as the valium of the nineteenth century, valerian is recognized worldwide for its relaxing effect on the body. Recent studies have substantiated valerian's ability to improve quality sleep and relieve insomnia.[13] Unlike many prescription drugs, valerian is not addictive and has no side effects, except for a bad taste. Forget the tea—take it in capsule form, 2 grams two hours before bedtime and another 2 grams at bedtime. Don't take valerian continuously for more than two weeks.

EXERCISE

Regular physical exercise improves sleeping habits and general well-being. It is best to avoid working out too close to bedtime, as it may be a long time before you feel relaxed enough to even get into bed. Relaxation techniques and a hot bath before bedtime may also be soothing.

Joint Pain and Arthritis

Aching hands, creaking knees, sore ankles, and a tired back are common complaints of menopausal women. Whether caused by age or hormones, body aches and pains seem to show up in midlife women who have not experienced them before, or to intensify in women who have. Arthritis is a condition that develops with advancing age. According to a national survey, arthritis affects approximately

3 percent of women under the age of twenty-five and more than half of those over age sixty-five.[14]

Inflammation of the joints has many causes, including injury and complications from another disease. It may occur sometimes as a side effect of medications, such as contraceptives, anticonvulsants, and major tranquilizers. A strong relationship apparently exists between arthritis and diet: Eating certain foods and eliminating others often results in relief from pain.

The two most common types of arthritis are rheumatoid arthritis (RA) and osteoarthritis (OA). RA is an autoimmune disease, in which the body attacks its own tissues. It strikes at any age and is characterized by inflammation, not only in the joints but also in the connective tissue throughout the body. The body replaces the damaged tissue with scar tissue, creating stiffness, swelling, fatigue, fever, weight loss, anemia, and often crippling pain. The onset of RA may be associated with physical or emotional stress; however, poor nutrition or bacterial infection may be factors as well.

OA is the most common form of arthritis and appears in later years. It is a degenerative disease related to the wear and tear of aging and involves deterioration of the cartilage at the ends of the bones. The joints most likely to be affected are those of the feet, toes, and fingers, and those of the weight-bearing bones, such as the knees, hips, ankles, and backbone. A sudden injury, such as a sprained ankle or finger, or a repetitive motion over time can lead to osteoarthritis, causing long-term damage. The onset of OA can be subtle, with morning joint stiffness often the first indication. As the disease progresses, there is pain when the joint is active that is worsened by prolonged motion and relieved by rest. Unlike the case with RA, disablement is usually minor and swelling minimal.

There is a relationship between lowered estrogen levels and the loss of cartilage. Research published in the *Annals of the Rheumatic Diseases* in 1997 showed that menopausal women taking ERT were three times less likely to suffer from osteoarthritis in their knees than women not taking hormones.[15] I am not advocating estrogen for the prevention or treatment of OA, but this is one more piece of information you may want to factor into your thought process as you decide whether or not to take hormones. Given that osteoarthritis and rheumatoid arthritis cannot be cured but can be controlled, prevention is vitally important.

MIND/BODY DISCIPLINES

It is well-known that stress can disrupt immune function and exacerbate symptoms of RA. Andrew Weil, M.D., internationally recognized expert on integrative medicine, has observed that RA often coincides with a patient's emotional highs and lows. He advises RA sufferers to incorporate some method of relaxation—such as breath work, meditation, or yoga—into their daily routine.[16] Other mind/body approaches, such as visualization, guided imagery, and hypnotherapy, may also ease the pain and frequency of RA flare-ups. In his February 2001 newsletter, Dr. Weil suggests a tape to help you learn about these techniques: Belleruth Naparstek's guided imagery tape for people with RA that is a part of her "Health Journeys" series (to order, call toll free 800-800-8661). You can also find practitioners to teach you these techniques or books and audiotapes for learning them on your own.

Releasing your frustrations on the written page produces both psychological and physical health benefits. Expressive writing is a technique that has been used successfully in several controlled studies to improve health and well-being in a variety of ways. In one randomized control trial, a volunteer sample of patients with asthma and rheumatoid arthritis who wrote about a stressful life experience demonstrated clinically relevant changes in health status after four months, compared with those in the control group.[17] Authors of the study concluded that these gains were beyond those attributable to the standard medical care that all participants were receiving. If you haven't already, you may want to start a daily or weekly journal to record your anxious thoughts, or sign up for a workshop that specifically addresses healing through writing.

Tai chi is a Chinese movement technique that some doctors now recommend for people with osteoarthritis as a way to reduce joint swelling and improve range of motion, flexibility, strength, and sense of balance. Tai chi has a long history stemming from the martial arts, but contemporary practices involve a series of fluid movements and postures in which the mind and body work interdependently. Tai chi is currently a subject of traditional medical research; meanwhile, it can complement medical treatment of musculoskeletal diseases and chronic pain.

A number of alternative healing systems are available if you are open to trying something new. In Judith Horstman's book, *The Arthritis Foundation's Guide to Alternative Therapies*, she discusses Chinese medicine, acupuncture, homeopathy, chiropractic manipulation, massage, and many other complementary treatments that may help with arthritis. She also provides postal addresses, phone numbers, website addresses, and advice on how to choose the right health professional. The book is a fantastic resource to help you on the road to recovery.

DIETARY RECOMMENDATIONS

Inadequate dietary intake of certain vitamins and minerals is associated with RA, although it is unclear whether poor nutrition is a cause or an effect of the disease. Some people, though, are clearly helped by a diet that minimizes saturated fat, sugar, meat, dairy, and alcohol and emphasizes complex carbohydrates from vegetables, beans, and whole grains. Fresh, unprocessed, raw fruits and vegetables are of paramount importance because they are rich sources of pain-relieving nutrients, including vitamin C, the carotenes, and bioflavonoids. Even if complete relief from pain is not realized, this diet will make you feel better in other ways and will improve the quality of your health.

In addition, the following dietary suggestions can help with joint pain:

Lose excess weight. Probably the best dietary advice for anyone with arthritis is to maintain a normal body weight for your age. Carrying unwanted pounds is one of the top predictors of osteoarthritis in the knees and other joints. Excess weight adds to stress on the weight-bearing joints, leading to increased pain. This recommendation alone can greatly ease discomfort and stiffness. Older people tend to gain weight because they are too sore to work out, but if you stop exercising, your joints can get stiffer and more painful. You may want to try swimming or water aerobics to ease the weight on your joints. Strength training with weights, yoga, tai chi, and qigong may be other types of exercise to consider.

Include sulfur-rich foods. A sulfur-bearing amino acid found in garlic, onion, eggs, beans, Brussels sprouts, and cabbage seems to alleviate pain and swelling of joints. Interestingly, a large study in the mid-1930s found the sulfur content of the fingernails of arthritis sufferers to be lower than that of nonsufferers.[18] This research has never been pursued, though others testify to its validity.

Recognize that some fats are good. We usually associate fat with ill health; however, some fats actually prevent and control the inflammation (and, subsequently, the pain) of arthritis. Prostaglandins are important contributors to the inflammatory process, and specific fatty acids can modulate their production. Diets rich in omega-3 fatty acids (fish oils), taken in supplemental form, have been shown to reduce inflammation in both OA and RA. When ten capsules of the fatty acid EPA (eicosapentaenoic acid) were given to patients with RA, noticeable improvement was found in joint tenderness and morning stiffness after twelve weeks, while the control group worsened.[19]

The recommended dosage of EPA is 2,000 to 3,000 mg daily. Diabetics should not take supplemental fish oils but can eat more cold-water fish such as salmon, tuna, trout, herring, and sardines. Another way to maintain essential fats is to incorporate more plant sources, such as flaxseed, pumpkin seeds, walnuts, and green leafy vegetables, into your diet. Fortified flax is particularly good; mix one tablespoon with water or juice, or add it to salads, yogurt, and cereals.

Some evidence has shown that gammalinolenic acid (GLA), an essential fat from the omega-6 family and found in evening primrose oil, may also be useful in some types of arthritis. It is thought that a lack of GLA may lead to a dysfunctional level of prostaglandins. The recommended dosage is 1 to 2 grams per day of GLA or evening primrose oil. These oils are found naturally in raw seeds and nuts, such as flaxseed, pumpkin seeds, sesame seeds, sunflower seeds, and walnuts.

Say "no" to the nightshade family. Sometimes it's not what you *do* eat but rather what you *don't* eat that can improve your health. Elimination of an entire food group is a simple dietary change that has worked for some arthritis sufferers. Some research suggests that susceptible people might develop arthritis, as well as a variety of other complaints, from long-term, low-level consumption of the alkaloid-containing nightshade plants: tomatoes, potatoes, eggplant, peppers, and tobacco.[20] Presumably, alkaloids inhibit normal collagen repair in the joints or promote the inflammatory degeneration of the joints. It may be worth experimenting with eliminating these foods if you suffer from OA or RA.

FOOD ALLERGIES AND ARTHRITIS

It has long been suspected that RA may result from or be exacerbated by a food allergy or sensitivity. Therefore, completely eliminating or minimizing certain common foods may also reduce symptoms. Food allergies have been tested and found to aggravate many of the aches and pains associated with arthritis. In a well-controlled experiment, a hypoallergenic diet produced marked improvements in 75 percent of the subjects.[21]

An allergy is an inappropriate response by the body's immune system to a substance that is not normally harmful. The manifestations of such an overreaction are varied: diarrhea, gastric upset, bloating, fatigue, headache, hives, acne, itching, ear infections, rapid heartbeat, shortness of breath, muscle pain or weakness, hypoglycemia, anxiety, mental confusion, inability to concentrate, and vision changes. What strikes me as I read over this list is the number of symptoms that are also thought to be menopausal. Wouldn't it be ironic if all we had were allergies, which flared up at this particular time?

Any food is a potential allergen, but the most common are wheat, milk, corn, soy, yeast, chocolate, tea, coffee, beef, citrus fruits, shellfish, eggs, and potatoes. To determine if you are sensitive to any of these, first consider how often you eat the food in question. It is more than coincidental that the foods you crave may be the ones to which you are also sensitive. The body's reaction to food allergens is similar to addiction.

It is possible to test for allergies without expensive treatments. The most effective method is to fast without food or juices for three to five days and then reintroduce one food at a time into your diet. Symptoms are usually obvious, leaving little doubt as to the offending food or foods. If going without food is not an option, try plan B. Eliminate a suspected food, such as dairy or wheat products, for two weeks or more, then reintroduce it into your diet and watch for symptoms. It is best to test one food at a time, as you may be sensitive to more than one.

There is another way of detecting a possible food intolerance. First, take your pulse several different times for one full minute to determine your resting pulse rate. Then, eat the potential offender, wait twenty minutes, and take your pulse again. If your pulse rate increases by more than ten beats per minute, you have uncovered a possible allergen. Drop the food from your diet, and test again in a month to confirm. During that time, you may notice withdrawal symptoms followed by a greater sense of health.

SPECIFIC NUTRIENTS

Dietary deficiencies are often found in people who suffer from arthritis. Blood levels of the following nutrients are often low in individuals with joint pain, and their symptoms improve when supplemented: vitamins C, E, B-3 (niacin), B-5 (pantothenic acid), and B-6, and the minerals calcium, magnesium, selenium, and zinc. Other nutrients likely play supporting roles as well. I will mention some that have been studied.

Vitamin C and vitamin E. Deficiency of vitamin C results in altered collagen synthesis and compromised connective-tissue repair. Several studies have reported that vitamin C has a positive effect on cartilage; moreover, cartilage erosion and overall changes in and around the arthritic joints were found to occur much less in animals kept on high doses of vitamin C.[22] This same study indicated that vitamin E appears to possess a synergistic action with vitamin C; thus, the researchers concluded that judicious use of these vitamins, either alone or in combination with other therapies, may be of great benefit to people suffering from OA. Additionally, a clinical trial of vitamin E (600 IU) alone in patients with OA demonstrated that vitamin E was significantly more effective than a placebo in relieving pain.[23]

Vitamin B-5 (pantothenic acid). In an older study, megadoses (2 grams daily) of vitamin B-5 relieved symptoms of RA.[24] Stopping treatment caused symptoms to return. Improvements in OA symptoms have been reported using smaller doses (12.5 mg daily) of vitamin B-5, and although it often took one to two weeks before progress was noted, it did work.[25] Recommended dosages of vitamin B-5

Basic Daily Supplements for Arthritis

Multivitamin and mineral complex (without iron).

Check the B-complex vitamins (B-1, B-2, B-6) for a range of 25–100 mg each, making sure to include between 100–500 mcg of B-12.

Add vitamins and minerals to reach the following totals:

Calcium	1,500 mg
Magnesium	750 mg
Vitamin C plus bioflavonoids	1,000–2,000 mg, 1–3 times daily
Pantothenic acid	50–2,000 mg
Vitamin E	600 IU
Zinc	15–50 mg
Selenium	200 mcg

Additional Daily Supplements for Arthritis

Fish oil or EPA capsules	2–3 capsules
Evening primrose oil	6–8 capsules
Glucosamine sulfate	1,000–1,500 mg
Chondroitin sulfate	800–1,200 mg
SAMe	400–800 mg
MSM	500–1,500 mg

Herbs for Arthritis

Feverfew, yucca extract, alfalfa, kelp, black cohosh, celery seed, parsley tea, valerian root, devil's claw tea.

Also Helpful for Arthritis

Exercise to reduce pain and retard joint deterioration (except when in pain).

Drink 1–2 quarts of water daily to hydrate joints.

Rest when in pain.

Take hot tubs and baths for pain relief.

Expose yourself to sunlight for 20 minutes per day to help pain and stiffness.

range from 15 mg to 2,000 mg per day. Start with the lowest dose only, and increase if necessary. Good sources of vitamin B-5 include beef liver, egg, avocado, milk, chicken, peanut butter, bananas, and potatoes. (For the precise amount of this nutrient contained in certain foods, consult Appendix C. Because the amounts found naturally in foods are so low, you may need to supplement.)

Niacin (vitamin B-3). Niacin has been tested with hundreds of patients and found valuable in treating OA and RA. Since the doses used were in the upper range (4 g) and may cause drug-like reactions, it is advisable to take this amount only under medical supervision. Side effects include glucose intolerance and liver damage in sensitive people. Daily doses of up to 1,000 mg of niacin appear to be safe and can be taken in a multivitamin supplement or B-complex tablet. A characteristic flushing of the skin will occur with this dosage of niacin; however, the niacinamide form does not produce this sensation.

Zinc. Zinc is a possible contributor to the nutritional treatment of arthritis. Sufferers usually have lower than normal zinc levels in their blood and, when supplemented, show noticeable improvements in morning stiffness, joint swelling, and the patients' own impression of their condition.[26] Zinc, along with vitamins A, B-6, and E and the mineral copper, are required for the synthesis of normal collagen and the maintenance of cartilage structure. A deficiency of any one would allow for accelerated joint degeneration. Recommended dosage of zinc is 15 to 50 mg daily. Good sources of zinc include oysters, turkey, lima beans, yogurt, and wheat germ. (For the precise amount of this nutrient contained in certain foods, consult Appendix C.)

Selenium. Selenium is a trace mineral with antioxidant properties. Together with vitamin E, it exerts an anti-inflammatory effect on the body and has the potential of reducing the natural decline of immune function that comes with aging. Sources include whole-grain cereals, seafood, chicken, egg yolk, red meat, and garlic.

NATURAL TREATMENTS

Increasing numbers of people are turning from drugs with harmful side effects to natural treatments. Conventional doctors are beginning to take the natural products seriously, because the public is choosing them regardless of the bias against them from traditional medicine. Before you decide to take any remedy, regardless of the "natural" label, read all you can about it, and make sure the claims have some scientific basis or the person recommending it is credible.

The following four supplements have received much attention, both anecdotally and scientifically, for the treatment of arthritis. They are worth looking into. A special note to those of you who have never tried natural remedies: They are not fast-acting, like drugs are, so be patient as they work to heal your body.

Glucosamine sulfate and chondroitin sulfate. One of the best natural treatments for OA may be glucosamine sulfate, found in high concentration in our joint tissues. It stimulates the manufacture of cartilage components necessary for joint repair and exerts a protective effect against joint destruction. Glucosamine sulfate can be derived from the muscle tissue of lobsters, crabs, and mussels.

Numerous double-blind studies have shown that glucosamine sulfate is more effective and better tolerated than the common arthritis pain relievers, including aspirin and the nonsteroidal anti-inflammatory drugs (NSAIDs) such as Nalfon, Motrin, Advil, Nuprin, Indocin, Naprosyn, Feldene, and Clinoril.[27] These drugs may have significant side effects, including damage to the intestinal tract, allergic reactions, easy bleeding and bruising, ringing in the ears, fluid retention, and, in extreme cases, kidney and liver damage. Although NSAIDs are fairly effective in suppressing pain and inflammation, when taken for long periods of time, they

actually worsen the condition by inhibiting cartilage formation and accelerating cartilage destruction (effects not frequently disclosed).[28] NSAIDs offer temporary relief, but glucosamine sulfate addresses the cause of OA—without contraindications or possible and worrisome drug interactions.

In his book, *Maximizing the Arthritis Cure*, preventive-medicine advocate Dr. Jason Theodosakis predicted that glucosamine sulfate and chondroitin sulfate would cause a revolution in the treatment of arthritis. Even though many other countries regularly used these products, U.S. physicians were slow to accept the research and experience of the world's scientists. Now, major newspapers and TV networks report on the benefits of these supplements, and even the prestigious Osteoarthritis Research Society, in its recent consensus statement, has acknowledged that these long-ignored agents may be beneficial in the treatment of arthritis.[29]

Chondroitin sulfate works well with glucosamine sulfate. Made from bovine or shark cartilage, it helps to lubricate the joints and provides elasticity to the tendons and ligaments. For the most part, both products are safe, the most common reaction being gas and softened stool. Neither children nor pregnant women should take these supplements, since there have been no studies yet to determine safety. Diabetics should monitor their blood-sugar levels when taking glucosamine sulfate because it is an amino sugar and could affect blood levels. As a final caveat, do not take chondroitin sulfate with a blood-thinning medication, daily aspirin, or ginkgo biloba, because the combination may cause excessive bleeding.

You can find these substances at health-food stores. The dosages for both are based on body weight. If you weigh up to 120 pounds, take 1,000 mg of glucosamine sulfate and 800 mg of chondroitin sulfate. If you weigh over 120 pounds, take 1,500 mg of glucosamine sulfate and 1,200 mg of chondroitin sulfate. If they upset your stomach, as some supplements do in sensitive people, take them with meals.

SAM-e. S-adenosylmethionine is a popular alternative to antidepressants and is more recently being heralded as a treatment for arthritis sufferers. Studies from both Europe and the United States are finding that it relieves joint pain just as well as nonsteroidal anti-inflammatories. SAM-e is an amino acid that occurs naturally in our bodies. Like many other substances we produce, it decreases with age. While scientists are still determining the exact method by which it works, we do know it is important to the building and rebuilding of cartilage and cell membranes. When searching for SAM-e, look for a coated tablet packaged in a lightproof container and labeled "butanedisulfonate." SAM-e is extremely unstable when exposed to heat, light, or moisture, so you want to make sure it is protected. A therapeutic dose is 200–400 mg twice per day with meals. To increase its effectiveness, take it with vitamin B-12 (50–100 mcg) and folic acid (400 mcg).

MSM. Methylsulfonymethane is derived from foods and can be used as an antacid, analgesic, and anti-inflammatory. It increases blood flow and brings nutrients, especially sulfur, to injured cartilage tissue. Sulfur is plentiful in fresh fruits and vegetables, whole grains, fish, and milk but is quickly destroyed with processing. Skeptics quickly point out that there are no valid human studies to back up the claims that MSM works, but those who have found relief maintain that it works better than prescription drugs. Most sources recommend starting with a low dose of 500 mg and gradually building up to 1,500 mg. If you don't feel relief in two months, try something else. Higher doses may result in stomach cramps and diarrhea, which should signal that other, better-tolerated remedies may exist for you.

ORAL ENZYME THERAPY

Enzymes work as catalysts in living cells, which means they facilitate every single chemical reaction in the body. Basically protein in composition, enzymes exist in all fruits, vegetables, grains, and animal products and provide a multitude of functions within the human body. One of their roles involves moderating the complex phenomenon called *inflammation*, which is said to be responsible for initial stages of heart disease and rheumatoid arthritis. Enzyme therapy has been shown to equal the anti-inflammatory drugs, such as NSAIDs, in treating arthritis and other conditions. According to Dr. Theodosakis, the enzyme combinations that have undergone the most extensive study and work the best are bromelain and trypsin, though there are many mixed formulations that also prove effective. He recommends starting with a larger dose during the first week or two of therapy and then cutting down to a maintenance dose. Divide the total daily dose into two or three servings and take the supplement thirty to forty minutes before meals. Daily starting and maintenance levels of oral enzyme preparations are as follows[30]:

bromelain: 650 mg/450 mg

trypsin: 350 mg/250 mg

chymotrypsin: 15 mg/10 mg

papain: 900 mg/500 mg

Some people only require enzymes for a few weeks or months, and others continue using them for years.

NOTES

PART II

PREPARING
FOR THE LATER YEARS

CHAPTER 9

HEART DISEASE

Heart disease is by and large a self-inflicted malady. You don't catch it.

— KENNETH COOPER, M.D., MPH

omen tend to think of heart disease as a men's issue, but it is the leading cause of death for women as well. Heart disease affects more women than the five leading causes of cancer deaths in women combined. While 40,000 women die of breast cancer each year, 250,000 die from heart attacks and another 250,000 succumb to other diseases of the heart and blood vessels.[1] Because women are "protected" by estrogen before menopause, the incidence of heart disease in women trails behind that in men by ten to fifteen years. According to the American Heart Association, one in nine women aged forty-five to sixty-four has some form of heart or blood-vessel disease; this ratio soars to one in three by age sixty-five and beyond.

Heart attacks may strike older women as frequently as they do older men, but women's prospects for a lasting return to normalcy are much gloomier. About 25 percent more women than men die within a year of having a heart attack.[2] This may be because female heart-attack victims are generally older, hence are more likely to experience complications from other illnesses, but this is speculation. Also, women do not respond as well as men do to treatments prescribed during or after a heart attack. For example, the death rate for women undergoing coronary-bypass surgery is twice that of men. Women are less likely to survive angioplasty, a treatment used to remove the plaque in arteries that is obstructing the flow of blood to the heart, and are twice as likely to have a second heart attack.

Women and their doctors often do not take women's heart symptoms seriously. Women tend to overlook the classic signs of a heart attack: chest pains or tightness, heartburn, shortness of breath, numbness or tingling in the arms or jaw, and sweating. Physicians hesitate to act on such symptoms in women and postpone referring them for diagnostic testing, which may be one reason why women don't fare as well in surgery, the disease being more advanced by the time they reach surgery.[3]

≋ What Is Heart Disease? ≋

Heart disease is a broad term used to describe many different diseases of the heart and blood vessels. The blood vessels of the heart, also called *coronary arteries*, supply the heart muscles with vital oxygen and nutrients. If the flow of blood is restricted or blocked, severe damage to the heart can occur—the heart attack.

Some thickening and hardening of the arteries, a process called *arteriosclerosis*, is normal. A more insidious and advanced stage, called *atherosclerosis*, occurs when the condition accelerates and the artery linings build up to the point of obstruction. The substance responsible for clogging the arteries—made up of fatty material, cholesterol, cellular waste products, calcium, and fibrin—is collectively referred to as *plaque.*

Atherosclerosis doesn't happen overnight, not even at menopause. It is a gradual process that takes almost a lifetime. Preventing the accumulation of plaque must start in the early years, maybe as early as childhood. Even children have been found to have fat deposits in their arteries that may later form into artery-clogging plaque. Fortunately, for those who are willing to be proactive in caring for their hearts, much information is now available. It is essential, however, to understand that women's heart-care issues differ from men's, a diversity finally being acknowledged in the medical community. In line with my desire to inform women and to provide practical options, I've written a book specifically on this topic, *Her Healthy Heart: A Woman's Guide to Preventing and Reversing Heart Disease Naturally* (see Resources).

≋ Hormones and the Heart ≋

The jury is in, the research definitive. Conventional HRT (hormone replacement therapy) does not reduce the risk of heart attacks and death from coronary events in older women with existing heart disease. I reported this news in 2000, in the fourth edition of this book, based on the landmark Heart and Estrogen/Progestin Replacement Study (HERS). The HERS study found that postmenopausal women with existing coronary heart disease received no benefit from HRT. This study was the first randomized, double-blind, placebo-controlled trial of HRT (the so-called gold standard of scientific research) that seriously questioned the value of HRT in preventing heart attacks in postmenopausal women with existing heart disease. Results were reported in the *Journal of the American Medical Association* in 1998.

A total of 2,763 women with coronary disease, ages forty-four to seventy-nine, were given either Prempro (estrogen plus progestin) or a placebo for four years. In the first year of testing, more coronary heart disease events occurred in the hormone group than in the placebo group. This same group of women also experienced more

gallbladder disease, increased blood clotting in the legs and lungs, and raised levels of triglycerides (a type of unhealthy fat that can harm the heart). The researchers involved in the HERS study suggested a cautionary approach to HRT for the purpose of preventing heart disease.[4]

No one seemed to heed the warnings of the HERS study, certainly not the eminent physicians who frequent the morning TV shows. When I tuned in to specials on women and heart disease, each network recited a similar mantra, the same one I heard from the various doctors I saw around that time: "If you're not on estrogen, your heart will suffer." No one paid attention in 1998, and I'm still wondering why.

Fast-forward to the summer of 2002, when the results were announced from two long-awaited research trials, HERS II and the Women's Health Initiative (WHI). HERS II, the follow-up study to the one mentioned above, measured results after a total of almost seven years, and the repeat performance showed similar results: Women with existing heart disease who were on HRT for an extended period of time were just as likely to have heart attacks and die of heart disease as women not on hormones.[5] Commenting on the trial findings, Dr. Nieca Golderg, chief of the Cardiac Rehabilitation and Prevention Center at Lenox Hill Hospital in New York, said, "While hormone treatment does have positive effects, like raising good cholesterol, reducing bad cholesterol and relaxing the blood vessels, it can also have negative side effects, like causing inflammation of blood vessels and increasing the likelihood of blood clots."[6]

The Women's Health Initiative was the second bombshell to blast HRT, and it happened in the same month. Significantly, whereas the HERS study focused on postmenopausal women with existing heart disease, the WHI studied healthy postmenopausal women. Broader in scope, the WHI focused on defining the risks and benefits of strategies that could potentially reduce the incidence of heart disease, breast and colorectal cancers, and fractures in postmenopausal women. As it turned out, researchers were forced to suddenly discontinue the study, because the overall health risks of using combined estrogen (conjugated equine estrogen) plus progestin (medroxyprogesterone acetate) exceeded the benefits. The results also indicated that this regimen should not be initiated or continued for the primary prevention of coronary heart disease.[7] (For more about the WHI study, see Chapter 2.)

It is clear now that conventional HRT—or, more specifically, Prempo—is not protective for heart disease. It's too bad that no long-term studies have yet been conducted to determine the effects on the heart of bioidentical, or natural, hormones in smaller doses. Until such studies are done, we can educate ourselves about the many known risk factors and lifestyle choices that affect the incidence of coronary heart disease and on which we can take action.

≈ Risk Factors for Heart Disease ≈

Risk factors are traits or habits that make a person more susceptible to disease. Some risk factors for heart-related problems, such as age and genetic inheritance, cannot be altered; however, most are conditions over which we have a great deal of control.

GENETICS

The fact that there is a link between families and incidence of heart disease is undeniable, but the question remains, is it nature or nurture? Just because heart disease runs in families doesn't necessarily mean that increased risk is genetic in origin, according to researchers at the Center for Inherited Diseases at the University of Washington, in Seattle. They found that the wives of their male heart-disease patients also had a greater risk for heart disease, suggesting that the spouses indulged in some of the same unhealthy habits as their sick husbands.[8]

AGE

Women tend to manifest heart problems about ten to fifteen years later in life than men, but as mentioned above, by the age of sixty-five to seventy-four years, the incidence is the same in both sexes. Also, the older a woman is, the more apt she is to develop high blood pressure and high blood-cholesterol levels, and to be diabetic, overweight, and more sedentary—all additional risk factors.

ETHNICITY

The risk of heart disease varies appreciably with race and ethnicity. For example, African-American women tend to have the highest incidence of heart disease, nearly 35 percent higher than Caucasian women.[9] Moreover, several risk factors for heart disease are also apparent in African-American women. For example, they have almost twice the rates of diabetes and obesity. Hypertension is more common in black women of all ages, and they experience it earlier in life, suffer more severely, and die from hypertension-related causes more frequently. Paying close attention to the lifestyle factors that regulate high blood pressure, diabetes, and excess weight is crucial for the young black woman.

Sadly, the plight of the black woman with symptoms of heart disease is even more unfortunate. Emergency-room physicians generally miss signs of a heart attack in women more often than in men, and this is especially true in the case of minority or nonwhite women. A study tracking over ten thousand patients at ten hospitals in the East and Midwest found that emergency-room physicians missed signs of a heart attack more often in blacks and young or middle-aged women.[10] In trying to explain why this occurs, the researchers said that the signature symptom of a heart attack, severe chest pain, is not characteristically present in women like it is in men. Women are more likely to exhibit nontraditional warning signs, such as shortness of breath or nausea. They also noticed that black patients are younger overall, which makes a diagnosis of heart attack highly unlikely. Study researchers confessed two more causes they cannot rule out as possibilities for the neglect: sexism and racism.

The lowest rates of CHD (coronary heart disease) in the United States are found in Asian-American women, although when they adopt a more Western lifestyle, their numbers begin to climb. Latina, American-Indian, and Alaska-Native women experience rates of CHD that are slightly lower than those of Caucasian women.

CIGARETTES

Women who smoke are two to six times more likely to suffer a heart attack than nonsmokers, and the risk increases with the number of cigarettes smoked per day.[11] Smoking is more of a risk factor for women than for men; a fifty-five-year-old woman who smokes is in greater danger of suffering a heart attack than a male smoker of the same age.[12] Surprisingly, women in the United States who smoke die almost as often from heart disease as from lung cancer.

Smoking affects the circulatory system in a number of ways. The carbon monoxide in cigarette smoke reduces the blood's oxygen-carrying ability, so less oxygen is available to the heart and other organs. Smoking decreases HDLs and raises LDLs. It damages the lining of the arteries, setting the stage for the development of coronary lesions. Smoking also increases the likelihood of clot formation, irregular heart rhythms, and coronary spasms. And as if that's not enough, women who smoke experience menopause an average of two to three years earlier than nonsmokers, which itself is another risk factor for heart disease.

No matter how many years you have smoked, when you quit, your risk of heart disease declines. Within two years of stopping, your chances of having a heart attack will be cut in half; ten years after stopping, your risk of dying from a heart attack will be almost the same as if you'd never smoked at all.[13]

Most women know this already, but do not take oral contraceptives if you smoke. If you do, your risk of a heart attack escalates forty times.[14]

ALCOHOL

Most people are well aware that moderate alcohol consumption is heart-healthy. The Nurses' Health Study found that women who drank one glass a day of wine, beer, or a shot of hard alcohol had a 40 percent lower risk of heart disease than non-drinkers.[15] The relationship between moderate alcohol consumption and risk of heart disease is largely unknown, but several theories exist. Alcohol appears to help the heart by raising HDLs, decreasing the stickiness of blood platelets, and lowering the levels of fibrinogen, a potent risk factor for heart disease. European researchers have found that red wine contains phenolic compounds, which have strong antioxidant properties that limit the oxidation of LDLs; it is these compounds that may be responsible for the apparent health benefits of red wine.[16] Initial reports on red wine encouraged many of us to switch from chardonnay to merlot, but guess what? Your choices have opened up. The news to date is that it's not red wine alone but all the different types of alcoholic beverages (beer, wine, liquor) that are associated with similar reductions in heart-failure risk, suggesting that pure alcohol rather than one type of beverage provides the benefits.[17]

Drinking alcohol brings risks with the benefits, so moderation is the operative word. Heavy drinking, or more than three glasses a day, can reduce blood flow to the heart and upset its rhythm, causing irregular heart beats, higher blood pressure and blood triglyceride levels, and eventually damage to the heart muscle. Some studies suggest a connection between alcohol intake and breast cancer; until we know more, it may be wise to substitute mineral water for wine part of the time. Keep in mind that alcohol provides no nutrition—only extra calories. Women who are trying to control their weight may want to save alcohol, just as they do dessert, for special occasions.

DIABETES

A diabetic woman with heart disease is more at risk for dying of a heart attack than a diabetic man.[18] Total blood cholesterol is frequently higher in diabetic women, and HDL cholesterol lower. Elevated blood-sugar levels also damage the lining of the arterial walls, increasing their vulnerability to plaque formation. Heart disease is just one of the many complications associated with diabetes. Be as diligent as you can about reducing other risk factors if you are diabetic.

EXCESS WEIGHT

Mildly to moderately overweight midlife women have up to forty times the risk of coronary disease as women of normal weight, according to a Harvard University School of Medicine study.[19] Also, women who gain weight during the middle years are at twice the risk of developing heart disease as women who have been overweight all their lives. The researchers involved in this study predict that as much as 40 percent of coronary disease in women could be prevented by weight loss alone.

Where you store your extra fat can be an additional hazard. If you thicken up in the waist and abdomen, your risk increases more than if you accumulate fat in the hips and thighs.

SEDENTARY LIVING

At the top of the risk-factor pyramid, along with cigarette smoking and high blood cholesterol, is sedentary living. There exists a significant relationship between physical inactivity and the risk for coronary heart disease.[20] In 1987, Kenneth Powell and his colleagues from the Centers for Disease Control, in Atlanta, scrutinized the findings of forty major studies of this relationship. They concluded that inactivity is as great a risk factor for death from heart disease as any of the better-known factors.

A study conducted in the late 1980s at the Cooper Aerobics Center, in Dallas, Texas, shows that even a moderate level of physical activity, such as a brisk walk of thirty to sixty minutes each day, significantly reduces the risk of dying from heart disease.[21] No matter what your age, an active lifestyle and a regular exercise program can keep your heart healthy. Exercise burns fat, thus regulating weight; it raises protective HDLs and lowers LDL cholesterol levels; it lowers blood pressure and heart rate; and it promotes more efficient use of insulin, which helps to control blood-sugar levels. If there is a magic pill for heart disease, exercise is it.

STRESS

We are all aware of the connection between stress and disease. Years ago many of us read the 1974 bestseller *Type A Behavior and Your Heart*, by Meyer Friedman and Ray Rosenman, and learned how men who have an aggressive "type A" personality are more prone to heart disease. More research has since refined this information. Not all aspects of the type A personality prove equally detrimental; only those related to chronic anger and hostility are harmful. Being ambitious, competitive, and hardworking are no longer considered toxic to the heart for either women or men. However, failing to learn how to express anger and thus either engaging in repeated explosive outbursts or submerging hostile feelings over time can be deadly and increase our risk of heart disease. Another factor that has been linked to women's stress and increased heart problems is working outside the home. The famous Framingham Heart Study that began in 1948 finds flaws here as well, as no connection appears to exist between heart disease and working in or out of the home.

Recent research into the effects of stress on the body means that the role played by stress in the heart-disease formula is becoming clearer. Continued emotional crises, which trigger the fight-or-flight response, produce chronically elevated levels of stress-related hormones, most notably cortisol. Chronically elevated cortisol levels eventually lead to permanent elevation in blood pressure, heart rate, and blood cholesterol levels. In addition, our typical responses to the effects of stress—such as overeating, overdrinking, and becoming overweight—stack the cards against us. We must learn how to counter the effects of a stress-filled life. Proven ways to ease tension include exercise, relaxation techniques, yoga, meditation, massages, hot baths, long walks, recreational reading, and movies. Whatever works to relax you will also protect your heart.

SOCIAL ISOLATION AND SELF-INVOLVEMENT

Many studies show that people who live alone and have no social network sustain a higher risk of dying early. A report reviewing several studies found evidence that social isolation heightens people's susceptibility to illness and disease. It suggests that lacking someone to share private feelings or have close contact with is as significant a risk factor as all the others we know.[22] Anything that develops intimacy and feelings of connection can be healing in all senses of the word.

People who live alone are prone to self-involvement. Interviews from a nine-year research study involving almost thirteen thousand men found that the participants who talked more about themselves developed heart disease more often than those who talked less about themselves.[23] Most striking was the even greater degree of self-involvement of those who ultimately died.

Midlife women often find themselves alone because of divorce or death. Keeping active in social groups, clubs, and other supportive groups may provide more than a fun evening; doing so may protect the heart.

HIGH BLOOD PRESSURE

Elevated blood pressure, also known as *hypertension*, contributes to cardiovascular disease and stroke. Even slight elevations double the risk. High blood pressure (HBP) is symptomless; you may feel great and lack any clue that the condition is silently damaging your body. Left untreated, hypertension can lead to kidney disease and vision loss. It is imperative to have your blood pressure checked regularly.

The term *hypertension* refers to a higher than normal force exerted by the blood against the elastic walls of the arteries. The heart generates pressure to pump blood throughout the body, and the muscular arteries contract to help it along. Each time the heart contracts, pressure in the arteries increases; each time the heart relaxes between beats, the pressure drops. Thus, there are two pressures that are

Natural Treatments for Reducing High Blood Pressure

- Lose weight if necessary (overweight women are two to three times more likely to develop high blood pressure).

- Decrease chronic stress (repeated stress may temporarily or permanently elevate blood pressure).[24]

- Exercise regularly (exercise has a beneficial effect on blood pressure regardless of any change in body weight).

- Maintain a low-stress diet (low in salt, sugar, coffee, tea, and saturated fats).

- Avoid oral contraceptives, especially if you smoke.

- Eat foods high in potassium (fresh vegetables, bananas, orange juice, beans, nuts, and molasses).

- Supplement daily with the following:
  - calcium (1,000 mg)
  - magnesium (500 mg)
  - zinc (30 mg)
  - vitamin C (1,000–2,000 mg)
  - B-complex (B-1, B-2, B-6 20–50 mg)

- Eat garlic (minced in foods or in capsule form).

measured to evaluate the heart's condition: an upper (systolic) pressure and a lower (diastolic) pressure.

As a general rule, systolic pressure, the first number, falls between 100 and 140, and diastolic pressure falls between 60 and 90. Many charts cite 120/80 as the optimum for a healthy adult, but it is possible to have a different reading and still be quite healthy. By taking several readings over a period of time, you can determine what is normal for you.

Are You at Risk for Hypertension?

According to the National Heart and Lung Institute, certain women fall into a higher risk category for hypertension.[25] Those women most susceptible to hypertension include

- older women (more than half of all women over age fifty-five suffer)

- women taking the Pill (one in twenty women who take estrogen have an elevated blood pressure)[26]

- women near the end of pregnancy (hypertension usually subsides after the birth of the child)

- women of color (especially African Americans)

Although high blood pressure can rarely be cured, it responds well to lifestyle changes. Good nutrition, exercise, weight control, and relaxation techniques bring blood pressure down safely and effectively. This natural treatment is particularly desirable when you weigh it against the side effects of the common antihypertensive drugs (vasodilators, diuretics, and beta-blockers): depression, heart palpitations, dizziness, muscle spasms, menstrual irregularity, nausea, weakness, dry mouth, mental confusion, insomnia, headaches, drowsiness, nightmares, twitching, loss of sexual desire, rash, and swelling of the breasts.

Women who experience adverse reactions to drugs for hypertension will be encouraged to know that recent studies show that nutritional therapy to treat high blood pressure can substitute for drugs in most cases or, if drugs are still needed, can lessen some side effects.[27]

≈ The Role Of Cholesterol ≈

High levels of total cholesterol in the blood contribute to the development of plaque in the arteries and thus raise one's risk for coronary heart disease. Cholesterol itself is not harmful; on the contrary, it is vital to our existence. It plays multiple roles in our biological functioning: It lines our cells and helps carry out basic functions of life; it insulates the nerves and allows normal transmission of nerve impulses; and it participates in the manufacture of certain hormones and hormonelike vitamins, such as estrogen and vitamin D. We can get cholesterol from food, but our body manufactures all it requires.

Some people confuse cholesterol with fat, yet it really isn't a fat at all, but a lipid: a waxy substance carried in the bloodstream along with several types of fat and proteins. Since fat and water don't mix, the liver combines fat and cholesterol with protein carriers called *lipoproteins*, so they can travel through the blood to be deposited in the cells. Lipoproteins in turn can help prevent or contribute to heart disease.

LOW-DENSITY LIPOPROTEINS (LDLS)

The chief carriers of cholesterol to the cells are the LDLs, also referred to as the "bad" cholesterol. Their reputation stems from studies showing that a 1 percent greater LDL value is associated with a slightly more than 2 percent increase in coronary artery disease over a six-year period.[28] The higher the LDL levels in the blood, the more cholesterol is available to clog the coronary arteries and bring on atherosclerosis. LDLs remain longer in the bloodstream in some people than in others; the more LDLs there are and the longer they linger, the greater the risk. One reason postmenopausal women are more susceptible to heart disease is that LDL levels rise after menopause.

LDL values are strongly influenced by diet. And here is a clue as to what works: Vegetarians have much lower LDL levels than omnivores.

HIGH-DENSITY LIPOPROTEINS (HDLS)

The "good" carriers of cholesterol are the HDLs. HDLs seem to pull cholesterol out of the arteries and carry it to the liver, where it is converted into bile and excreted. People with very low levels of HDLs are more prone to heart attacks: A 1 percent lower HDL value is associated with a 3 to 4 percent increase in coronary artery disease.[29] Even when total cholesterol levels are below 200 mg/dl, decreased HDL levels are associated with a greater incidence of heart attacks in both men and women.

Blood Cholesterol Levels: What Do the Numbers Mean?

Below 200 mg/dl	Desirable
200–239	Borderline
240 or above	High risk

LDL Levels

Below 100 mg/dl*	Desirable
100–159	Borderline
160 or above	High risk

HDL Levels

50 mg/dl or above	Desirable
35–50	Borderline
Below 35	High risk

Triglycerides

20–140 mg/dl	Normal
140–190	Monitor
Above 190	High risk

Ratio of Total Cholesterol to HDL

Below 4.5	Desirable
Above 4.5	Higher risk

*recently reduced from 130 mg/dl

The levels of HDL in the bloodstream are determined partly by genetic code and partly by lifestyle factors such as weight, exercise, smoking, and diet. Before menopause, women's HDLs are generally higher then men's, and this may account for their lowered incidence of heart disease. Women also have higher levels of a subfamily called *cholesterol HDL-2*, a factor that is critical in lowering the risk of heart disease. Combine the effects of both HDL and HDL-2, and we can come up with another valid explanation for why women are somewhat protected from heart disease. Estrogen may not be the only reason women tend to avoid heart problems until later in life.

Researchers suggest that HDL levels are a more powerful predictor of heart disease in women than in men. Even if your total cholesterol level is below 200 mg/dl, lowered HDL levels increase the probability of a heart attack. To help you appreciate its significance as a risk factor, those who have an HDL blood count lower than 35 mg/dl sustain the same risk as someone who is a moderate to heavy smoker—and we all know that is not good. Even at or below an HDL level of 45 mg/dl, you will want to pay attention to your food choices, exercise levels, and stress levels.

TRIGLYCERIDES

Triglycerides (TGs) are fatty substances formed in the liver from the food we eat and by the body's own synthesis of internal fat, to be used for energy or storage. Some researchers have found that elevated TGs are predictors of heart disease, especially in women over fifty. TGs rise with age, are higher in overweight people, and can be increased by taking the Pill or ERT.

TESTING FOR CHOLESTEROL LEVELS

Women need to be as conscientious about their blood cholesterol as men. For an accurate assessment, it is essential that you undergo a blood test to get the complete lipid profile—that is, not just your total cholesterol reading, but the individual levels of HDL, LDL, and TGs, and the ratio of total cholesterol to HDL. Data from the mid-1990s suggest that the total cholesterol-to-HDL ratio is a better measure of risk for coronary heart disease than either total cholesterol or LDL levels.[30]

Toxic Blood Components

High levels of certain blood components—including homocysteine, fibrinogen, c-reactive protein, and lipoprotein (a)—can prove damaging to the heart and are a greater concern for women than men.[31] Dr. Stephen Sinatra, a cardiologist who coined the term *toxic blood components*, suggests that women should ask for specialized blood tests to determine their levels of these neglected factors. Having this knowledge may offer significant clues concerning your future heart health.

HOMOCYSTEINE

High homocysteine levels in the blood can be more deadly than elevated cholesterol levels. Homocysteine does its damage by eroding the lining of blood vessels and triggering the growth of cells, thus setting the stage for plaque buildup in the artery walls. This amino acid, which is natural to the body, turns against us partly because of a deficiency in three common B vitamins: B-6, B-12, and folic acid. Taking the B vitamins in a multivitamin tablet is sufficient for most women as a prevention against high homocysteine levels, but women with excessively elevated homocysteine may require a higher dose to bring it down. A group of international experts recommends the following regimen to reduce and normalize high homocysteine levels in individuals with heart disease:

- folic acid: 1–5 mg

- B-6: 10–50 mg

- B-12: up to 1,000 mcg[32]

FIBRINOGEN

An elevated fibrinogen level is an independent risk factor for heart disease and stroke, meaning that it can increase your risk without any other risk factors present. Fibrinogen is a protein produced in the body to ensure proper "stickiness" of the blood. When a person has elevated fibrinogen levels, the blood clots too easily. For some reason, fibrinogen levels soar after menopause, especially in women who smoke. If you have a history of coronary artery disease, this is one instance

when you want to consider supplemental estrogen, which can bring your fibrinogen levels under control. Natural blood thinners that can offset blood stickiness include garlic, fish oil, vitamin E, ginkgo biloba, ginger, and bromelain. Don't take them all at once.

C-REACTIVE PROTEIN

Headlines released in the summer of 2002 from Boston to California proclaimed that cholesterol was about to be trumped by what doctors say is an even bigger trigger of heart attacks—inflammation. Researchers have found that persistent low-level inflammation in the arteries, triggered by infection or irritants, promotes the formation of plaque and leaves them more vulnerable to ruptures and blood clots that cause heart attacks.[33] Scientists looking for ways to determine inflammation have found that a blood test measuring c-reactive protein (CRP) may be the answer. A report in the March 2000 *New England Journal of Medicine* concluded that, compared with twelve standard risk factors, CRP was the best predictor of coronary events. This study of over twenty-eight thousand healthy women (notice that the study did not include men) found that high CRP levels increased the risk even for those with healthy LDL cholesterol levels.[34]

While cholesterol screening has been the primary predictor of heart-attack risk, half of all heart attacks occur in people who don't have high cholesterol. Dr. Paul Ridker of Brigham and Women's Hospital, Boston, and Harvard Medical School showed that CRP is a better indicator of heart-attack risk in women than the measure of total cholesterol, LDL, homocysteine, or lipoprotein (a).[35] Women taking HRT often have elevated levels of CRP, a factor to weigh if you are considering supplemental hormones.

LIPOPROTEIN (A)

Lipoprotein (a), or Lp(a), is a type of LDL cholesterol that runs in families and is abundant in many people whose coronary disease cannot be attributed to other causes. It appears to rise with the fall of estrogen and can be brought back to normal levels with supplemental hormone therapy. It is primarily because of my elevated Lp(a) levels that I decided to try natural hormones. Along with natural HRT, my cardiologist suggested I take coenzyme Q10 (100–300 mg/day), which is a higher dose than one would normally take for health. He has also suggested that I could try a therapeutic dose of vitamin B-3, or niacin, (1–2 grams/day). Since I don't like to start too many new treatments at once, I will wait and see how my present protocol is working before embarking on another.

❧ Diet for a Healthy Heart ❧

An extensive body of studies, laboratory findings, and clinical evidence has established an association, if not a causative link, between diet and heart disease. For the most part, attention has been focused on fat and fiber intake, although a variety of other foods and a host of nutrients are now known to aggravate or protect against various heart problems.

FAT

Of all the nutritional factors involved in circulatory problems, total dietary fat has consistently been implicated as the most important. Lower your overall fat intake, and your risk drops markedly. Control saturated fat, and you lower blood cholesterol and decrease your risk even further. Indeed, fat in all forms has emerged as the primary troublemaker for anything wrong with the body. Heart disease, cancer, and other diseases are caused by too much fat in the diet. We have become a fat-obsessed nation.

But is the subject that clear-cut? Have we overlooked other evidence? A handful of researchers suggest something else: that the *amount* of fat consumed may be less important than the *kind* of fat consumed regularly.

The reigning low-fat, high-fiber diet evolved from research that began decades ago. Pioneer researchers studied cultures in which heart problems were virtually nonexistent and noticed that their diets included very little fat and considerably more complex carbohydrates than the traditional American diet. But what else do these populations do on a regular basis that may be beneficial to their health? Rural Chinese and Japanese, for instance, eat an abundance of fruits, vegetables, seafood, and tofu, and they are highly active. So why do we focus on fat intake alone when other elements of their lifestyles may contribute equally to a lower risk of heart disease?

When we look closer, apparent paradoxes emerge. The Greenland Eskimos, for instance, consume an enormous amount of whale and seal fat, yet they have strong, healthy hearts. If the amount of fat were the only criterion for determining heart health, this group would be extinct. It's easy to want to find simple answers to "fix" a frightening phenomenon such as heart disease, but the issue is complex, and it is potentially dangerous to focus on the single factor of fat consumption.

The type and amount of fat eaten by certain populations is being reexamined, and many scientists are suggesting that maybe they have carried the recommendation of fat restriction too far in their quest for answers. For women, the issue is particularly crucial and timely. Many women are reducing their fat intakes to

super-low levels, thinking they are following heart-healthy guidelines. Not only may this be unnecessary; for women it may be harmful. Evidence shows that the low-fat diet that works so well to lower total cholesterol and LDL cholesterol comes with a downside—it drags down the protective HDL cholesterol levels, which for women, as we have discussed, may be a more hazardous risk than extra dietary fat.

Defending the Low-Fat Diet

Over the last decade or so, exciting news has emerged: proof that heart disease can be not only prevented with dietary changes, but actually reversed. A well-known study by Dean Ornish, director of the Preventive Medicine Research Institute in Sausalito, California, has shown that in only one year, patients with severe arterial blockages began to unclog when they followed a comprehensive lifestyle program.[36] Better yet, the only known side effects of the program are positive ones.

I wish to emphasize that as Ornish himself has said, a low-fat diet doesn't mean Snack Well cookies and tea. And it must also be noted that fat reduction was not the exclusive variable in this trial. The Ornish program includes giving up smoking, exercising moderately, following daily stress-management classes—including meditation—and drastically changing dietary habits, especially reducing fat intake. The plan's diet is primarily vegetarian and consists of 10 percent of calories from fats, 15 to 20 percent from protein, and up to 75 percent from complex carbohydrates. The basic difference between this and a generally healthy food plan is the lowered level of fat, but treating a disease state usually involves some stringent measures. At the end of one year, Ornish's patients showed significant overall reduction of atherosclerosis and coronary heart disease. The program is outlined in his book, *Reversing Heart Disease.*

Additionally, a low-fat diet can reduce high blood pressure, which in turn lowers the risk for coronary disease. Studies have shown beneficial effects on blood pressure from a diet obtaining 27 percent of its calories from fat. (The American Heart Association recommends getting no more than 30 percent of calories from fat.)

This raises a pertinent question: How do we account for the vast difference between Dr. Ornish's recommendation of 8 to 10 percent of calories from fat and the American Heart Association's (and other experts') guidelines of 25 to 30 percent? The key is to distinguish between reversing an already existing condition of heart disease and preventing heart disease. A diet to reverse heart disease will generally be more stringent than one designed to prevent it. If you have survived a heart attack and you know your arteries are thick with plaque, then shoot for the low end of the scale until you have seen a major improvement in your arteries and blood work. Then you can gradually add healthy fats to your diet while incorporating lifesaving nutrients, exercise, and stress reducers.

For those of us concerned with maintaining healthy hearts, obtaining 30 percent of our calories from the right kinds of fats is a reasonable goal. The different kinds of fats and their effects are discussed below.

Women and the Very Low Fat Diet

A diet that is very low in fat, as has already been mentioned, has one major drawback: Besides lowering the "baddies"—total cholesterol and LDLs—it also lowers the protective "goody," HDLs. This may be fine for men, because their circulatory system is strongly influenced by LDL levels. But women's hearts respond more favorably to the good effects of high levels of HDLs. One alternative for women, then, is to avoid going too low in their overall dietary fat intake.

According to Margo Denke, M.D., of the American Heart Association's Nutrition Committee, it is only when one reduces total fat consumption to below 25 percent of calories that HDL levels fall. When fat makes up between 25 and 30 percent of total calories consumed, HDL levels are maintained. For most of us, this is a healthy range to stay within for our whole lives. But if you have suffered a heart attack and are under the care of a physician who has you on a very low fat diet (10 to 15 percent of calories), you can bump up those HDLs with exercise, more fiber, omega-3 fatty acids (found in certain fish oils and vegetable oils), and specific nutrients.

Questioning the Low-Fat Diet

Prevailing wisdom says that all we must do to lose weight is cut out fat and stock up on carbohydrates: breads, rice, pasta, and cereal. What a great eating plan, we may think, but unfortunately it isn't working for a lot of women. Substituting carbohydrates for fat, popularly thought to be a healthy way to eat, has not proven to beneficially affect serum lipids (blood fats) or long-term weight management. Despite the abundance of fat-free foods on the market, Americans are not getting thinner. According to a USDA survey, although Americans' fat intake is edging down—from the high of 43 percent to 33 percent in 1994—we're still getting fatter by eleven pounds per person on average.[37] According to the Centers for Disease Control and Prevention, the percentage of overweight Americans increased from 25 percent of the population in 1980 to 55 percent in 1998.

How can this be? If we are following advice and filling up on all the fat-free carbs we want in place of fried foods and marbled meats, why aren't we losing weight? The answer lies in a condition called *insulin resistance*, thought by some health experts to affect 50 to 75 percent of the population. For these people, high levels of dietary carbohydrates—especially simple sugars and refined carbs such as

191

are found in white pasta, white rice, and white breads—hike up weight and serum lipids, putting them at risk for cardiovascular disease.

Insulin resistance—which can accompany one from birth or develop over time—essentially means that insulin stays in the bloodstream longer than it should. Insulin is the hormone from the pancreas that metabolizes carbohydrates. The chain of events works like this: You overeat carbohydrates, which provokes a very high blood-sugar level, which in turn leads to insulin overload in your system. The body cannot utilize the excess sugar, so it gets stored as fat. If you have found that you are not losing weight on a high-carbohydrate diet, this may be the reason why.

In addition to adding pounds to your frame, maintaining high levels of both glucose and insulin in the blood can have a devastating effect on the heart. It can cause blood clots, raise triglyceride levels, lower HDLs, make the blood vessels narrower and less pliable, and elevate blood pressure. This cluster of heart-disease risk factors triggered by insulin resistance is gaining acceptance by mainstream medicine as a major cause of heart disease. If you suspect that this scenario describes you, then the ultra-low-fat, high-carbohydrate diet is not recommended.

Contrary to the myth that no diet can be too low in fat, low-fat diets generally are not based on whole foods and thus are low in essential fatty acids (EFAs). Not only are women shunning red meat and cream sauces, we exclude nuts, oils, and fatty fish from our menus. We women need some fat in our diets. Since we cannot manufacture EFAs, we must get them from our diets. EFAs aid in numerous body functions, including the relaxation and contraction of blood vessels, keeping our platelets from clumping together, and keeping inflammation down, to name just a few.

Extremely low-fat diets may also produce deficiencies in fat-soluble nutrients such as beta-carotene and vitamins D and E, leading to an increased incidence of atherosclerotic disease and many other health problems. Many women may be severely hampering their nutrition—literally starving themselves on pasta and bagels and not getting enough protein and fat. As always, the best advice is to listen to your body. Do you have symptoms that may be sending you a signal, such as low energy, an insatiable appetite, uncontrolled sugar binges, loss of hair, acne, bloating, food allergies, mental confusion, irritability, thin skin, brittle nails, and menstrual problems? If so, it's time to temper your carb intake and add some protein and fat to your diet.

Remember, no one diet is right for everyone. It has been clinically demonstrated—and it just makes common sense—that individual patients may respond differently to the same eating plan, no matter what the diet gurus tell us. The "perfect" diet that lowers cholesterol and strips the fat off one group of people may not benefit others in the same way. Remember the Eskimos.

All Fats Are Not Created Equal

So, let's say you diligently study package labels and other resources for the fat content of your favorite foods, and you've managed to get your total fat intake consistently into the optimal range for your condition: 25 to 30 percent of calories for prevention of heart disease, or perhaps lower if you're trying to reverse heart disease. Now it's time to bone up on the various types of fat that exist in the foods you love, because they have different effects on your body.

Saturated fat. The worst single dietary offender in heart disease is saturated fat. Saturated fats clog the arteries and raise blood-cholesterol levels. They are generally solid at room temperature and come primarily from animal products such as red meat, poultry (especially the skin), whole milk, cheese, butter, and cream. Many people confuse saturated fat with cholesterol. While they may be found together in many animal products, they are different substances. Prime rib contains both saturated fat and cholesterol; lobster is full of cholesterol but has no saturated fat. Which is worse for the heart? Both are thought to raise blood-cholesterol levels, but if there were a contest, saturated fat would win hands down.

A few vegetable oils are also saturated and carry the same risks, even though they do not contain cholesterol (which comes only from animal-based foods). Palm kernel and coconut oils are highly saturated fats—in fact, even more saturated than beef fat. These oils are commonly used by manufacturers in making every snack imaginable, from crackers and chips to cookies, cakes, whipped dessert toppings, and granola bars.

Trans fatty acids. Trans fatty acids are found in the margarines, shortenings, and cooking fats commonly used to prepare french fries, corn chips, commercial baked goods, and dozens of other processed products. Using a chemical process called *hydrogenation*, naturally occurring oils, such as peanut oil and coconut oil, are converted into saturated fats that are solid at room temperature and do not turn rancid quickly.

Early studies showed that trans fatty acids could raise cholesterol levels; recent research from Harvard Medical School has linked them to a higher risk for heart disease. Epidemiologist Walter Willet calculated the intake of trans fatty acids from a questionnaire completed by over 87,000 women as part of the Nurses' Health Study. During the eight years following the questionnaire, 431 of the nurses had heart attacks. Those who consumed the most trans fatty acids sustained a 50 percent higher rate of heart disease than those who ate less of these substances.[38] Women who ate margarine four or more times a day had a 66 percent higher risk of heart disease than those who ate it less than once a month.

Can you believe it? McDonald's is planing to cut the levels of trans-fat oils in its Chicken McNuggets and french fries by half.[39] We would all like to think that the global hamburger chain is concerned about worldwide health, but the announcement came shortly after a New Yorker sued McDonald's and others, claiming that their food made him obese. Just in case you are planning to incorporate more burgers into your diet, be aware that the fat and caloric content of the food will remain the same as before, no matter what kind of oil it's cooked in. A large order of fries will still come packed with 540 calories and twenty-six grams of fat. The one saving grace is that the oil they're cooked in will be only partially of the trans-fatty-acid variety.

Food manufacturers are not currently required to list the amounts of trans fatty acids in their products, so there is no way of knowing how much is hidden in the items you buy. This will change soon, though, because this information will be required by law as of January 2006. Check labels for the term "partially hydrogenated vegetable oils." If they are one of the first three ingredients listed, you can be certain you are getting a high-fat food. A quick measure for total fats is that if the product has more than three grams of fat per hundred calories, it falls over the 30 percent limit. The main point to remember is that we must minimize both saturated fats and trans fatty acids in our diets.

Polyunsaturated fats. Polyunsaturated fats, generally liquid at room temperature, are derived from vegetable sources such as corn, safflower, and soybean. Most vegetable oils, except for coconut and palm oils, are not saturated and have been shown to lower blood cholesterol levels. Evidence is mounting, however, that these fats may lower the "good" as well as the "bad" cholesterol and may also be implicated in the development of breast cancer. Although the research is still speculative, there are enough data to recommend substituting for these oils with the oils considered safest to eat, the monounsaturated fats.

Monounsaturated oils. The Greeks and Italians thrive on a diet low in saturated fats and plentiful in both complex carbohydrates and monounsaturated oils. The fact that inhabitants of these countries suffer half as many fatal heart attacks as we do in the United States is thought to be due to their fondness for olive oil, but we cannot forget that more than one factor may be producing such heart-healthy people. A diet rich in monounsaturated oils such as olive oil, peanut oil, and canola oil makes LDLs more resistant to oxidation than a diet high in polyunsaturated oils such as corn and most other vegetable oils.[40] This is a plus, because oxidized fats may be potent artery cloggers. If your recipe calls for oil, go for the monounsaturates.

Fish oils. The health benefits of fish oils have been widely investigated since it became known that Eskimos enjoy a low incidence of heart disease despite their traditional diet of whale and seal fat. Further studies noted that the Japanese also eat a diet rich in fish and show a similarly reduced rate of heart disease. In 1985, after twenty years of following a group of men, scientists from the Netherlands concluded that there was in fact an inverse relationship between fish consumption and death from coronary artery disease and that as little as one or two fish dishes a week may be valuable for prevention.[41]

Fish and fish oils, which contain omega-3 fatty acids, have been ascribed a broad spectrum of biological benefits. They are reported to lower blood pressure, reduce blood lipids, improve blood flow, and prevent blood platelets (which aid in blood clotting) from forming. As platelet inhibitors, they may even be more effective than aspirin, the most commonly used agent thus far.[42]

The active ingredients in fish oils are eicosapentaenoic acid (EPA) and docosahexaenoic acid (DHA). EPA originates in plants and algae; fish eat them and store the EPA in their muscles and liver. No food sources of EPA in a vegetarian diet can match the concentration in fish. The best fish sources are high-fat fish such as salmon, mackerel, sablefish, Florida pompano, bluefin tuna, swordfish, bluefish, shark, and herring. If you do not regularly eat fish, you can supplement with 1,000 to 3,000 mg of EPA or omega-3 fatty acid capsules several times a week.

FIBER

There is strong evidence that oat bran and other foods high in soluble fiber can lower blood cholesterol. An analysis of twenty studies concluded that approximately three grams of soluble fiber per day from oat products can lower the total cholesterol level five to six mg/dl and that the reduction is greater in those with initially high blood-cholesterol levels.[43] Oat bran should not be used to replace a low-fat diet but should be added to one. You should also be aware that many of the oat muffins and crackers on the market are swimming in fat, which negates any cholesterol-lowering effect from the bran.

Nature has provided us with a wide variety of fibrous foods: black-eyed peas; kidney, navy, lima, and pinto beans; carrots; green peas; corn; prunes; sweet potatoes; zucchini; bananas; apples; pears; and oranges are some of the best. If you like these foods, add them to your daily menu and lower your cholesterol levels.

Supplemental fiber is an effective way to lower blood-cholesterol levels when total dietary intake is low or dietary modification is not working. A supplement containing 4 grams of guar gum and 3.5 grams of pectin mixed with three types of insoluble fiber was given to patients with a history of mild to high cholesterol. After

Sources of Oat Bran

Oat Source	Grams of Oat Bran
Oat bran (1 tbsp)	15
Oat bran muffin (1)	10–15
Oat bran cereal (1 oz)	4–5
Oat bran bread (1 slice)	2.5–3

fifteen weeks, total cholesterol, LDL, and the ratio of LDL to HDL were significantly reduced.[44] Other kinds of supplemental fiber proved equally beneficial. Daily dietary supplements of 15 grams of grapefruit pectin significantly lowered plasma cholesterol and improved LDL-to-HDL ratio in patients with high cholesterol levels who were unable or unwilling to follow a low-risk diet.[45] Adding 7.3 grams of psyllium, an edible fibrous seed, to cereal reduced total serum cholesterol concentration after two weeks.[46] I would not recommend fiber supplementation as your first line of defense, but as an adjunct to a broader program it can prove useful.

SOY PROTEIN

Although a diet high in animal protein promotes elevated cholesterol, plant protein may inhibit or reduce cholesterol synthesis in the liver. Soy protein, in particular, helps maintain strong arterial walls and promotes resorption of plaque that builds up in the coronary arteries. Additionally, soy proteins are part of a group of plant chemicals called *phytosterols* that have the ability to inhibit the absorption of cholesterol, thus keeping down cholesterol levels in the blood.

Evidence has mounted for decades that indicates that soy protein significantly lowers blood cholesterol and aids the heart in several ways. An exhaustive analysis of thirty-eight studies examining the effect of soy protein on serum lipid (blood fat) levels showed the following average reductions in cholesterol:

⊙ Total cholesterol declined 23.2 mg/dl (9.3 percent).

⊙ LDL cholesterol dropped 21.7 mg/dl (12.9 percent).

⊙ Triglycerides declined 13.3 mg/dl (10.5 percent).

The authors of the same review concluded that soy can reduce the risk of coronary heart disease by 18 to 28 percent. Specifically, their analysis indicated the following:

⊙ A daily intake of 25 grams of soy protein over several months could reduce blood cholesterol by 8.9 mg/dl.

⊙ An intake of 50 grams of soy protein could reduce it by 17.4 mg/dl.

⊙ An intake of 75 grams could reduce it by 26.3 mg/dl.

If a low-fat diet has failed to lower your cholesterol, try soy. In a study at the University of Illinois, sixty-six postmenopausal women with cholesterol levels above 200 mg/dl were put on either a low-fat diet using nonfat milk as the protein source or a diet containing soy. Both groups experienced a reduction in total cholesterol, but only the soy group saw a significant reduction in LDLs plus a rise in HDLs.[47] (HDLs are most significant for women, remember?) However, the researchers pointed out that these results were seen in women with high cholesterol levels. If your cholesterol levels lie within the average range, you may not notice similar effects.

Soy's Many Heart-Healthy Effects

Soy proteins have several heart-healthy effects in addition to lowering cholesterol. Consider the following:

- Soy isoflavones, phytates, and saponins have strong antioxidant activity and help curb the formation of toxic free-radicals, which contribute to arterial damage.

- Genistein, the principal phytoestrogen in soy, may work in the early stages of atherosclerosis by hindering the overgrowth of epithelial cells lining the arteries. Overgrowth of these cells promotes plaque buildup and clogged arteries.

- Genistein appears to prevent blood clots, which can lead to heart attack and stroke, by inhibiting the formation of an enzyme called thrombin.

- Genistein may increase the flexibility of blood vessels, helping to prevent spasms that can trigger a heart attack.

- Soy modulates blood-sugar levels. Glycine and arginine, two of the amino acids in soy, decrease insulin levels in the blood, thus stabilizing blood-sugar levels. Keeping blood sugar fairly stable is important for women, because the combination of high estrogen levels and high insulin levels has a doubly negative effect on both the heart and breasts.

FLAXSEED

Flaxseed, the plant kingdom's primary source of healthy omega-3 fatty acids, lowers cholesterol. Although not as potent as the fat of cold-water fish, flaxseed oil does provide its own benefits for circulatory health. And it houses another essential fatty acid, alpha linolenic acid, that may protect against stroke. This particular EFA can

reduce the dangerous clotting tendencies of the blood's platelets. Flaxseed itself (not the oil) also proves to be a fair source of both soluble and insoluble fiber; $1/8$ cup offers 10 grams of fiber. Finally, it contains lignan precursors that are converted during digestion into phytoestrogens. Boasting all these advantages, flaxseed has been shown to lower cholesterol by between 5 and 15 percent, when ingested at amounts between 5 and 50 grams per day.

⇒ Antioxidants ⇐

One of the most important recent discoveries in research on nutrition and aging is that oxygen, our basic source of energy and life, has a dark side. At the molecular level, oxygen can form highly reactive biochemical compounds, called *free radicals*. When not tempered by antioxidants, free radicals can start branching chain reactions that reproduce uncontrollably, attacking the cells in the body, destroying cell membranes, and contributing to accelerated aging and age-related diseases. Some of the conditions studied so far that may be related to damage from free radicals are cancer, heart disease, emphysema, rheumatoid arthritis, and Parkinson's disease.[48]

Oxidation is triggered by environmental pollutants as well as by our metabolism. We are bombarded with influences from the outside and from substances we absorb—ultraviolet light, radiation (including X rays), air pollution, cigarette smoke, pesticides, alcohol, rancid fats—that promote free-radical activation and cellular damage. Many of the external influences lie beyond our control, but not all.

The body houses a complex antioxidant system composed of enzymes, vitamins, and minerals, which neutralize free radicals before they damage tissues. These self-manufactured and food-derived antioxidants may or may not serve us adequately, depending on a number of factors, such as what we eat and whether we smoke or drink alcohol. By middle age our ability to maintain this defense system declines, and the antioxidants we obtain from food cannot make up for the lack in our system. By resupplying the body with the full range of antioxidants, we may be able to safeguard against the diseases of aging.

Antioxidants have hit the media with a bang. Television commercials and magazine advertisements extol the benefits of these miracle nutrients—but what exactly are they? Antioxidants have been used commercially for years. The food industry adds synthetic antioxidants like BHT and BHA, or the vitamins C and E, to cooking oils and canned meats to prevent the fats in them from oxidizing and turning rancid. The use of antioxidants to prevent aging and disease is a relatively novel concept, however, though research does go back several decades. Below are

explanations of some of the antioxidants, what they do, where to find them in food sources, and how much of them we need.

VITAMIN E

Vitamin E, along with other antioxidants such as vitamin C, beta-carotene, and selenium, are being acclaimed as protectors of the body's cells. Individually and collectively, they appear to help specifically by preventing oxidation of LDLs, thereby inhibiting the formation of plaque and the destruction of the blood-vessel linings. The susceptibility of LDLs to oxidation is inversely related to the presence of antioxidants in the blood, most notably, vitamin E. In simpler terms: When vitamin E intake is high, LDL levels and, thus, the risk of heart disease are lowered. Many studies confirm that low vitamin E intake is a better predictor of heart disease than elevated cholesterol levels.

Two large-scale studies, one of men and one of women, have shown that large daily doses of vitamin E (100 IU) lower the risk of heart disease. The more than eighty thousand women studied were followed for eight years. Both studies found that vitamin E, when obtained only through diet or even when supplemented as part of a basic multivitamin and mineral tablet, offered little or no protection; therapeutic doses were needed for a protective effect.[49]

Vitamin E is most known for its antioxidant role, but it also protects the heart by inhibiting platelet formation. In one test, after two weeks of 200 IU/day of vitamin E, platelet adhesion was reduced by 75 percent; after two weeks of 400 IU/day, platelet adhesion was reduced 82 percent.[50] Researchers noted that the inhibitory activity of alpha-tocopherol (our main form of vitamin E) was dose-dependent; higher doses offered greater benefits. You should supplement if you feel you are at high risk for heart disease or if you just want the best possible protection. Good sources of vitamin E include sunflower seeds, almonds, crab, sweet potatoes, vegetable oils, fish, and wheat germ. (For the precise amount of this nutrient contained in certain foods, consult Appendix C.)

VITAMIN C

In a study of both men and women, it was found that high levels of vitamin C concentration in the blood may lower the risk for heart disease.[51] The researchers concluded that even in a well-nourished population with perfectly adequate concentrations of plasma vitamin C and at intakes well above the RDA of 60 mg, there is still an association between vitamin C levels and HDL. What this means is that the previous RDA levels were not enough to result in antioxidizing effects. (It

should be noted that the RDA for vitamin C has since been increased to 75 mg for adult women and 90 mg for adult men.)

The Nurses' Health Study, which examined eighty-seven thousand women between thirty-four and fifty-four years of age, found the risk of developing heart disease was more than 42 percent lower for women who took high doses of vitamin C compared with women with low vitamin C intakes. Sources of vitamin C include raw green peppers, orange juice, broccoli, cantaloupe, strawberries, fresh tomatoes, and potatoes. (For the precise amount of this nutrient contained in certain foods, consult Appendix C.)

BETA-CAROTENE

Researchers at Harvard Medical School set out to study the relationship between beta-carotene and cancer and whether aspirin had any protective effect against heart disease. Surprisingly, they found that in the men taking beta-carotene, incidents of heart disease and strokes were cut in half.[52] Another study from the nineties found that beta-carotene, along with vitamin E, can reduce the risk of a first heart attack.[53] Individually, but even more so collectively, antioxidants have been proven to guard against this killer, and many more studies concerning the roles and benefits of antioxidants are in progress.

The recommended dosage for beta-carotene as an antioxidant ranges between 15 to 50 mg per day and can be met with less effort than some of the other antioxidants. Good sources of beta-carotene include spinach, carrots, sweet potatoes, winter squash, cantaloupe, and broccoli.

SELENIUM

Selenium is another vital antioxidant that protects cell membranes from damage by highly reactive oxygen fragments. Regional studies on the incidence of cardiovascular disease and soil levels of selenium show a higher rate of heart attacks and stroke in areas of the United States where soil is low in selenium.[54] The so-called "stroke belt" in Georgia and the Carolinas are areas of very low selenium soil content, and these areas correspondingly have the highest levels of heart disease and stroke in the country.

There is sufficient reason to supplement the diet with 50 to 200 mcg of selenium daily as a protection against heart disease. Many researchers prefer the organic forms, derived from a special type of brewer's yeast, to the inorganic sodium selenite. Inorganic selenium cannot be taken with vitamin C because it decreases its absorption; it has also been reported to be toxic at high levels when taken for a long time. Neither is true of organic selenium. Because of its synergistic effects with vitamin E, it is good to take them together as part of a multivitamin and mineral formula.

The selenium content of food is dependent on the amount of selenium found in the soil in which the food was grown and can vary as much as 200-fold. Grains such as whole wheat, brown rice, and oatmeal are fairly good sources if the soil is rich in selenium. Meats, poultry, and fish contain higher amounts, but these may not be preferred sources for many people. Good sources of selenium include lobster, tuna, shrimp, ham, eggs, chicken, whole-wheat bread, and whole-grain cereal. (For the precise amount of this nutrient contained in certain foods, consult Appendix C.)

B Vitamins

The antioxidants must share the spotlight with the B vitamins, which play an entirely different role but are potentially just as important in reducing cardiovascular risk. In the absence of vitamins B-6, B-12, and folic acid, the amino acid methionine is converted to a substance known as homocysteine. As discussed earlier in the chapter, convincing proof exists that an elevated homocysteine level is an independent risk factor for vascular diseases. (Homoscysteine appears to be elevated in postmenopausal women.)[55] Several investigators have demonstrated that homocysteine can be normalized with supplementation of these three B vitamins.[56] (See the section "Toxic Blood Components," on page 187, for recommended intake levels.)

Coenzyme Q10

Coenzyme Q10 (CoQ10, for short) is a substance the body needs to survive. Scientists have branded this vitamin-like antioxidant a miracle nutrient because of its link to oxygen and ultimately to life itself. Experts estimate that once the body becomes more than 25 percent deficient of CoQ10, it suffers in several ways, resulting in a wide variety of diseases that range from high blood pressure and a lowered immune system to heart failure and cancer. Deficiency has been found in 50 to 75 percent of individuals with heart disease.[57]

WHERE IS IT FOUND?

A variety of foods contain coenzyme Q10, most notably beef (especially the heart), chicken, fish (primarily salmon, sardines, and mackerel), eggs, nuts (especially peanuts), vegetable oils (especially rapeseed oil), broccoli, spinach, and wheat germ. The body also manufactures CoQ10 with the help of specific vitamins, such as

B-2, niacin (B-3), panthothenic acid (B-5), B-6, C, and folic acid. With its abundance in nature, you may wonder how people can become deficient in CoQ10, but they do, for a number of reasons. Some people suffer a genetic error or an acquired defect in CoQ10 synthesis. Or they simply may not ingest the foods that offer either adequate CoQ10 or the cofactors needed to produce it. And, as with most nutrients, as we age we are less likely to efficiently absorb CoQ10.

WHAT DOES IT DO?

Coenzyme Q10 helps to create energy within each cell. It is an essential component of the mitochondria, known as the powerhouse of the cell, and its primary job is to protect the cell from oxidative stress. It rescues tissues by regulating the flow of oxygen into the cells. It can help repair organs or tissues that have been damaged by oxidative stress, and it is especially useful in reenergizing heart cells and rejuvenating weakened heart muscles so that they pump blood more efficiently. Studies from both the United States and Japan show that supplemental CoQ10 can lower the blood pressure of high-risk patients without additional medication. Many conditions associated with heart disease—heart failure, angina, hypertension, mitral valve prolapse, enlarged heart, and ischemic heart disease—show marked improvement with increased CoQ10.

INTERNATIONAL RESEARCH

Studies from around the world have confirmed that CoQ10 reduces major and minor symptoms of heart disease. Yet in the United States, most doctors remain uninformed about its potential healing qualities. Extensive Japanese research has shown that about 70 percent of heart patients are helped with supplemental CoQ10.[58] An Italian study involving 2,664 patients with heart failure showed that after three months of taking an average of 100 mg of CoQ10 daily, improvements were measured in the classic signs and symptoms of congestive heart failure: less edema, relaxed breathing, normal coloring, fewer heart palpitations, and better sleeping patterns.[59]

In the United States, Dr. Karl Folkers, director of the Institute for Biomedical Research at the University of Texas, is considered one of the pioneers in the field for his work on CoQ10 here and in Japan and Europe. In one of his many studies, he found that three-fourths of patients with congestive heart failure who took CoQ10 survived for three years, while only one-fourth lived that long with conventional therapy.[60] Such dramatic results cause researchers to boldly suggest that heart disease can be a direct result of CoQ10 deficiency.

DOSAGE

Cardiologists have been utilizing CoQ10 for years to treat people with major heart conditions or who are at risk for heart disease. Stephen Sinatra, M.D., of the New England Heart Center in Manchester, Connecticut, over his twenty years of administering CoQ10 has found that it works more than 70 percent of the time. He reports that some patients taking CoQ10 cut their dosage of other medications in half after a few months.[61]

If you have a heart condition, do not stop taking your medication to try CoQ10 or any other nutritional remedy. Talk to your doctor first and work together with him or her. You may want to use CoQ10 as an adjunct to your standard treatment, but do not replace your treatment without first discussing it with your doctor.

Dr. Sinatra suggests a dosage range between 90 mg and 180 mg CoQ10 for patients with angina, cardiac arrhythmia, or hypertension and for those who have undergone angioplasty. He ups the dosage to between 180 mg and 360 mg for people with more severe problems of coronary heart failure or cardiomyopathy.[62] As part of a healthy-heart preventive program, a safe dosage lies between 30 mg and 60 mg per day. You do not need to check with your doctor for this "insurance" support, as long as you don't use it to replace your regular treatment. This is a very safe compound; no toxicity has been reported in the literature, even at levels considerably higher than the ones recommended.

Because CoQ10 is a fat-soluble nutrient, it is best taken with meals. Divide the daily dosage into portions of 10 mg to 20 mg. CoQ10 comes in both a dry form and a soft-gel, oil-based preparation. The latter is preferred because it enhances bioavailability throughout the body.

Daily Supplements for a Healthy Heart

Beta-carotene (vitamin A)
cuts heart disease and strokes in half . . . . 30 mg

Vitamins B-6, B-12, and folic acid
deficiency raises homocysteine level, which
has a toxic effect on arterial cells . . . . 50 mg

Vitamin C . . . . 2,000–3000 mg

Vitamin E
increases HDL cholesterol and decreases
risk of heart disease . . . . 100–400 IU

Selenium
a protective antioxidant . . . . 200 mcg

Calcium
reduces high blood pressure . . . . 1,000 mg

Magnesium
reduces high blood pressure and lowers the
incidence of arrhythmia and sudden death by
more than 50 percent . . . . 500 mg

Chromium (picolinate)
lowers total cholesterol and raises HDLs . . . . . . 200 mcg

Lecithin
lowers cholesterol, reduces triglycerides,
and raises HDLs . . . . 23 tbsps

Omega-3 fatty acids
increases HDLs and lowers TGs . . . . 1 g

Garlic
reduces total cholesterol . . . . 1 clove or 2 capsules

L-carnitine
reduces angina pain . . . . 2,000 mg

CoQ10
a protective antioxidant . . . . 30–60 mg

COQ10'S PROMISE

The ubiquitous CoQ10 is a versatile nutrient and might be useful for other conditions as well as for heart disease. It has been shown to protect against tissue inflammation, such as that found in periodontal disease; it bolsters the immune system; it thwarts the damaging effects of aging; it may be helpful in weight loss; and it is currently being studied as a treatment for breast cancer, Huntington's disease, Parkinson's disease, and multiple sclerosis.

CHAPTER 10

BREAST CANCER

Health is the state about which medicine has nothing to say.

— W. H. AUDEN

There is no disease that women fear as much as breast cancer—and justifiably so. Breast cancer has become the leading cause of death among women between the ages of thirty-two and fifty-two. Statistics tell us that one out of eight women (or about 12 percent) have a chance of developing breast cancer sometime during the course of their lifetime. Every three minutes a woman is diagnosed, and every eleven minutes a woman dies from the disease.[1] Approximately 80 percent of all breast cancers occur in postmenopausal women, and these rates continue to rise. At one time Caucasian women were at a higher risk than African-American women, but this has changed; the rates for blacks have doubled, so the incidence is now higher than that in young Caucasian women.

The Risks of Conventional HRT

The question of conventional HRT and breast cancer is now crystal clear. Federal officials announced early in July 2002 that Prempo, the type of HRT most U.S. women take, raises the risk of breast cancer. Cut short due to frightening results, the Women's Health Initiative trial showed that 26 percent more women on the combination of Premarin (conjugated equine estrogens) plus a synthetic progestin (medroxyprogesterone acetate) developed invasive breast cancer than women on placebo. These women had participated in the study for an average of 5.2 years.[2] (For a closer look at the results of the WHI study, see Chapter 2.)

Following the announcement of these findings, panic spread via every newspaper and TV talk show. But why the shock? This is not new information. Many of us who have been following the research trail did not blink an eye at the headlines, because similar facts have been recorded for decades. Excessive doses of estrogen along with the toxic effects of synthetic progestins can be harmful to breast tissue.

Eminent researchers who specialize in hormones and breast cancer have been warning women for years.

Three years ago, in the fourth edition of this book, I reported that another major study, conducted by the National Cancer Institute, confirmed that HRT can harm the breast, at least under some circumstances. The NCI study, which involved 46,355 postmenopausal women (making it one of the largest ever of its kind), showed that the combination of the hormones estrogen and progestin substantially increased a woman's risk of developing breast cancer if taken for several years. For each year of therapy combining estrogen and progestin, a woman's risk of breast cancer was found to increase by 8 percent, compared with a 1 percent increase per year in women taking estrogen alone. These results occurred only in thin women who had used HRT in the previous four years.[3] An earlier study indicated that women with a family history of breast cancer who have taken postmenopausal hormones sustained a twofold greater risk for developing breast cancer than women who have never taken them at all.[4] There exists a wealth of literature supporting the link between conventional HRT and breast cancer that was obviously not taken seriously until the final blow of 2002.

Articles appearing since the fateful WHI study seem to be pointing all the blame for breast cancer on progestins; and yes, there seems to be a larger risk attached to the coupling of estrogen and progestin in HRT than there is to estrogen alone. But again, overwhelming evidence shows that excess estrogen exposure is a contributing factor to breast cancer. Fifty to 60 percent of all breast cancers are estrogen sensitive, meaning the cancer grows faster in the presence of estrogen.[5] In a review of the relationship between estrogen levels and breast cancer, the National Cancer Institute records that a plethora of population studies suggest a positive relationship between estrogen levels, estrogen exposure, and an increased risk of breast cancer.[6]

Estrogen is a growth-promoting hormone that stimulates cells in the uterine lining and in the breast to divide and multiply in preparation for pregnancy and lactation. Estrogen can get out of hand in a woman's body even if she doesn't take replacement therapy. She may be exposed to more continuous estrogen over her life by starting her periods early, arriving at menopause late, and not having children (which provides protective progesterone during pregnancy). Excess estrogen can be the result of increased body fat or overexposure to environmental estrogens. Moreover, the data suggests that several types of pollutants may contribute to an oversupply of estrogen, particularly organochlorines, such as DDT analogues and polychlorinated biphenyls (PCBs).[7]

The longer the exposure to estrogen, no matter its source, the greater the potential harm. When studies of the estrogen–breast cancer link from 1985 to 1990 were collectively examined and reported in 1991, researchers calculated that the risk of breast cancer increased with ERT use: The more years a woman was on hormones, the greater the risk. For women who had been on estrogen for fifteen years, the researchers cited a 30 percent increase in breast cancer.[8]

Women have been told and continue to be assured that Premarin and Prempro are safe for short-term use—which is not necessarily true. At a meeting in late October 2002 sponsored by the National Institutes of Health, Dr. Rowan Chlebowski reported that even women from the WHI study who stopped taking the hormones had more breast cancer than those who never took the hormones.[9] *New York Times* medical writer Gina Kolata, who covered the NIH meeting, noted that the scientific evidence has failed to show that women can avoid breast cancer risk by taking HRT for a short time. Furthermore, research also has failed to show that the risk disappears once the drugs are stopped. It appears that the synthetic hormones used in the study are not safe under any conditions.

The Hope of Natural HRT

Some researchers believe that the negative effects of conventional HRT are due to the fact that the drugs used are synthetic products and therefore poorly received by the human body. It is thought that natural, or bioidentical, hormones may avoid such troublesome outcomes because they are recognized by the body as identical to the substances produced by the body. (See Chapter 2 for a definition and detailed discussion of natural, or bioidentical, hormones.) Many women find that natural hormones do not produce the same offensive side effects as their synthetic counterparts and may therefore be a better option. After poring over the research, I am convinced that bioidentical hormones, which exactly match the ones native to our bodies, offer a viable alternative to the synthetic products most women have been ingesting. The question is, if these bioidentical hormones replicate our own hormones, and if we take them only if we need them and in small therapeutic doses, will they raise the risk of breast cancer and blood clots, like Prempro does? The research is scant, because natural hormones are not profitable enough to fund studies, but we do have a sampling of research indicating that estriol (a safer form of estrogen) and progesterone (*not* synthetic progestin) may be cancer protective.

If breast cancer is a major concern to you, and you want to make an informed decision about hormone therapy, there is a wonderful book on this topic titled *What Your Doctor May Not Tell You about Breast Cancer*, by John R. Lee, M.D., a renowned pioneer and expert in natural hormone replacement therapy, David Zava, Ph.D., a biochemist with extensive experience in breast cancer research, and Virginia Hopkins. If you have never explored the natural-hormone route for treating menopausal symptoms or for protecting against osteoporosis or for modulating any other hormone imbalance, and if you are especially concerned about breast cancer, pick up this book. It will open your world to options. In it, Zava shares his most recent findings, which result from analyzing a huge computerized database of saliva hormone levels at ZRT Laboratory. (Dr. Zava is director of ZRT Labs, in Oregon.) Working with Dr. Rebecca Glaser, a breast surgeon from Ohio who sends saliva samples from women who have been recently diagnosed with breast cancer to his lab, Dr. Zava observed a pattern in the samples. He refers to the pattern as a "breast cancer hormone profile." He noticed that women with breast cancer have similar hormone readings on their saliva tests: high estradiol levels, even if they've had a hysterectomy; extremely low progesterone levels; high testosterone levels; and very low DHEA-S, which he remarks is a hallmark of most cancers.[10] Could it be that a saliva test may be predictive of breast cancer? Perhaps such testing methods could be used right now, as an adjunct to tumor-imaging procedures. Your doctor may be unaware of saliva testing. (Read more about saliva testing in Chapter 2.)

Bottom line: Some forms of ERT may be safer than others. There are actually three forms of estrogen active in women: estradiol, estrone, and estriol. Estradiol is the primary estrogen produced by the ovary. It is converted first into the weaker form, estrone, and then into its weakest dilution, estriol. Estradiol and estrone are thought to be the estrogens primarily responsible for facilitating breast cancer. Estriol not only does not stimulate breast tissue growth, it is actually protective against breast cancer.[11] Although your doctor may be unaware of ERT or HRT options that utilize estriol, this third estrogen has been studied and used in Europe for well over sixty years.

Some prominent physicians and cancer specialists are offering to their patients what they believe is a safer version of ERT: a combination of 80 percent estriol, 10 percent estrone, and 10 percent estradiol. This formula is not patented but can be formulated by any compounding pharmacy at your doctor's request. (See Chapter 2 for a further discussion of conventional versus natural hormonal therapies; see also the Resources section, at the end of the book, for more information on these potentially gentler forms of hormonal therapy.)

≈ Risk Factors ≈

Being aware of the risks that predispose you to any disease can save your life if you use the information to take aggressive precautionary measures. It is estimated that about 30 percent of women who develop breast cancer have at least one of the risk factors listed in the sidebar to the right. However, it is the 70 percent of women who do not identify themselves as potential cancer victims that concerns me: They may harbor a false sense of security. It is important for all women to learn how best to protect their bodies.

When a disease is as mysterious as cancer and has so many risk factors, we may freeze at the seemingly impossible task of prevention. It is true that a variety of things we eat, breathe, and come into contact with have carcinogenic (cancer-causing) potential. It has been estimated that 90 percent of all cancers are environmentally caused. The good news is we can identify many of those potentially harmful substances and thus adopt some safeguards to keep cancer from invading our bodies.

Risk Factors for Breast Cancer

- **Heredity:** Risk is greater for those whose mothers, aunts, or sisters have had it.
- **Age:** Older women are more at risk.
- **Country of birth:** North American and northern European women have increased risk.
- **Socioeconomic class:** Higher-income families have increased risk.
- **Marital status:** Never-married women have higher risk.
- **Menarche:** Early menarche (under twelve years) increases risk.
- **Menopause:** Late menopause (over fifty-five years) increases risk.
- **Childbearing experience:** Having had no children or having a first child after age thirty increases risk.
- **Weight:** Being overweight increases risk.
- **Shape:** Having extra weight distributed in the upper body and stomach, rather than in the hips and thighs, increases risk.
- **Diet:** A poor diet (high fat, low fiber, low intake of vitamins A, E, C, and selenium) increases risk.

Diet

One of the breakthroughs of the 1980s was the finding that diet leads other factors in beating cancer. Hard data now exist to prove that specific nutrients can appreciably lower cancer risk.

The conservative American Dietetic Association estimates that 30 to 60 percent of all cancer is nutrition related.[12] Most of the support for these findings comes from years of population studies. Scientists have long suspected a link as they observed that countries in which people primarily eat high-fat diets—such as the United States, the United Kingdom, and the Netherlands—suffer the world's highest rates of breast cancer, while countries with leaner diets—such as Japan, Thailand, and Poland—have much lower rates. At one time heredity was thought to explain this difference, but the data have since proved otherwise. A landmark 1973 study conducted by a division of the National Cancer Institute showed that second-generation Japanese women who had lived in California all their lives had breast cancer rates similar to European Americans. Studies from many other countries reach the same conclusion.

Research shows that eating properly may help to prevent breast cancer and may make the cancer more amenable to treatment if it does occur. According to Sherwood Gorbach, a researcher at Tufts University School of Medicine, in Boston, all other risk factors taken together do not appear to bear anywhere near the importance of lifestyle factors, such as diet.

The evidence is indisputable: Poor diet is a major contributor to cancer. Henry Dreher, former senior writer at the Cancer Research Institute, states, "Scientists from the National Academy of Sciences, the National Cancer Institute, and the American Cancer Society now estimate that 35 percent of all cancers are directly related to diet and the rest may be influenced by it."[13]

The diet that experts now agree will reduce the risk of breast cancer can also reduce the risk of heart disease—and probably many other disease states as well. It is the diet that many nutritionists have advocated for years as the foundation for basic healthy living: Eat foods that are low in fat and high in fiber, and supplement when you are lacking in any nutrients.

If you are seriously concerned about breast cancer because you have several risk factors, or if you want to ensure optimum health, there are precautions you can take. Paying attention to the specific types of fat and fiber you eat and incorporating anticancer nutrients into your program can provide protection from cancer in general and breast cancer in particular.

FAT

Studies examining the relationship between dietary fat and breast cancer are conflicting and thus can be quite confusing. For decades most material suggested that the amount of fat in the diet was causally related to breast cancer, as earlier editions of this book stated. Then in 1996, a classic study of 350,000 women, reported in the *New England Journal of Medicine*, debunked the theory that a high-fat diet increased the risk of breast cancer.[14] Some experts now suggest that the *type* of fat women eat, rather than the *total amount* of dietary fat, can possibly promote or prevent breast cancer.

Animal fat seems to be more directly related to a higher incidence of breast cancer than does fat from vegetables, as studies over the last three decades have consistently found. Going back to the 1970s, to a study conducted by the National Cancer Institute, we find that women who lived in countries with the highest intake of animal fat had the highest rates of breast cancer.[15] Research from the 1980s added credence to this theory, although researchers were at a loss to fully explain why this occurs.[16] A study from the early 1990s also found that breast cancer is associated with a diet high in saturated fat.[17]

While there may not be a clear explanation of the link between animal fat and an increased risk of breast cancer, there is some speculation. Animal fat stimulates bacteria in the colon to synthesize estrogen from cholesterol in the body, thus contributing to excess estrogen in the body. The human body itself manufactures a type of estrogen from its own stores; the more fat one houses, the more estrogen the body can produce. Commercially raised animals contain estrogenic hormones given to them to promote growth, so if our diet is rich in meat and poultry loaded with female hormones, there again lies a potential for excess.

Asian women who consume a native diet including vegetable and soy proteins excrete estrogen at a higher rate than women who do not eat this way; they also have a much lower rate of breast cancer.[18] Soy products as well as other plant foods tend to block estrogen receptors on the cells, minimizing the effect of the more toxic estrogens (see page 217 for more on soy in the prevention of breast cancer). Another way to modulate hyperestrogenism is to eat a high-fiber diet, because dietary fiber increases the excretion of estrogen.[19]

We often attribute Asian women's lower rates of cancer to their lower-fat, higher-soy diets. However, another point needs to be mentioned concerning this population group: Asian women have a higher ratio of estriol in their blood than Western women. One of the pioneers in breast cancer research discovered that women who produce very little estriol relative to estradiol and estrone are at increased risk of developing breast cancer.[20] Sometimes we're too quick to ascribe one factor, such as soy in the Asian diet, to the health of an entire race or population. Let us be reminded that health factors are not generally that clear-cut.

More support exists for the theory that the proportion of the different types of estrogen in a woman's body may affect her risk for breast cancer. An analysis of thirteen dietary fat intervention studies implies that dietary fat reduction can result in lowered serum levels of estradiol (the strongest form of estrogen), which may aid in breast-cancer prevention.[21]

So what should one do with this sometimes confusing array of information? What follows are some pointers for modifying your dietary fat intake—both the total amount and the types.

It is a good idea to limit total dietary fat to no more than 25 to 30 percent of calories. Figuring out how much fat you eat is not too difficult, given all the books available that list fat grams in common foods and the current food-labeling guidelines for packaged products. If you know approximately how many calories you consume in a day, multiply that number by 0.30 for the upper limit of total calories that should come from fat. To arrive at the maximum number of daily fat grams you should eat, divide your answer by nine (there are nine calories in one gram of

fat). Record every bite of food you eat for a week to get an idea of how much fat you actually are taking in. The comparison of your maximum fat-gram intake to your actual intake may surprise you.

Example: 2,000 calories x .30 = 600 calories from fat (maximum recommended intake).

600/9 = no more than 67 fat grams per day.

As I have stated elsewhere in this book, all fats are not created equal. Although limiting total dietary fat is prudent, it is also important to take advantage of the research indicating that the type of fat eaten may be more important than merely the amount eaten.

Animal fats and saturated fats, the ones so convincingly linked to breast cancer in the studies cited above, are not the only fats to avoid. Vegetable oils that have been transformed into margarine and shortening are no better for you. The process of hydrogenation, which converts the oils to solids, creates trans fatty acids, and they, too, cause damage to cells and potentially promote disease. You can find hydrogenated and partially hydrogenated fats in cookies, pies, cakes, french fries, chips, crackers, and dozens of other packaged foods. Check food labels before you buy, and avoid products that include "hydrogenated" or "partially hydrogenated vegetable oils" among their list of ingredients.

Our bodies need certain types and amounts of fat to remain healthy, and certain fats do exist that apparently promote optimum health. Essential fatty acids (EFAs), fats that the body cannot make, are needed for the functioning of nerve cells, cellular membranes, and hormonelike substances known as prostaglandins. Most vegetable oils supply EFAs, and some of these have even been found to promote anticancer activity. According to some scientific literature, the safest oils are believed to be olive oil and canola oil, two monounsaturated oils. A recent Swiss study of over sixty thousand women reported that eating monounsaturated fat reduced the risk of breast cancer by 45 percent.[22]

Omega-3 fatty acids are documented to inhibit tumor production and protect against breast cancer. Flaxseed oil is rich in omega-3 fatty acids.[23]

Other good sources of EFAs are fresh pumpkin seeds, soybean oil, walnut oil, wheat germ oil, and fish oils. Increasing fish in your diet also appears to protect against breast cancer. A study involving twenty-six countries found that an increase in fish consumption was associated with lower breast cancer rates.[24] Your best choices are salmon, mackerel, Florida pompano, herring, bluefish, bluefin tuna, swordfish, and shark.

FIBER

Adding foods high in fiber to your diet may be the second-best precaution you can take against breast cancer. Until recently, research on the role of fiber in relation to cancer had focused on colon cancer, because dietary fiber comes into direct contact with the lining of the digestive tract. Now the benefits of fiber have been shown to extend to breast and other types of cancer too.

Since the 1980s, studies have explored a possible link between fiber and breast cancer. Particularly noteworthy is the observation that Finnish women, who consume as much fat as American women but significantly more fiber, have only two-thirds the incidence of breast cancer.

Experimental evidence has further confirmed the important role of fiber in prevention of breast cancer. In a recent study conducted by the American Health Foundation, in New York, female rats on a high-fat, high-fiber diet were found to be one-third less likely to succumb to breast cancer from a drug-induced breast tumor than those on a high-fat diet alone.[25]

The amount of fiber a woman eats appears to play a part in regulating her estrogen level. Fiber enhances estrogen excretion, which means less of the hormone is reabsorbed into the bloodstream. Thus, the woman's breast tissue is exposed to lower amounts of estrogen. Fiber may also reduce the absorption of fat into the body, thereby also reducing estrogen production. A third possibility is that fiber may bind with and dispose of other carcinogens, keeping them from entering the bloodstream.

Fiber comes in two primary forms: soluble and insoluble. The insoluble, or indigestible, form (also known as bulk or roughage) fights cancer better. Health educators have told us for years that insoluble fiber prevents and treats constipation by sweeping food through the intestinal tract. What has not received publicity is the relationship between constipation and breast cancer. If it were a more acceptable topic of conversation, we would probably place greater stress on the necessity of regular bowel movements. Constipation can be a serious health risk. Women who have two or fewer bowel movements a week have four times the incidence of breast cancer as women who have one or more movements a day.[26]

Insoluble dietary fiber is found in large quantities in bran and whole grains and in smaller amounts in fruits and vegetables. The National Cancer Institute recommends that Americans eat up to thirty grams of dietary fiber a day; other groups suggest as high as forty grams a day. This is more than double what most women currently consume. Make it a priority to figure your fiber intake for a few days to see how close you get to the goal. (See Chapter 15 for a list of high-fiber foods that fight cancer.)

ANTIOXIDANTS

Antioxidant nutrients from fresh fruits and yellow and leafy green vegetables have been associated with a reduced risk for many cancers, including breast cancer. Unfortunately, most American women don't eat the recommended four to five servings of fruits and vegetables per day, so supplementation is essential. Supplementing even in low doses can reduce your risk of cancer. In a major study of fifteen thousand adults in China, a daily dose of antioxidants consisting of 15 mg of beta-carotene, 30 mg of vitamin E, and 50 mg of selenium over a five-year period resulted in a 13 percent reduction in total cancer rates.[27]

For over a decade, pioneer nutritionists have been advocating the use of supplementation, and within the last few years mainstream health practitioners have come out and publicly admitted that it may be a good idea to take additional antioxidants. The first public-health organization to officially recommend vitamin supplements for warding off illnesses such as heart disease and cancer is the Washington, D.C., advocacy group called the Alliance for Aging Research. It advises Americans to take the following antioxidants:

beta-carotene, 15–30 mg, or 17,000–50,000 IU

vitamin C, 250–1,000 mg

vitamin E, 100–400 IU[28]

VITAMIN A AND BETA-CAROTENE

No other nutrient has captured the attention of cancer researchers the way vitamin A or its precursor, beta-carotene, has. Once thought to be effective because it was converted to vitamin A in the body, beta-carotene apparently has an independent role as an antioxidant, as current research suggests.

Studies in the United States and England note a direct relationship between vitamin A intake and cancer rates.[29] At least seventy clinical studies have found that people who do not eat fruits and vegetables (which are high in beta-carotene and other antioxidants) have a greater incidence of cancer. Scientists leave no doubt that low beta-carotene states are associated with an increase in overall cancer death.[30]

Vitamin A requires caution when taken in supplement form, because it can be toxic in large doses. Beta-carotene, however, shows no apparent toxicity, even when used in high doses for therapeutic treatment of medical conditions. What is needed is absorbed, and what is not is excreted. The only hazard associated with taking too much beta-carotene is an orange tint to the skin. The color may clash with your outfit, but it is not harmful and will wear off after the dosage is lowered.

No RDA has yet been established for beta-carotene. A safe daily range is between 15 to 30 mg, or 17,000 to 50,000 IU. It is always a good idea to get what you can of any nutrient from food sources before adding supplements. This is easier for beta-carotene than for some of the other nutrients; good sources of beta-carotene include spinach, carrots, sweet potatoes, winter squash, cantaloupe, and broccoli. (For the precise amount of this nutrient contained in certain foods, consult Appendix C.)

VITAMIN C

Vitamin C is another powerful antioxidant that blocks free-radical damage. It is also a general detoxifier (it removes body toxins or poisons) and is a crucial anticarcinogen. Specifically, it prevents the formation of nitrosamines, potent carcinogens formed from nitrates and nitrites that are found in meats that are smoked, pickled, and salt-cured.

As with beta-carotene, low intakes of vitamin C are associated with increased cancer risk.[31] While no tests have looked directly at vitamin C and breast cancer, factors initiating one type of cancer may be associated with other cancers as well. Studies indicate a strong protective effect of vitamin C for non–hormone-dependent cancers. And an analysis of forty-six studies found that in thirty-three there was a statistically significant degree of protection with high intakes of vitamin C, approximately twice that associated with a low intake of the vitamin.[32]

How much vitamin C is enough to protect the body from disease without exceeding toxic limits? Reviews on the safety of vitamin C fill the literature. At the high end are those who support extreme doses, up to 10,000 mg daily. Therapeutic doses of this magnitude are indicated for some conditions; however, for preventive measures and relatively healthy individuals, the dosage need not reach the ceiling. You may want to experiment with amounts by taking up to 5,000 mg (the upper limit of the safety range) and noticing when your stools turn watery. Richard Cathcart, a noted vitamin C expert, came up with the concept of bowel tolerance. He feels that if your body needs vitamin C, it will absorb it; if not, the excess will be excreted. Some people may stop at 100 mg, some at 6,000 mg. Good sources of vitamin C include raw green peppers, orange juice, broccoli, cantaloupe, strawberries, potatoes, and raw tomatoes. (For the precise amount of this nutrient contained in certain foods, consult Appendix C.)

VITAMIN E

Vitamin E has been under study for several years as a major antioxidant. It is especially effective in blocking the free-radical formation that comes from the oxidation

of fats.[33] The process by which fatty foods and oils turn rancid in the presence of oxygen is thought to be a prime contributing cause of breast and colon cancer, and vitamin E is seen as a major ally against it. In addition to its role as a free-radical scavenger, vitamin E enhances the body's immune response and inhibits the conversion of nitrates to the cancer-producing nitrosamines.

Most data support the hypothesis that dietary vitamin E protects against cancer. Women with low blood levels of vitamin E have a much higher risk for breast cancer. In one study, blood levels of vitamin E were correlated with cancer incidence. The analysis revealed that individuals with low levels of vitamin E had about 1.5 times the risk of those who had a higher blood concentration.[34] In a fourteen-year study of more than five thousand women in the United Kingdom, low levels of vitamin E were found to increase the incidence of breast cancer by 500 percent.[35]

A reasonable and safe amount of vitamin E for optimum protection is between 400 and 600 IU daily. For those concerned with vitamin toxicity, a comprehensive review of the literature states that vitamin E is safe in doses up to 3,000 IU per day.[36] A word of caution for people with special problems: Vitamin E intake should always be monitored by a physician if you are taking an anticlotting drug or if you have high blood pressure, liver disease, biliary-tract obstruction, or malabsorption syndrome. Good sources of vitamin E include sunflower seeds, almonds, crab, sweet potatoes, fish, and wheat germ. (For the precise amount of this nutrient contained in certain foods, consult Appendix C.)

SELENIUM

Vitamin E works best to prevent cancer when it is teamed with the mineral selenium. Together, they form part of a potent anticancer enzyme system that wipes out renegade free radicals. When researchers in Finland examined cancer patients, they found that low levels of selenium increased the risk for cancer, but low selenium plus low vitamin E levels increased the risk even more.[37] More than fifty-five different studies conducted in eighteen countries show that the higher the selenium intake, the lower the incidence of breast, colon, and prostate cancer.[38] The National Academy of Sciences has recommended 50 to 200 mcg of selenium daily as a safe range. However, many other scientists feel this level is too low to offer protection. Professors at Cornell University, in New York, suggest 600 mcg as offering a greater degree of protection that is still safe.[39] When choosing supplemental selenium, look for an organic form, as it is better absorbed and less likely to cause toxicity than the inorganic sodium selenite form. Good sources of selenium include lobster, tuna, shrimp, fish, ham, eggs, chicken, and whole-grain bread. (For the precise amount of this nutrient contained in certain foods, consult Appendix C.)

SOY, FLAXSEED, AND OTHER ANTICANCER FOODS

Besides the benefits soy apparently conveys in reducing menopausal symptoms such as hot flashes (see Chapter 3), diets containing high amounts of soy-based phyto-hormones have been correlated with a substantial reduction in breast cancer risk. Soybean consumption is thought to be one of the primary reasons for the relatively low rates of breast cancer in Japan and China. In a case-controlled study of diet and breast cancer among Singapore Chinese, it was found that soy protein had a pro-tective effect.[40] Beta-carotene was also found protective in premenopausal women, and a high intake of animal protein and red meat was associated with increased risk.

Soy's major influence appears to be its antiestrogenic effect. Soy seems to lengthen the menstrual cycle by one to five days, thus reducing the body's exposure to estrogen and cutting the risk of breast cancer. Asian women are known to have longer menstrual cycles than Western women, as well as a lower risk of breast can-cer. An Australian study, after adjusting for possible mitigating factors such as age, parity (whether or not the woman had given birth), and alcohol and fat intake, like-wise found a substantial association between phytoestrogen intake (as measured by urinary excretion) and the risk of breast cancer. The researchers concluded that the reduction in risk they found among women who consumed significantly higher amounts of phytoestrogens was unlikely to have resulted from mere chance.[41]

Studies continue to mount that demonstrate that soy foods contribute to breast health. Two human studies show that the higher the levels of soy isoflavones in the body, when the isoflavones come from eating whole soy foods (rather than from swallowing pills), the smaller the chance that the individual will be diagnosed with breast cancer. Three more studies indicate that soy-isoflavone consumption exerts cancer-protective effects by decreasing estrogen synthesis and deactivating cancer-causing metabolites. Furthermore, evidence now shows that isoflavones can block proliferation of breast cancer cells caused by environmental estrogens. You can easily check out this research for yourself by accessing the Internet site www.doctors@revivalsoy.com, a website operated by Physicians Laboratories, a group of doctors who are researching the effects of soy and conducting double-blinded human clinical studies on soy. (Physicians Laboratories also develops and sells Revival brand soy products.)

A Physicians Laboratory product is being tested to treat potential breast can-cer patients and breast cancer survivors. Using a new type of breast imaging called B.E.S.T. (breast enhanced scintigraphy testing), doctors are able to distinguish between normal breast tissue, inflammation of the breast (a precursor to breast can-cer), and breast cancer. Women who had either signs of inflammation in breast tis-sue or breast cancer itself drank a Revival soy drink daily. The study data demonstrated

a statistically significant improvement in breast inflammation among twenty-five women who followed a daily regimen of soy protein for six months. Other than the supplementation with soy protein, no dietary or lifestyle changes were reported by the women during follow-up evaluation.

For women who want to supplement their diet with soy but can't tolerate tofu and tempeh, Revival is easy to use. One packet a day provides the same amount of isoflavones as a typical Asian diet, the amount recommended for therapeutic benefit.

Experts generally agree that when estrogen levels stay elevated for too long, a woman's risk of breast cancer increases. Reducing the effect of estrogen, it is widely believed, can produce a four- to five-fold reduction in breast cancer. One way to curtail estrogen production is to block the body's estrogen receptors before they can be filled with estradiol, the strongest form of estrogen. Genistein and daidzein, two isoflavones in soy, attach to the receptors in the breast and block estradiol, which is known to stimulate cancer cells in the breast. Two popular anti-cancer prescription drugs, tamoxifen and raloxifene, work the same way. But whereas tamoxifen also stimulates uterine cells, phytoestrogens actually appear to exert a positive influence on uterine cells. Phytoestrogen-containing foods, therefore, have also been studied in relation to uterine cancer. The Cancer Research Center of Hawaii studied 332 women from many different ethnic backgrounds and compared them to a control group. The study found that women who ate the most foods rich in phytoestrogens, including tofu and beans, saw a 54 percent reduction in the risk of uterine cancer.[42]

Good options for increasing soy in your diet are tofu, tempeh, soy milk, fresh or roasted soy beans, and soy flours. (See also Chapter 3 for a discussion of soy supplements, and Chapter 15 for more tips on adding soy to your diet.)

Soy and flaxseed (another food rich in phytoestrogens) both contain lignans, another plant compound thought to reduce both estrogen exposure and cancer risk. Lignans are substances that are changed by friendly bacteria in the intestines into compounds that fight cancer. Like phytohormones, they fill estrogen receptors and thus block normal estrogen activity. Studies have shown that breast cancer patients excrete lower amounts of lignans than healthy women. Lignans, though contained in many plants such as fruits, legumes, vegetables, and grains, are found in the greatest concentration in flaxseed (not the oil, just the seeds). The National Cancer Institute is reviewing flaxseed as a potential cancer fighter because it contains both lignans and omega-3 fatty acids, whose benefits we reviewed earlier in this chapter.

That we should eat a variety of foods is good basic nutritional advice. Although specific nutrients, such as phytohormones and lignans, have been singled out and studied in cancer prevention, other foods with unknown properties have also demonstrated cancer-fighting qualities. For example, cruciferous vegetables, a unique group of vegetables from the cabbage family, appear to inhibit the formation of cancer cells. These foods contain both sulfur and indoles, substances thought to deactivate carcinogens and protect against cell destruction. The plant chemical contained in the compound indole-3 carbinol also alters estrogen metabolism, possibly reducing cancer risk.[43] Cruciferous vegetables include broccoli, Brussels sprouts, cauliflower, and cabbage.

Studies on a variety of other foods continue to add to the research. Among the proposed cancer fighters are yogurt, seaweed, garlic, lima beans, green tea, licorice root, parsley, and rosemary.

⇒ Exercise ⇐

The first study specifically designed to investigate whether regular exercise can reduce a woman's risk of breast cancer was reported in 1994. Studying a group of more than one thousand women, researchers from the University of Southern California found that women who exercised at least four hours a week during their reproductive years had a 58 percent lower breast cancer risk. Those who spent one to three hours a week exercising cut their risk by 30 percent.[44] Even though the study focused on younger women, who are less likely to develop breast cancer, the results are exciting and substantiate what we know: Ways exist for women to take health care into their own hands and effect a change.

Previous studies have suggested that physical activity can modify menstrual-cycle patterns and reduce the frequency of ovulation, thus lessening a woman's exposure to estrogen.

⇒ Emotions ⇐

Women with breast cancer often share a similar emotional makeup as well as a physiological one. Of course variations occur, but, generally speaking, many women with breast cancer tend to suppress their emotions, often putting others' needs before their own. Sometimes women completely lose touch with themselves and their priorities because they get so wrapped up in the problems of others. Christiane Northrup, M.D., has noticed in her practice that the refusal to honor and express emotions can sometimes reach a pathological extreme.[45] I don't think we women have to give up our caregiving role entirely, but we do need to pay attention to when it becomes a negative rather than a positive force in our lives. Getting away from obligations for a day, weekend, or extended vacation can oftentimes provide the perspective we

need to see our relationships more clearly. Some women may require individual counseling or a support group to help them set realistic boundaries.

There are reams of scientific studies addressing one's emotional style and its impact on breast cancer. One such study included 119 women between the ages of twenty and seventy who were referred for a breast biopsy because of a suspicious lesion. They were asked to look into their most difficult life events (death, divorce, loss of job) for up to five years before discovery of the breast symptoms. After tallying the data, the authors arrived at what they termed a "key message." Women with breast cancer often endure severe life events in the five years before diagnosis, and the way they deal with these events may put them at risk for breast cancer.[46] The role played by stress is a thread that runs through all disease states. Learning how to cope with stress is a skill that requires serious attention. Another study verified something we women know is paramount to good health: having friends and acquaintances who encourage and support us. Patients with breast cancer who went to weekly group therapy for a year lived significantly longer (an average of eighteen months) than a similar control group.[47] Not only is social support important in coping with stress, it may be critical to survival itself.

Potential Sources of Cancer

- **pesticides** (the Environmental Protection Agency identifies sixty-four pesticides as potentially cancer-causing)
- **formaldehyde** (industrial solvent used in rugs and plastics)
- **coal tar**–based food colorings
- **nitrates and nitrites** (found in foods such as hot dogs, bacon, and luncheon meats)
- **smoked foods** (bacon, ham, fish, and cheese)
- **burned proteins** from charred meats
- **cyclamates;** saccharin (artificial sweeteners)
- **radiation** (low doses accumulate in the body)
- **tobacco** (including secondhand smoke)
- **alcohol** (taking more than nine drinks per week is associated with increased breast cancer risk)
- **aflatoxins** (found in moldy nuts, seeds, and grains)
- **DES** (diethylstilbestrol, a synthetic estrogen)
- **DDT** (although banned in the United States, other countries still use this pesticide and send their products to the United States)

Potential Carcinogens

It has been said that the majority of all cancers are caused by the environment and are thus preventable. Cancer has been linked to things we eat, breathe, and are exposed to for a length of time. Without becoming paranoid, we need to be aware of potential cancer promoters and avoid them when possible. For example, eating organically grown foods without the addition of synthetic chemicals, pesticides, and herbicides is seriously worth considering. For a list of potential carcinogens, see the sidebar.

≫ **Preventive Screening** ≪

Finally, sometimes our fear stops us from doing the very things that could save our lives. Early detection and treatment of breast cancer significantly reduces the probability of death, yet many of us either do not take the time for preventive care, or we just neglect simple measures. Within the last couple of years both breast self-examination and mammograms have come under fire because they supposedly do not reduce a woman's chances of dying from breast cancer. Maybe we need to look at these tests more realistically and agree that they are not foolproof; sometimes cancer sneaks in anyway. Still, I think that to check ourselves regularly and to learn about our bodies is an extremely powerful tool; no matter what the studies say, we can only benefit by continuing to pay attention to what and how we feel. For this reason, I encourage you to learn how to examine your breasts for lumps. Regarding mammograms, maybe we don't all need a yearly one after age fifty, but who is to say with certainty who does and who does not? As for myself, I try to hold off longer between X rays. Because I've been exposed to so much radiation in my lifetime, and since its effects are cumulative, each X ray I get increases the number on my risk-factor scorecard.

You must use your intuition and judgment and decide for yourself, but don't ignore preventive testing entirely. I've heard too many stories about women who went in for a routine exam and were saved because of it. There are a variety of options these days for detection of breast problems: mammography, sonograms/ultrasound, and possibly saliva testing. Consult with different experts and a breast-imaging specialist to find a diagnostic approach that makes sense to you.

CHAPTER 11

MORE THAN SKIN DEEP

I have some lines in my face from 50 years of life. They tell me of years in the sun, of sorrows and joys. They tell me of time. They tell me I have lived and that I am still alive. They can't be erased. They can be softened.... Do I long to be the smooth-skinned, freckle-faced kid I once was? No. I long for the same thing today that I longed for then: to be the best I am able to be.

— KAYLAN PICKFORD, *Always a Woman*

How many of us are willing to admit that we don't always share these lovely sentiments? As mature adults we would like to, but looking into the mirror each morning to find pillow creases etched on our cheeks, we wonder how long it will be until they last all day. What cream can we purchase to smooth out the newly formed lines? What miracle cure will erase these indelible furrows?

The first visible signs of aging appear in the largest and most public organ we have: our skin. A woman may feel young, think young, and act young, but if her face is lined, society will remind her that she has "crossed over" into middle age. And while men seem to profit by their character lines and graying temples, signs of aging are not admired in women.

A woman who is noticeably in the prime of her life may not appear on the cover of fashion and beauty magazines geared toward the young, but in the real world where we all live, I find that women are not as obsessed with fine lines and age spots as we are led to believe. We want to look our best, but the panic that fills the literature seems less pervasive in the majority of women I talk to at seminars. Hopefully, the time will come when we even appreciate the real beauty of the mature look, as they do in some foreign countries.

I am not suggesting we give up trying to look as good as we can. How I look has always been important to me, and I avail myself of many health and beauty tips. I am saying that we should do all we can to present our best image, then get on with the really important matters of life.

Knowing how our bodies change and how those changes affect the skin enables us to take precautions to prevent premature aging and maintain healthy skin.

⤳ Basic Skin Anatomy ⤶

The skin contains one-fourth of the body's blood supply, two million or so sweat glands, and even more nerve endings, hair follicles, and sebaceous glands. It performs many necessary functions: helping the body regulate temperature, eliminating waste products and toxins, and protecting the body from invading germs and harmful environmental conditions. It is an organ we must care for both inside and out.

From the moment we are born, the skin is continually renewing itself. At any given time, approximately one-fourth of the cells are developing, one-half are mature, and one-fourth are degenerating. It is said that the human body gets a new outer skin every twenty-seven days, from birth to death. That means that what you are doing to or for your body today will show up in your skin next month.

There are three basic layers and several sublayers of skin, and it is deep within the body that healthy skin is conceived. The underskin, filled with blood vessels, nerve endings, fat cells, hair follicles, and connective tissue, is the life-support system that transports nutrients to the visible external layer. Yet our outermost wrapping, or epidermis, is often the only part of the skin to which we pay attention.

As we approach menopause, and even sooner for some women, several changes occur in the skin: The underlying fat layer diminishes; collagen and elastin, the skin's structural support system, lose elasticity, gradually yielding less moisture; sweat glands function less vigorously; and the body's natural protection against the sun is reduced. If precautions are not taken internally and externally, a dry, sagging skin is likely to result.

Somewhere around age thirty-five, external evidence of aging begins to show on the face. Because skin cells are regenerating at a slower rate, as are all body cells, it takes more time for a fresh supply of cells to reach the surface. The dead outer covering that remains is now exposed to the elements for a longer time, resulting in a dehydrated texture. A general loss of oil and moisture makes the skin thinner and less flexible. Dryness develops; fine lines and wrinkles emerge.

⤳ Skin Changes with Age ⤶

How fast the skin ages depends primarily on heredity and partly on a person's lifestyle and skin-care regimen. We can accelerate or postpone signs of aging by manipulating both our external and internal environment. All we do to and for our bodies is eventually reflected in the skin, which is a mirror of our internal condition. If we choose to live in the fast lane—smoking, drinking to excess, eating junk foods, worshiping the sun—we will accelerate cellular destruction. If we avoid these excesses, or at least take precautions against their effects, and concentrate on nourishing and rebuilding healthy cells, we can greatly enhance a healthy appearance.

GENETICS

Our genetic makeup predetermines much of our aging pattern. People with darker, thicker, more oily skin show fewer wrinkles than people with fair skin, because the heavily pigmented outer layer protects the interior cells from the harmful effects of the sun. Men generally do not exhibit fine lines as early as women because their skin is normally thicker and because many of them follow a daily skin-care program that helps to remove dead skin cells: They shave.

ACNE

Most of us consider wrinkles and age spots the major skin problems of the midlife years, but some women experience a return to adolescence in the form of acne. Unsightly pimples sometimes occur in women during perimenopause, when hormones tend to fluctuate most unpredictably. Women who have enjoyed smooth complexions may complain of preteen skin problems. The situation usually takes care of itself in time, but who wants to wait? Some women find that a natural progesterone cream works to combat acne when applied during the second half of their cycles. Severe cases of acne can often be treated with a prescription of retinoic acid (a form of vitamin A). While retinoic acid is effective, it can irritate sensitive skin. Over-the-counter products containing glycolic and citric acids are less expensive and seem to work just as well.

COLOR CHANGES

The color of the skin changes with age. Skin pigmentation that was once uniform becomes variegated. Since the skin is susceptible to many influences, it is difficult to determine whether the cause is temporary hormonal imbalance, normal aging, or discoloration due to sun exposure. Age spots—or more appropriately, sun spots, since they are caused by overexposure to the sun—multiply with each passing year.

I wish we had all known thirty years ago, when we basked at the beach for hours, that our short-lived tans would come back to haunt us in unsightly patches on our hands and body.

☙ Hormones ❧

Estrogen receptors cover the skin; thus it seems reasonable that when estrogen dwindles, wrinkles appear. Estrogen participates in determining skin thickness as well as the amount of collagen our skin holds. As we age and lose estrogen, we notice a general loss of skin elasticity and increased dryness, not just on our face but all over the body. Given these hard facts, one would think that replacing the lost estrogen would turn back the clock and restore our youthful face and body. Many studies have looked at oral hormone replacement to see if it does prevent skin from aging, but the conclusion at this time is unclear. While some studies show that oral estrogen does prevent and restore loss of collagen, others have not found this to be true. Women taking estrogen are mixed on the results as well. Some swear they look better taking estrogen, and others haven't noticed an appreciable difference.

Estrogen creams and phytoestrogen creams reportedly work well when combined with common moisturizers, and many women subjectively feel these products enhance their appearance. Because wrinkle creams are highly profitable, studies using topical estrogens are vigorously being conducted throughout the world, some with favorable results. In one study in Austria, fifty-nine premenopausal women with noticeable aging skin took either 0.1 percent estradiol or 0.3 percent estriol for six months. In both groups researchers noted a marked improvement in elasticity and firmness of the skin; wrinkle depth and pore sizes decreased by 61 to 100 percent.[1] The authors commented that estradiol may cause systemic side effects, whereas the biologically weaker estriol did not. The conclusion of the study suggested that estriol represents a new and promising therapeutic approach toward aging skin in perimenopausal women.

☙ Caring for Your Skin from Within ❧

The condition of your skin is a fairly accurate gauge of how well you are treating your body. If you have been neglecting your health or have been under greater than normal pressure and tension, your skin will let you know. Fortunately, the skin will also respond to positive changes in lifestyle more quickly than any other organ. Learn to deal with your stress; refrain from eating highly processed foods; stop smoking, drinking too much alcohol, and basking in the sun; feed your body with good food and drink plenty of water; and see how your skin reacts.

A healthy lifestyle is basic to healthy skin. An imbalance or inadequate supply of nutrients can surface on the skin. Chronic dieters who are not eating adequate fat or protein often set themselves up for dry skin and dull hair. Women who are eating adequately and still notice these conditions need to consider other possibilities. They may have a genetic susceptibility to skin and hair problems. They may suffer some other medical condition, such as an allergy, that could cause an outward reaction. They may be taking medication that produces changes in the skin or hair as a side effect. Or they may not be absorbing the nutrients their bodies need for a healthy appearance. For example, alcohol hinders the body's ability to absorb several of the B vitamins and disrupts levels of magnesium, potassium, and zinc. Foods high in saturated fats and concentrated sugars demand greater nutrient requirements for absorption. When the diet consists primarily of these types of foods, there occurs a chance of undernutrition, which can show up on the skin. (See the sidebar to the right for more on what nutrients contribute to the health of your skin.)

⮕ Keeping Skin Healthy Inside and Out ⬅

MOISTURE IS ESSENTIAL

Any element that draws moisture out of the skin, internally or externally, will result in drying and wrinkling. Be aware of aspects of your environment—air conditioning, steam heating, smog, pollution, wind, and sunlight, for example—that affect your skin, and take steps to minimize their dehydrating effects. Avoid using harsh soaps and applying heavy makeup since these, too, reduce natural moisture. As women age, they tend to apply extra makeup. Not only is extra makeup ineffective for hiding lines and wrinkles; it actually accentuates them. Let the skin breathe by using more moisturizer and less cover-up.

There are many ways to add moisture to your home environment. For instance, you can keep your bathtub filled with water when you are at home; the evaporation of water molecules moistens the air and hydrates the skin. You may want to purchase a large aquarium or fill your home with large plants and bouquets of flowers in oversized vases, enhancing the loveliness of your surroundings while moisturizing your skin.

SKIN-CARE PRODUCTS

Adding moisturizer to your skin and protecting the innermost layers becomes more crucial with each passing year. Several safe products on the market can plump up the tissue under the surface of the skin, smooth out lines and wrinkles, and nourish beneath the external layers as well. Which moisturizers will work best for you? It depends on the ingredients and how sensitive your skin is. Don't assume that your moisturizer must be expensive. *Consumer Reports* tested forty-eight moisturizers and found that the most effective creams and lotions were the least expensive. Look for the one with the fewest ingredients. The more ingredients in a moisturizer—perfumes, colors, thickeners, emulsifiers—the greater the chance of an allergic reaction.

It was once thought that skin creams did not penetrate the epidermis; now we know this is not true. So before you put anything on your face, check the ingredients to make sure there is nothing harmful in the product, such as alcohol, preservatives, fragrances, coloring, mineral oil, lanolin, or petroleum.

Skin-care product labels are often confusing. Manufacturers are not required to list all ingredients or to indicate whether their sources are natural or synthetic. The use of synthetic ingredients, some of which are proven or suspected carcinogens (quaternium-15, formaldehyde, methylparaben, propylparaben, hexachloraphene, NDELA [nitrosodiethanolamine], TEA [triethanolamine]), is especially problematic in lotions or creams that are designed to stay on the body for long periods of time (twelve hours). Immediate allergic reactions and irritations are obvious dangers, but what about the effects of continuous absorption of a potentially harmful chemical over the course of several years?

Certain natural-product manufacturers have recently taken the initiative in developing safe skin-care products. A major improvement is the substitution of natural vegetable oils for mineral oil as the base for body and facial lotions. Mineral oil, a petroleum derivative, is difficult to remove from the skin and can actually clog

Nutrients and Skin Health

All vitamins, minerals, and amino acids guard in one way or another against cellular destruction, premature aging, and dry and wrinkled skin.

- **Vitamin A:** Keeps tissues soft and healthy; guards against scaling and drying; acts as an antioxidant. Vitamins A and D and the mineral zinc may be applied externally for acne-related problems.

- **B-complex vitamins:** Assist in tissue repair; prevent skin eruptions and hair loss; promote a healthy nervous system; improve circulation; regulate body secretions.

- **Vitamin B-6:** Aids in the utilization of DNA and RNA (basic to the process of cell reproduction).

- **Niacin:** Improves circulation and reduces cholesterol; keeps skin, gums, and digestive tissues healthy.

- **PABA (para-aminobenzoic acid):** Stimulates intestinal bacteria.

- **Vitamin C:** Acts as an antioxidant; essential for healing and the formation of collagen; prevents capillary breakage.

- **Vitamin E:** Acts as an antioxidant; maintains healthy cellular respiration within the muscles.

- **Essential fatty acids (EFAs):** Lubricate skin and hair; prevent dandruff, hair loss, and dry skin.

- **Iodine:** Essential for normal thyroid activity; necessary for healthy skin, hair, and nails.

- **Zinc:** Forms collagen for binding cells together as tissues.

- **Iron:** Vital for blood formation; a deficiency can cause dry skin.

pores and cause blemishes. As it inhibits the ability of the skin to produce its own oils, it can worsen an already dry skin condition. Olive, wheat germ, safflower, sesame, almond, apricot kernel, and avocado oils are closer in composition to the natural secretions of the skin. Most of them are also rich in linoleic acid, an essential fatty acid that aids in skin-cell renewal. Some manufacturers have also replaced synthetic coloring and scents with herbal extracts and powdered flowers, such as rose, iris, orange blossom, lavender, and chamomile.

Plant products that gently exfoliate the top layer of the skin smooth fine lines and lighten the brown spots that crop up as we age. Alpha-hydroxy acids are natural fruit-sugar acids that sometimes come mixed with progesterone cream or moisturizing lotions. They are available in various concentrations; most require an 8 to 10 percent dosage in order to be effective.

EXERCISE

Exercise is vital to vibrant skin and a healthy body. A strenuous workout will increase your circulation, enhance the absorption of nutrients, and stimulate collagen production. Go out for an early morning walk and notice how pink and healthy your skin looks throughout the day.

UNCONSCIOUS FACIAL EXPRESSIONS

Many of the facial cracks and creases we develop are due less to aging than to habitual facial expressions and unconscious grimaces. Constant squinting, scowling, smiling, or frowning eventually will leave permanent imprints on the face. To avoid this, some women have even learned to control their smiles. In a television interview, actress Morgan Fairchild demonstrated how she had taught herself to "laugh down" so that crow's feet and other laugh lines would not form on her face. I tried her exercise in front of a mirror and it was not easy. On a more practical level, try to avoid unnecessary squinting (especially when outside or reading) and frowning. The furrowed brows and tight lips characteristic of scowlers are among the most unpleasant of all permanent expressions.

SMOKING

Over a period of years, lines form around the lips of cigarette smokers because every puff on a cigarette causes the muscles around the mouth to contract. More important, smoking reduces the body's oxygen level, which affects circulation—the primary source of nutrition for all cells. Some authorities suggest that the lower estrogen levels associated with both cigarette smoking and perimenopausal women may further accelerate premature wrinkling. The more heavily you smoke, the more quickly and severely your skin will age. Probably the best all-around good health advice, for a variety of reasons, is to quit smoking.

ALCOHOL

Alcohol in excess impairs the functioning of the liver, which, in turn, affects every other organ in the body. In the skin, it can contribute to broken or enlarged capillaries near the surface. If you are drinking too much, you will have facial redness or blotchiness, particularly on the cheeks and nose; dullness or poor texture; and excessive wrinkles from the drying effect.

STRESS

Stress obviously touches every organ and system in the body, and no skin treatment—aside from massage—will alleviate it. Lack of sleep, overwork, and unresolved issues can manifest on the face and eyes. We have all had times in our lives when no amount of makeup could hide the turbulence. Stress inhibits our digestive processes, prevents absorption of nutrients, and creates a greater need for good nutrition and eating habits. Be kind to your body when it is going through emotional stress, and you will be less likely to see the strain mirrored on your face.

THE SUN

Up to 90 percent of the skin changes we once associated with normal aging—including wrinkling, sagging, and a leathery appearance—may actually be a result of damage from the sun and ultraviolet (UV) radiation.[2] UV radiation damages the skin's elastic fibers and causes them to thicken while reducing the amount of collagen in the skin, thereby decreasing the skin's ability to hold water. Wrinkling, broken capillaries, age spots, and darker pigmentation may all be more visible with increased exposure to UV radiation.

To protect yourself from premature aging from the sun, avoid direct exposure between the hours of 10:00 A.M. and 3:00 P.M. Wear a hat and long sleeves, and apply a sunscreen anytime you are out for more than half an hour. You are subject to the sun's rays even when you ride in a car, sit in the shade, or are out on a hazy day.

Sunscreens offer the best protection against both UVA (ultraviolet A) and UVB (ultraviolet B) radiation, but read labels and find one that assures both UVA and UVB, or broad-spectrum, protection. The shorter UVA rays do the most visible damage, cause sunburn, and can be more dangerous, causing skin cancer. UVA effects are heightened during the midday hours from May to September. The longer

UVB rays are present all day long whenever there is visible light. They may not result in a burn, but when combined with UVA, they can also lead to skin cancer.

Experts vary on the best sun protective factor (SPF) rating to use; suggestions range from fifteen to fifty. If you are fair skinned or have a tendency to burn, a higher number will be more protective.

There is recent debate about whether sunscreen blocks the conversion of vitamin D in the body. This may be of concern if you are cautiously avoiding the sun and fully covering up when you are outside. If no part of your body sees natural light, consider taking a multiple-vitamin supplement with 400 IU of vitamin D.

When you are in the sun, do not use perfume, drink alcohol, or take diuretics, antibiotics, or hormones of any kind. Tetracycline and sulfa drugs produce rashes in the sun; cortisone can cause inflammation around the hair follicles; birth-control pills and hormones can discolor the skin; and Valium can bring on measle-like eruptions if the skin is overexposed. Many other photosensitive drugs and chemicals can cause scales, pimples, or rashes on the skin.

Sun rays are very harmful to the skin and body and can cause skin cancer and melanomas. Heed the warnings and cautiously enjoy your outdoor activities.

A Basic Skin-Care Regimen

To learn about treating the aging skin externally, I interviewed Vera Brown, noted beauty and skin-care expert and owner of Vera's Natural Beauty Retreat and Vera's in the Glen, in Beverly Glen, California. During our afternoon together, Vera explained the fundamentals that all women should follow to keep their skin healthy, as well as the special problems that arise at menopause.

Not only did Vera teach me the basics of skin care, she also offered personal insights into some of the concerns of menopausal women. Many midlife women she sees are extremely unhappy with themselves. They feel their skin and their bodies don't look like they used to, and they feel so badly that it colors their entire life.

Vera gently tells the midlife women who walk through her door that now is the time to start pampering themselves, to give themselves strokes, to be nice to themselves. Instead of looking in the mirror in the morning and being unhappy with what you see, she says, change your outlook. Look at yourself and realize how lucky you are to be alive, how wonderful it is that we now have information about how to feel better and look better, and how blessed we are to live in a time of so many discoveries that will help us through the change. Skin care is vitally important, but don't lose sight of the true meaning of life.

Vera is past eighty now and more lovely both inside and out than the day I first interviewed her. Her skin radiates the beauty within her soul. Vera gave me a book, *Amazing Women, Amazing World*, by Marsh Engle. In one section the book speaks about what it means to be beautiful. Engle writes, "Simply by looking into her spirit, I can see beauty in every woman." Wouldn't it be great if we all shared that sentiment and recognized each other's inward beauty, rather than crow's feet and brown spots.

One of the secrets Vera teaches is that skin care isn't just about applying one cream after another. It's about closing the door in the morning and evening to create privacy, to create a time when you will do something only for yourself. Think about your day: You arise, dress, wash your face, eat breakfast, talk on the phone, make appointments, see people—and all your energy is going out, out, out. How often do you sit down, take a deep breath, wash your hands, rub them together, bring the energy back into your face, and do a simple skin-care routine? It may be just washing your face, but use loving strokes, bringing the circulation back into your skin. You will feel better—physically and emotionally—and you will look better. You will be doing something for yourself.

What follows are Vera's recommendations for a daily skin-care routine.

CLEANSING THE SKIN

Any basic skin-care program starts with a cleanser void of lanolin or mineral oil. You want to use a cleanser that penetrates the skin, because the most important thing about skin care is to keep the skin clean. Nothing is more important. Many women who wear makeup just use soap and water to remove it, and they are not getting a deep enough cleansing. You need a cleanser that actually penetrates the pores. Use a glycerine soap for the face or another mild soap made without lye, synthetic fragrance, synthetic colors, or preservatives. Fancy soaps are best reserved to impress guests.

FRESHENERS

After cleansing, use a freshener, void of alcohol, to remove any residue left on the skin. If you don't want to fill your bathroom with skin products, you can apply pure aloe vera or aloe combined with a few drops of lemon juice. There is no need to rinse after the freshener.

FACIAL MISTS

Next, use a facial mist to return moisture to the skin. Vera uses one made of minerals and rose water, but mineral water will do as well. This step is especially important for dry skin and fine lines. Mineral water reintroduces moisture into the skin, then the cream seeps underneath the skin's surface and pushes out the indentations

231

Masque for Tightening

1 tablespoon avocado, mashed

2 tablespoons raw honey

2 egg whites

Place ingredients in a blender and process until smooth. Pat onto face. Relax, with feet raised, while masque acts to tighten skin and increase circulation, about 20 to 30 minutes. Rinse and freshen.

Masques for Dry Skin

Massage some yogurt into clean skin. Add mashed avocado. Leave on the skin for about 20 minutes. Rinse with warm water.

Mash a banana well. Add honey until a creamy consistency is obtained. Apply to a clean face for 20 minutes. Rinse well.

Mash a ripe papaya. Add the white of an egg, and mix until creamy. Apply to the face for 20 minutes. Rinse well.

caused by dehydration. The cream also acts as a seal to keep in moisture. Deep wrinkles you will probably have to live with, unless, of course, you have a face-lift; even then, the surgery is not permanent. You will need another in about five years.

MOISTURIZERS

Apply moisture creams, sparingly, on the dampened face. Use just a little cream, especially at night. So many women going through menopause have extreme sweats; they put lots of cream on at night and all this does is treat their pillowcases. You want your pores to be clean. Let them breathe. You are constantly getting new cells: You slough off the old cells and make new ones. But as one gets older, the cycle slows down. If your cells are clogged, it slows down even more. This is vitally important: When going through menopause, use less cream at night so your pores will stay open. Never go to bed feeling cream on your face.

The steps, then, are to cleanse, freshen, mist, and moisturize.

MASQUES

It is very important to slough off the top layer of dead skin so that the new healthy cells can surface. Do this weekly by using facial scrubs, masks, and, in extreme conditions, peels. Many products on the market will work, and you can even make ones at home that are equally effective. Presented above are a couple of "kitchen facials" from *Vera's Natural Beauty Book*.

≋ Caring for the Rest of Your Body ≋

So far, we have focused on facial skin, but we should not neglect the rest of the body. When it comes to total body relaxation, nothing compares to a long, hot soak in the tub. Baths can be relaxing and invigorating for the mind as well as the body. Some experts claim that baths are too drying for the skin, but they need not be if you moisturize afterward.

To make your bath special, add natural ingredients to the water for various effects. Cleopatra used milk in her bath; you might want to try adding a quart of milk to your bath water. For very dry skin, try one-half cup of sesame oil. Some women like the fragrance and feeling that freshly brewed herbs offer. Brew your favorite combination (try rosemary, thyme, and lavender flowers) in a bowl, steep for about 20 minutes, strain, and add the liquid to your bath. If you are in the mood for an invigorating bath, if your muscles are aching from aerobics, or if you are tired or have a sunburn, try one cup of natural apple-cider vinegar in your water. To really energize your body as well as your spirits, shower after soaking, alternating hot and cold sprays.

After soaking, use a loofah sponge to remove the dry, dead cells from the outer layer of skin. The scrub will invigorate you, as it increases blood circulation and tones the skin.

⇒ Hair Care ⇐

Hair is an extension of the skin, and it responds to changing hormones and normal aging in characteristic ways. Like the skin, hair reflects your state of health. Philip Kingsley, a British specialist in scalp and hair science, writes, "If you're not eating properly, or exercising regularly, or if you've been under a great deal of stress, the effects are bound to show up on your hair."[3]

Hair follicles are nourished deep beneath the surface of the skin, so if you have problems with dull, dry, or limp hair, check your diet and daily habits before spending your entire paycheck on external conditioners and treatments. External treatments may enhance the hair's manageability and work with the nutritional treatments recommended here—and they need not always be expensive.

HORMONAL CHANGES AND HAIR GROWTH

At menopause, some women experience hair loss from their heads and pubic area, while others find new growth in places where they have never seen it before: the chin, upper lip, chest, and abdomen. While facial hair may be unsightly and embarrassing, it is not a sign of emerging masculine tendencies. It indicates only a reversal in the ratio of female to male hormones, both of which we all—men and women—share. Since estrogen is not dominant following menopause, hair follicles tend to follow a male growth and distribution pattern.

Logical reasoning would suggest that taking more estrogen would reestablish the ratio of hormones and therefore the hair-growth pattern. Unfortunately, estrogen does not reverse the process, but it may prevent further hair growth. Progesterone cream also seems to be of some benefit in slowing down the growth

233

The Bottom Line for Healthy Skin and Hair

- ⊚ Keep out of the direct sun, and protect your skin with hats and sunscreen.
- ⊚ Don't smoke.
- ⊚ Minimize chemical drinks (coffee, tea, cola, diet drinks, and alcohol).
- ⊚ Drink plenty of water—at least two quarts per day.
- ⊚ Don't lose weight too rapidly (two pounds a week at the most).
- ⊚ Eat high-quality protein and complex carbohydrates.
- ⊚ Minimize your intake of excess oil, saturated fats, and hydrogenated spreads.
- ⊚ Reduce sugar and refined and enriched flours and grains in your diet.
- ⊚ Keep the air in your home moist (especially if you live in a dry climate, work in an air-conditioned building, or fly often). Spray mists of water to help bring moisture back to your face.
- ⊚ Supplement your diet, emphasizing antioxidants (vitamins A, C, and E and the mineral selenium) and essential oils, such as flaxseed oil.
- ⊚ Exercise regularly.

of facial and body hair, but it takes time, up to six months. The best alternative may be topical: to bleach the hair if it is dark, or remove it through shaving, waxing, depilatories, electrolysis, or laser treatments.

NUTRITIONAL FACTORS RELATED TO PROBLEM HAIR

Sudden hair loss or hair that is dry, greasy, or lusterless may not always be hormonally related; it may be nutritionally induced. Healthy hair depends on a delicate balance of protein within the hair shaft and oil outside the hair shaft. If the follicles are inadequately nourished, any number of symptoms might emerge. For example, if your hair feels unusually greasy, it may indicate a diet too rich in animal fat. Eliminating red meat, butter, fried foods, and pastries from your diet may be all that is necessary to reestablish chemical equilibrium. Dry hair frequently responds to foods rich in B vitamins, vitamin E, vitamin A, and a daily dose (two teaspoons) of vegetable oil. Hair loss may be checked by adding high-quality protein to and eliminating junk foods from your diet and supplementing with iron and zinc.

Fasting and fad dieting over the years often lead to hair thinning and loss. Past years of depletion can intensify a woman's present needs for nutrients; she will need greater amounts of all vitamins and minerals than if she had been adequately nourished all along.

It is easy to overlook certain nutrients in your diet. For example, a subtle complication of the vegetarian diet, especially one that does not include egg and milk products, is the lack of the amino acid methionine.[4] Even a slight deficiency in this nutrient over a period of time may result in loss of hair.

Certain drugs, most notably birth-control pills, have been implicated in hair loss. If you are taking hormonal drugs, it would be wise to increase your intake of foods containing sulfur, the B-complex vitamins, and zinc.

Essential fatty acids are especially important to menopausal women, since they provide lubrication to all tissues of the body as well as to the skin and hair. Incorporate more whole, raw seeds and nuts into your diet; eat fresh fish several times a week; and for supplementation, add one to two teaspoons of flaxseed oil to salads or vegetables. Flaxseed oil also comes in capsules; two to eight a day will replace moisture in your skin and hair and may make an appreciable difference in the way you look and feel.

Stress endured over a long period of time or a sudden traumatic experience may cause sudden hair loss or scalp disorders. However, the hair will usually return to normal when the situation has subsided. You can aid the process by making your diet rich in B-complex vitamins, vitamins E and C, and folic acid.

CHAPTER 12

WEIGHT CONTROL

*The sad thing is that too many people ignore the basics
in the search for the esoteric.*

— COVERT BAILEY

f we are not careful, middle-age spread can creep up on any of us. After thirty, the body starts to change metabolically; muscle tissue decreases, and the body's basal metabolic rate (BMR), the rate at which we burn calories in sustaining basic life functions, slows down. By some estimates, the BMR decreases about 2 percent each decade, which means by age eighty, we need to take in two hundred fewer calories each day then we do at midlife (see Figure 5). For most women, this will not be enough of a reduction. Because their activity level has also lessened, maintaining the same weight requires further reduction in food intake. There is no way around it: To maintain our weight, we must alter our eating habits and remain physically active.

Obviously, monitoring your weight throughout your life is better than discovering at menopause that you have a serious problem. Menopause brings enough issues to contend with; you don't need to compound the situation by having to diet as well. Sometimes I think the best way to maintain your figure is to vow never to buy a larger size in clothes. You may not be eating more than you normally do, but your body will tell you the time has come to make adjustments.

A bathroom scale is not an accurate indicator of fitness or optimum weight. In fact, I suggest you throw out your scale. It does not tell you how your body should look or how healthy you are. Worst of all, it can become a constant source of anxiety and guilt.

How important is keeping our weight down after fifty? Certainly, a few additional pounds won't harm most women, but I think the operative word here is *few*. Studies show that the pounds you put on in midlife may be more harmful than any extra weight you carried in your early adult years. Women who gain weight later in life are at a higher risk for heart disease than those who have carried the weight all their lives. Being overweight to the point of obesity is extremely high risk and is associated with heart disease, high blood pressure, adult-onset diabetes, and certain types of cancer (notably breast, endometrial, and colon cancers).

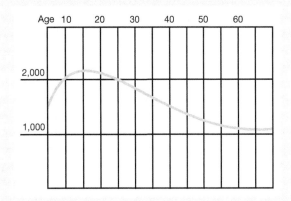

Figure 5. Women's Changing Energy Needs

Half of all adult women in the United States are currently overweight, and trends show that with each successive generation we are becoming an increasingly overweight society.[1] Why is this, given the explosion of weight-loss programs, diet drinks, low-fat foods, and exercise clubs? The basic reason is simple: Diets that are very different from your natural way of eating do not work.

During the early 1990s, I worked for two major diet enterprises, one a medically supervised fasting program and the other a popular food-control weight-loss center. People did lose weight in record amounts, and I felt gratified that I had been helpful in their efforts. When they regained their weight—often with several additional pounds—the excitement subsided. From this experience and my studies of the literature for answers, I think I have found some reasons why people cannot maintain weight loss.

Most Diets Don't Work

Anyone who has agonized over successive diets knows that diets do not help keep the weight off permanently. You lose pounds, but the loss is temporary; once you resume your normal eating habits, the fat finds its way back.

There are two primary reasons why diets fail. First, most diets are foreign to the way people normally eat. Many dieters carefully follow strict low-calorie menus or concoct special drinks until the scale shows the right numbers, then they go back to potato chips, croissants, and hot-fudge sundaes because they cannot maintain the unnatural rigidity of the diet. A diet must change your approach to eating in the long term, or you will not maintain weight loss.

Second, very low caloric intake changes the body's metabolism in a way that promotes weight gain. When you go on a crash diet of, say, nothing but grapefruit and hard-boiled eggs, you actually encourage the storage of fat. As caloric intake is drastically reduced, the body does everything it can to conserve energy. It lowers the metabolic rate to protect you from starving. The more quickly pounds dissolve

Why Americans Are Overweight and Overfat

- Unhealthy eating habits (eating high-fat foods, overeating, and skipping meals) can promote weight gain and prevent weight loss.
- Most people miscalculate what they eat by 18 percent.
- The more you diet and regain weight, the harder it is to lose weight subsequently. Your metabolic rate may decrease by as much as 15 to 20 percent after only a 6 percent decrease in weight, so it becomes harder for you to burn off calories the next time around.
- There may be a link between yo-yo dieting and choosing a high-fat diet.
- A survey of the recreational habits of Americans found that the first thirteen most popular activities listed—among them, watching TV or videos and reading books—are inactive. The fourteenth is walking.
- It is harder for women to lose weight and easier for them to gain weight than it is for men. Estrogen is pro-fat: The more fat you store, the more estrogen you make; the more estrogen you make, the more fat you store.

(especially if you lose more than two pounds a week), the more intensely the body hoards its fat. You may lose weight initially, but the pounds you are burning are from your lean muscle tissue rather than from fat stores. Biochemically, your body changes. When muscle mass is decreased, the basal metabolic rate slows down. This means you are burning fewer calories than you did before you started dieting. So, when you return to "normal" eating, it is even easier to gain weight than it was before.

Crash diets are counterproductive in more ways than one. Reducing calories to bare-minimum levels usually means reducing nutrient stores as well. When the system is depleted of its vitamins and minerals, it triggers the appetite mechanism in the brain to replenish its supply. Result? You are starved, so you eat. Bingeing and compulsive eating are common among habitual dieters.

When women "blitz," they often cut fat out of their plans entirely. This, too, is both unhealthy and ineffective. A good rule is never to follow any diet that eliminates an entire food group—fats, carbohydrates, or proteins. If you eliminate fats completely, you may develop dry and brittle hair, dandruff, swelling in the hands and feet, acne, and loss of sex drive. Ironically, one essential fatty acid, linoleic acid, helps to burn fat. Restrict your intake of fats—but do not eliminate them entirely.

Frequent and drastic dieting is an emotional nightmare for many women. The Mayo Clinic studied a group of young, healthy women—women who had no reason to lose weight but who volunteered for the sake of research. They lived together in the clinic, ate a restricted diet, and were tested continually for side effects. "Before three months had passed, the women's personalities underwent startling changes. They began to quarrel endlessly with one another, experienced unprovoked feelings of anxiety, persecution, and hostility. Some suffered nightmares; others felt extreme panic at times.... Their memories became faulty; they were clumsy and had trouble paying attention to assigned tasks."[2] Remember, before the experiment these women were emotionally healthy and not overweight; they were exposed to only one reducing diet, yet they suffered great anxiety. (Other factors, such as living in the clinic together, could also have contributed to these changes.)

Repeated dieting can be dangerous. Analyzing thirty-two years of data from the Framingham Heart Study in Massachusetts, researchers looked at weight changes in more than three thousand men and women. They found that people whose weight fluctuated often or dramatically doubled their risk for developing heart disease and increased their rate of premature death.[3] Equally startling was the finding that relatively thin people were as much at risk as the overweight. This study does not suggest that weight loss is harmful, but that it should be taken seriously.

Dieting is a stress on the body, both physically and emotionally. Individuals who experiment with one diet after another are forced to deal not only with the normal anxiety of dieting but with the psychological repercussions of failing, the feelings of guilt, frustration, and ego deflation. Crash diets, fad diets, and minimum-calorie diets are unhealthful for the mind as well as for the body. Their benefits are temporary at best; their side effects are multiple and potentially dangerous. So what's the solution?

⤳ The Proper Attitude ⤳

The place to begin is with one's basic attitude toward dieting and good health. We live in a society in which we are conditioned to expect instant results. Over-the-counter remedies are available for almost every ache and pain. For a headache, an upset stomach, or a runny nose, we simply take a pill. If we are overweight, our response is no different. Where's that magic solution—the pill that promises to dissolve our unwanted bulges while we sleep? Clearly, the dollars we shell out for such overnight cures would be far better spent on whole, nutritious foods and a pair of walking shoes.

You cannot keep pounds off your body permanently until you realize that the foods you eat on your "weight-loss program" must be similar to the foods you will choose for the rest of your life. A diet is not temporary; it is a way of living that you maintain on a regular basis. The emphasis needs to be changed from short-term deprivation to long-term change.

It is necessary to retrain your mind to focus on "eating for life" those foods that cause you to feel good, alive, energetic, young, and positive about yourself. It is an attitude of "what is good for my wonderful body" rather than "what do I have to give up so I can lose ten pounds by Saturday night."

All eating behaviors are learned and can be unlearned. Therefore, unhealthy eating habits can be replaced with more constructive patterns. This sounds easier than it is, however. Destructive thoughts and practices concerning food and eating have become so much a part of our lives that we don't even realize they exist. Before making changes, we need to take some time, make a personal inventory, and evaluate our attitudes and behaviors about food. We need to examine why we eat or overeat, when we eat, and what we may be doing in terms of our eating that may be preventing us from losing weight.

I discussed the reasons for failed diets with psychologist and weight-loss expert Bobbe Sommer, and it is her belief that our present-day thought patterns concerning food originate in early childhood. Dr. Sommer suggested that much of what we believe to be true may be, in fact, lies. For example, when we were young and experienced actual hunger, we knew crying would get us prompt attention. Someone would come along and shove a warm bottle into our mouth, and we were soon sated. At the same time, we were also cuddled and held close. Now examine this association between food, security, and love—only forty years later. We may still be responding to this associative conditioning. Sometimes, when we think we are hungry, we are really experiencing another emotion that is triggering feelings of uneasiness in our abdominal area. We reach for our famous tension reducer, because it worked so well forty years ago. We have misconstrued the feelings of anxiety in the "pit of our stomach" as hunger pangs and have acted inappropriately.

Dr. Sommer's theory is that "being fat may be the result of faulty problem solving, at least in some people." Many people attempt to solve their current problems with methods that were appropriate once but no longer serve them well—and they will remain caught in this syndrome until they identify their true emotions. Once they bring the hidden feelings to the level of awareness, they can take action. By unraveling childhood emotions and associations, they can be free of the old compulsion to eat whenever they feel a pang in the tummy.

For some people, accepting that their weight problem may lie within the subconscious is frightening. But, if this is a primary source of the problem, other programs probably will not work. Not everyone requires extensive therapy, but some people will greatly benefit. For the majority, just raising their own awareness of when they eat or overeat is enough. There are place cues (movies = buttered popcorn and candy), activity cues (watching television = leftovers and cake), and time cues (the hour before dinner = munchies and glasses of wine). Overweight people are much more susceptible to external or environmental cues. Dr. Sommer strongly recommends a daily journal as a tool for bringing one's feelings to the surface and ultimately taking control of behaviors that interfere with our lives.

⮡ The Stress–Fat Connection ⮢

Stress makes you fat. Prolonged, unrelenting stress, especially in your later years, can result in excess weight. It's scientifically proven that how you cope with stress determines where your fat is deposited, as well as determining how, when, and what you eat. In her book *Fight Fat after Forty*, Dr. Pamela Peeke, a physician, nutritionist, and researcher with the National Institutes of Health, explains the connection between toxic stress and toxic fat—the kind of fat that accumulates inside your abdomen and places you at a higher risk for heart disease, diabetes, and cancer. Even if you are not overweight, the fat that builds up in the belly around menopause can be life-threatening to the body. Stress-related fat often starts to accumulate after a major life event, but Dr. Peeke highlights a number of common circumstances that arise in women over forty: the resurfacing of childhood trauma, perfectionism, divorce, caregiving, career challenges, illness, dieting, and menopause.[4] Peeke's book makes it obvious that the more situations we experience from this list, the more likely we will be to find fat hovering below our belts.

Stress is a survival mechanism that is supposed to protect us from harm—not turn against us. But because most of us can't or don't blunt the effects of a continual outpouring of stress hormones, they accumulate in unhealthy places and turn toxic. Two hormones are activated when we perceive a stressful situation: adrenaline and cortisol. Together these adrenal hormones prepare our body for action by raising blood pressure, bringing more oxygen to the lungs, slowing down digestion, and diverting energy to the muscles. They instantly bring sugar that has been stored in our muscles and liver into the bloodstream for quick energy. Once this supply is used up, our auxiliary fat tank is tapped. The fat that is used for this purpose comes from our internal organs, specifically the stomach. Dr. Peeke explains that fat cells have special stress-hormone receptors for cortisol, and that there seem to be more of these receptors on the intra-abdominal fat cells than on fat cells in other parts of the body.[5] When the emergency is over the body seeks to replenish both the depleted hormones and the fuel. It craves nourishment, but in our haste to refuel we do not usually search for an apple or carrot. The foods we seek in the wake of an episode of stress are typically ice cream, cookies, and chips—high-sugar and high-fat foods that quickly restore the diminished reserves. And the fat cells from the abdomen get restocked first, which is why continual stress creates this vicious cycle that leads to stomach fat.

Stress hormones operate according to a well-defined biorhythm throughout the day and night. For most people they tend to peak in the early morning, waking us up and keeping us energized and attentive to greet the challenges of the day.

Becoming Aware of Unconscious Messages and Attitudes Regarding Food

Certain universal attitudes or childhood messages concerning food can unconsciously destroy our best intentions:

◉ I must eat everything on my plate. (What if you're full?)

◉ It's wasteful to throw food away. (What if you really don't like it? or Would you rather have it go to waste on your body than in the trash can?)

◉ I can't imagine myself thin. (Keep practicing.)

◉ I'm just a fast eater. (You will enjoy your food longer if you savor each bite.)

◉ I won't enjoy eating if I have to change. (Try it first and see.)

◉ I've never kept my weight off. I was meant to be fat. (There are reasons the weight has returned after dieting. Find out what they are.)

Left unchallenged, all of these messages defeat permanent weight loss. If you believe any of them, you need to replace them with new, positive thought patterns—such as those accompanying the negative messages above.

By late morning they start to decline, until they reach their lowest levels between midnight and 2:00 A.M., at which point they start climbing again in preparation for the next day. As the levels of these hormones drop during the day, generally our attention span, focus, and energy do, too. To rejuvenate and restore our stressed adrenal glands, it is wise to pay attention to this predesigned body rhythm. Make sure to get quality sleep, especially during the repair hours before 2:00 A.M. Eat lightly in the evening. Late-night eating and drinking prevents us from restful sleep and keeps stress levels elevated, adding pounds of toxic fat to our body. Physical exercise is another easy way to minimize oversecretion of stress hormones and thus keep the pounds under control.

Most perimenopausal women notice that their belts get tighter and their pants don't feel quite as comfortable around the waist as they did before the change. Even if they are exercising and maintaining their weight, that little stomach pooches out where once it was flat. This does not necessarily mean that you are at an increased risk for heart disease and stroke, but if you are concerned, there is a quick and easy way to check. First, if you are overweight and your waist measures thirty-five inches or greater, your risk is increased. If your waist is less than thirty-five inches, the ratio of your waist to hips will determine risk. Measure your waistline at the smallest part, just above the hipbone; then measure your hips at the widest point. Divide your waist circumference by your hip circumference. A ratio less than 0.80 is optimal; one greater than 0.85 indicates an increased risk for heart disease, high blood pressure, stroke, breast cancer, uterine cancer, diabetes, kidney stones, arthritis, gallstones, polycystic ovary disease, and incontinence.

Some lifestyle factors are specifically associated with an unhealthy waist-to-hip ratio. Too little physical activity, excessive alcohol intake, and smoking seem to exacerbate central obesity. Changing these habits results in marked improvement and subsequently less potential risk. A list of other possible detrimental factors has been studied and found harmful as well, including social and emotional distresses, such as frequent absence from work, use of psychotropic agents, sleep-related difficulties, dissatisfaction with life, low social support, depression, anxiety, mental fatigue, anger, and hostility.[6]

The stress–fat connection is obviously an extremely complicated process that needs more study. The bottom line is this: Chronic stress and overexposure to adrenal hormones plus an inability to recover all make it easier to gain weight and harder to lose weight.

Evaluating Your Eating Habits

People eat for countless reasons that have nothing to do with hunger. We eat to be sociable or to be accepted. We eat to recover from stress—to restore hormone levels and fuel supply. We eat out of boredom, frustration, anger, a need for acceptance, and habit—most of all habit. And often we are not even conscious of what we are doing. How many cups of coffee and halves of doughnuts did you devour when you were pouring out your soul to your neighbor? As you wait for dinner to be served, do you keep track of the rolls and butter you accept or the glasses of wine poured for you?

Research has shown that many overweight women have completely lost the sensation of hunger: They cannot differentiate it from other feelings. Eating has become their universal response to all stimulation. Therefore, no matter what or how they feel, they seek to satisfy themselves with food. One of the first aspects of food control is to determine when you are eating out of genuine hunger and when you are eating to fulfill a secondary need.

I find charting eating habits to be the best way to record caloric intake as well as to track faulty eating patterns. I sense your reluctance at the mere thought of all that work, and I hear your response: I know what I eat and I don't have the time. Well, several studies have proven you wrong. Diet histories show that women underestimate their daily intake by five hundred to nine hundred calories. When I am struggling with zippers and wondering why, I go back to charting and find the dietary culprits in no time.

To use the charting method, write down—and be specific—everything you eat and drink for three weeks. (See the sample chart on page 245.) This time frame is necessary to cover a variety of occasions and experiences—your period, social situations, family get-togethers—that can affect your eating habits. You will be amazed at the different kinds of foods you select when you are alone or with

relatives, at parties, and during your period. Most people eat about fifteen foods regularly, so the task won't take that long. It is not what you eat occasionally that adds up; it is what you do on a daily basis.

In addition to the kinds and amounts of food you eat, record the time that you ate and what you were doing (watching TV, reading the paper, getting dressed, feeding the baby). Often, when we are involved in another activity, we forget that we have eaten and repeat the process shortly thereafter. Finally, record how you felt while you were eating: relaxed, bored, angry, upset, nervous, or nothing in particular? Were you really hungry, or did you have some other need to meet?

By the time you complete three weeks of entries, you will know a great deal more about your day-to-day eating patterns. How much of your diet is nutrient-rich food and how much is junk food? You will have a greater appreciation of the nutrient density of your diet, how many fruits and vegetables you eat, and the amount of fiber you get in a day or week. It is an exercise that is well worth your time.

Just as important as what, where, and why you eat is how often you eat. Do you go all day without eating and then gorge before going to bed? Barbara Edelstein, author of *The Woman Doctor's Medical Guide for Women*, believes strongly in eating balanced meals throughout the day. In her opinion, the female body cannot metabolize more than a certain number of calories per meal; if this amount is exceeded, the excess will be stored as fat.[7] While the idea of eating several meals may sound counterproductive to losing weight, it really is not. The following study cited by Dr. Edelstein illustrates this important concept.

Volunteers were divided into four groups and given a basic calorie-restricted diet. The first group balanced 1,000 calories among three meals throughout the day and lost two pounds per week. The second group ate no breakfast, had 250 calories for lunch, and 500 calories for dinner. They, too, lost two pounds, though they consumed only 750 calories. The third group ate only 500 calories—all for dinner—and lost the same amount. Personally, I would rather have the freedom to eat twice as much if the weight loss is the same. The fourth group consumed 1,000 calories, all at dinner, and lost less weight than the other groups. So it does appear that small but frequent meals spread throughout the day are more conducive to weight loss and health.

If you have a weight challenge, it is vital to examine the whats, whens, and whys of your eating behavior. Until you know exactly what your eating habits are, you cannot make informed choices and changes. Once you have determined what you are eating or doing that promotes weight gain, you can develop a plan for change. Start by considering foods on your chart that do not add either nutritional or emotional value to your eating pleasure. Are there any you can totally eliminate?

Daily Eating Behavior Diary

Time	Food (type and quantity)	Activity while eating	Location	Thoughts and feelings	Action plan
6:00 AM	juice	getting dressed	bedroom	no time to eat	wake up 15 minutes earlier tomorrow
10:00 AM	2 doughnuts; coffee	talking to coworker	lunchroom	low energy; needed a pickup; ate too fast	(1) eat one doughnut more slowly (2) get muffin or bring bagel
1:00 PM	tostada with sour cream and guacamole; cola; cheesecake	reading newspaper and eating alone	restaurant	eat something healthful; need dessert	(1) take sour cream off food and just taste guacamole (2) don't eat shell (3) take mints to satisfy sweet tooth
3:00 PM	diet soda	working	work	thirsty; just want something	water is a better choice
8:00 PM	3–4 glasses white wine; chips; vegetables and dip; salad with dressing; 2 rolls with butter; chicken in cream sauce; steamed vegetables; rice; chocolate cake; coffee with cream	dinner meeting	hotel banquet room	these people make me nervous; look, busy, eat; I paid for this food so I'm going to eat it	(1) wine spritzer (2) sip wine more slowly (3) eat vegetables without dip (4) just taste roll and butter (5) scrape most of cream sauce off food (6) just taste cake (7) take coffee black

What about placing some in a special-occasion category? Don't choose something you can't go one day without. Make it easy for yourself. For example, forego that fifth cookie or predinner wine and munchies. Another way of cutting down calories and fat is to substitute lower-calorie foods for things you regularly eat. Sometimes this works and sometimes it doesn't. If the taste and sensual pleasure are missing from a substitution, pass it up. Don't force yourself to eat foods you don't like; it won't work.

Too many of us have tried to lose weight through stringent dieting or unrealistic exercise programs. When goals are not met, discouragement and depression follow. Changing our mindset to realistic lifestyle changes may not come naturally, as we have grown up thinking that we must starve or eat strange things to lose weight. But I have seen how small, seemingly insignificant modifications in food patterns, combined with moderate physical activity, can alter women's lives dramatically. Not only do they feel better physically, but the fact they did it themselves boosts their self-image. You really can do it yourself—with little time and effort.

It is important to start slowly—just the opposite of commercial programs, which promise instant results. Actually, the faster you lose, the faster you regain. Get used to the idea that you are making permanent changes, by charting and thinking about what might realistically work for you. Changing habits permanently is never easy; consider one modification at a time, and when you feel comfortable with one success, move on to the next goal.

Is Fat the Only Culprit?

Calories in Food

Food	Calories/Gram
Protein	4
Carbohydrates	4
Fat	9

No doubt: Fat in the diet is one of the keys to both weight loss and weight gain. Since fat contains more calories per gram than either protein or carbohydrates, when you reduce fat intake, you substantially cut down on calories.

Fat further encourages fatness by its metabolic effect. While it takes 25 percent of the energy in protein and carbohydrates to transform them into substances the body uses, a similar conversion only takes 3 percent of the energy in fat. This means that 97 percent of fat calories can be stored immediately. "A minute on the lips, forever on the hips" is oh, so true for fat.

An average woman consumes eighty to one hundred grams of fat per day. An optimal level for good health as well as weight loss is between twenty-five and fifty grams per day. If you want a more specific number, you can calculate your optimal daily fat intake from the total number of calories you ingest in a day. Multiply your total daily caloric intake by the optimal percentage of fat calories (25–30 percent) and divide the result by nine (the calories in one gram of fat). (See Chapter 10 for an example.)

Fat intake is relatively easy to monitor given the number of books on the market listing fat grams for every kind of food. More detailed food labels have greatly enhanced our awareness. But you will need the three-week food records first. You don't have to continue keeping these records for the rest of your life, only until you get a feeling for what you are eating and those areas that need revamping.

You will find that when you start eating lower-fat foods, you can increase your quantities and still not gain weight—within reason, that is. If you replace the fat calories with the same amount of calories from carbohydrates or proteins, you will still add pounds. Excess calories, or more than *your* body can utilize immediately, will be stored as fat. Obviously the amount varies with the individual. To give you some appreciation for the amount of food you can eat that may equal a high-fat food, look at the chart to the right, "What Could You Eat If You Gave Up a Bacon Cheeseburger?" I love to demonstrate this with plates of all these items, but I think you will get the idea.

What Could You Eat If You Gave Up a Bacon Cheeseburger?

Food	Fat Grams
Bacon cheeseburger	63
Charbroiled chicken sandwich	7
Bagel	12
Potato	0
Apple	0
Banana	0
1 cup spaghetti	1
1/2 cup marinara sauce	4
Chicken leg	9
Turkey sandwich (no mayo)	7
1 slice pizza (small)	5
Corn tortilla	1
Flour tortilla	3
1 oz cheese	9
1 egg	7
1/2 cup cereal	2
3 pancakes (small)	2
2 low-fat cupcakes	4
Total	**63**

But focusing on dietary fat tells only part of the story. After years of following advice to lose weight by eliminating fat from our diets, why are so many of us still overweight? One of the culprits is likely a condition called *insulin resistance*, thought by some health experts to affect 50 to 75 percent of the population. If you suffer from insulin resistance, then high levels of dietary carbohydrate—which is the food most often increased when fat is reduced in the diet—can result in weight gain and increased risk of heart disease. The worst culprits are simple sugars and refined carbohydrates, such as those in white pasta, white rice, and white breads.

Insulin is the hormone from the pancreas that metabolizes carbohydrates. If you're insulin resistant, when you overeat carbohydrates, a very high blood-sugar level results. The body cannot utilize the excess sugar, so it gets stored as fat. If you fail to lose weight on a low-fat, high-carbohydrate diet, you may be insulin resistant.

(Read more about how dietary fat and insulin resistance participate in the big picture of our health in Chapter 9's section on a heart-healthy diet.)

⇒ Are You Following the Wrong Diet? ⇐

There is no generic perfect diet. You may think that your high-protein diet or vege-tarian lifestyle is the only diet for you, and maybe it is. But too often we follow the plan of the month when in fact it is all wrong for our specific body type and chem-istry. Whatever your diet of choice is today, consider how you feel most of the time. Are you energetic, clear thinking, motivated, and free from nagging complaints? If you can't say yes, then consider that you may be eating foods that are failing to nourish your body, no matter how healthy they are or how committed you are to your program. To provide further insight and direction into what's not working, look at the following lists of symptoms that can be triggered by particular diets when they're not appropriate, and see if you need to make some changes:

High protein, high fat, low carbohydrate: loss of appetite, nausea, loss of water weight, bad breath, carbohydrate cravings, weakness, dizziness, diarrhea, headaches, high uric acid, kidney disease.

Reduce Amounts of High-Fat Foods

Food	Calories	Fat Grams
Butter (1 tbsp)	100	12
Cheese (1 oz)	100	9
Mayonnaise (1 tbsp)	100	11
Potato chips (1 oz)	150	11
Nuts (1 cup)	850	80
Hershey's chocolate (2.6 oz)	390	20

Low protein: loss of hair, fatigue, mental confu-sion, irritability, thin skin, brittle nails, lack of sex drive, food cravings, bloating, anemia, poor mus-cle tone, loss of muscle mass, slowed metabolism.

High carbohydrate, low fat: bloated feeling after eating, hunger cravings, lack of stamina, fatigue in late morning or early afternoon, PMS, bleed-ing, cramps, bruising easily, bone pain, loss of hair, flaky skin, extreme thirst, allergies, yeast infections, sinus infections, headaches, earaches, stomach problems.

⇒ Minor Lifestyle Changes Make Major Differences ⇐

The goal of weight loss is to take it off slowly and then to maintain it. If you elimi-nate one tablespoon of butter a day, an amount that easily covers two slices of toast, in one year you would lose ten pounds. Consider the charts titled "Reduce Amounts of High-Fat Foods" (above) and "Replace with Lower-Calorie, Lower-Fat Foods" (on the next page), as you think about what to cut out of your diet to pro-duce lasting results.

≈ Exercise Is a Must ≈

Exercise is a major factor for long-term weight loss.[8] Studies confirm that maintaining a regular exercise program is the surest way of determining future success. Cutting calories and fat without adding exercise may cause you to lose as much lean muscle tissue as you do fat. A person who drops twenty pounds from dieting alone will often lose as much as ten pounds of muscle. While this looks good on the scales, the muscle loss lowers metabolic rate and thus increases the chances of regaining the weight.

Exercise builds muscle mass, thereby raising the BMR. Even moderate exercise increases the metabolic rate three to eight times. And there is a residual effect of regular exercise that keeps the metabolic rate higher than normal for several hours afterward, allowing you to burn more calories even when you are not working at it.

Exercise can change the body's chemistry. When biopsies from endurance athletes were compared to those of untrained college students, it was found that the athletes had a greater number of fat-burning enzymes. After the untrained person engaged in endurance exercise for several months, his or her enzymes increased too. Apparently, in people who exercise regularly, the body "revs up" the metabolic system to burn fat more efficiently while protecting the muscle tissue.

Exercise affects many hormonal systems in the body. It increases the responsiveness of cells to insulin so that the insulin does not cause increased fat storage. Stress-related hormones such as adrenaline and cortisol are metabolized by exercise, which decreases their effect on fat storage. Endorphins secreted in the brain as a result of endurance exercise create a feeling of well-being and alleviate depression. Many chemical reactions occur from continued exercise that change the body from one that likes to store fat to one that likes to burn fat.

There is no alternative to a sound exercise program for burning fat. It must be included in any weight-loss program.

Replace with Lower-Calorie, Lower-Fat Foods	
TRY	**INSTEAD OF**
1 slice whole-wheat toast (71 calories/1 fat gram)	1 croissant (300 calories/ 12 fat grams)
4 cups air-cooked popcorn (109/0)	2 oz potato chips (300/22)
7 oz broiled fish (175/2)	7 oz fried fish (525/18)
1/2 cup Dreyer's Lite (100/4)	1/2 cup Haagen-Daz (270/17)
1 corn tortilla (50/1)	1 flour tortilla (150/4)
2 tbsp broth (0/0)	2 tbsp cooking oil (240/27)
3 oz turkey sausage (150/0)	3 oz pork sausage (300/25)
3 oz skinless baked chicken (160/4)	3 oz fried chicken (230/14)

⇒ A Few More Tips ⇐

A few other tips may be helpful as you plan your weight-loss strategy and try to create new eating habits. No advice is universal, so take what works for you from the list below and throw out the rest.

- ⊙ Eat at least three meals a day. Skipping meals promotes the starvation response and the storage of fat.

- ⊙ Get into the habit of talking to your food. Before eating, ask, "Do I want you? Do I need you? Are you going to make me feel good or bad when I'm finished?"

- ⊙ Eat without distractions: no TV, radio, newspaper, or book. Concentrate on the food.

- ⊙ Create a relaxing, positive eating environment.

- ⊙ Eat slowly, enjoying the aroma, color, taste, and texture of the food.

- ⊙ Eat sitting down. You will be less likely to forget what has gone into your mouth.

- ⊙ Practice leaving a few bites on your plate at each meal. This teaches self-control.

- ⊙ Eat with friends, family, or coworkers. Overweight people often feel they must prove to others they are trying to lose weight, so they limit their selections to lettuce and cottage cheese in public, only to binge in solitude. Eat your favorite foods with your friends. Chances are you won't feel the need to overeat later.

- ⊙ Make a list of activities that make you feel good and that you can do in place of eating: reading a novel; going to a concert, play, or movie; calling a friend; watching soap operas; getting a facial or massage; going shopping.

- ⊙ If you must have a hot-fudge sundae, go ahead. But don't chastise yourself. There's no place for guilt in weight management.

- ⊙ Start a support group or find a friend who will walk with you and listen to your struggles. Social support has been associated with success in weight loss.

CHAPTER 13

EXERCISE FOR LIFE

I don't bust my buns working out every day for nothing.

— CHER

Exercise is as important to a healthy body as good food is. Preventing menopausal symptoms and dealing with the associated problems of aging involves more than what we do or don't eat. To be well prepared for midlife, we must engage in some form of physical exercise. "Virtually all the evidence we have points in the same direction," says Jack Wilmore, director of the Exercise and Sport Sciences Laboratory at the University of Arizona. "Exercise makes you healthier and may impact longevity. It's time to become more aggressive in using exercise to improve overall health."[1]

Exercise literally can save your life; without it, your body deteriorates. If you are inactive during your adult years, your bones will decalcify, leading to osteoporosis. Taking time out of your day to attend an exercise class, take a walk, or jog is not frivolous; it is essential.

If you want strong bones to support your frame and firm muscles to protect your internal organs when you reach fifty, you should start your program early. However, it is never too late to benefit from exercise; quite the contrary, with conditioning, you can have stronger muscles at fifty than you did at thirty. I do, and Jane Fonda says her body was in better shape at forty-nine than at twenty. But optimum results come from planned preparation, not last-minute desperation.

Most people are aware of the role exercise plays in weight loss. We are also familiar with its influence on the muscle-bone system. But there is more—much more—that exercise can do for your body, mind, and spirit. When you are working the entire body, the effects radiate throughout every organ, tissue, and cell. The following are some of the benefits of sustained, regular exercise:

⊙ When you exercise vigorously, you bring oxygen to every cell of the body, improving circulation, reducing fatigue, creating energy, and increasing your capacity for handling stress.

⊙ Harvard studies show that aerobic exercise is a practical way to treat the emotional stress of daily living. It can reduce depression and give you a feeling of well-being.

⊙ Regular exercise can prolong life, according to Ralph Passenbarger, Jr., of the Stanford University School of Medicine: "For each hour of physical activity, you can expect to live that hour over—and live one or two more hours to boot."[2]

⊙ Physical activity stimulates digestion and increases the absorption of nutrients. A study performed by Gail Butterfield of the University of Southern California showed that active women had appreciably more vitamin C and iron in their bloodstream than did sedentary women.[3]

⊙ Exercise guards against constipation.

⊙ Exercise helps you to sleep soundly.

⊙ For women, exercise can help bring the hormones to a normal level, greatly reducing menstrual cramps, PMS, and hot flashes.

⊙ Exercise helps the adrenal glands to convert androstenadione into estrone, the major source of estrogen after menopause, allowing for a smoother transition.

⊙ Exercise is vital to weight control: It diminishes appetite, burns calories, builds muscle, and speeds up body metabolism.

⊙ Aerobic exercise stimulates new bone formation, thus warding off osteoporosis.

⊙ Exercise greatly reduces the risk of heart disease. Researchers at the University of North Carolina have found that inactive women are three times more likely to die prematurely from heart disease than the physically active.[4]

⊙ Exercise lowers the incidence of cancer. In a landmark study at Harvard University, female athletes were found to have 50 percent less incidence of breast cancer and 60 percent less cancer of the uterus, ovaries, cervix, and vagina than nonathletes.

⊙ Exercise reduces the risk of adult-onset diabetes by improving one's ability to utilize sugar in the blood.

⊙ Exercise helps prevent joint stiffness, arthritis, and lower-back pain.

Exercise comes in many forms. The kind that's best for you depends on your age, level of fitness, and interests. Evaluate your goals before you buy shoes or equipment or join a health club. Make sure that what you choose is something you want to pursue and can easily incorporate into your life. Your exercise program should not be approached like a fad diet—a temporary inconvenience you tolerate until you reach a desired goal. It should be something you can enjoy. To derive permanent benefits, you need to continue a regular program for the rest of your life. The kind of exercise you choose today may change as you expand your goals and improve your level of fitness, and you should keep adjusting your routines to accommodate your changing needs.

Women approaching menopause have specific fitness needs that can best be met by three basic forms of exercise: aerobic conditioning, muscle strengthening, and stretching. Within these groups, however, are endless variations; you can choose the ones you like and that best fit your schedule.

Aerobic Exercise

The great thing about aerobic activity is that it can be completely individual, matched to your state of health. You do not have to join an arduous dance class or run ten miles to get into shape. If you are middle-aged, or even a young but unfit woman, simply walking briskly will elevate your heart rate and give you the training effect you require.

Aerobic exercise involves the large muscles of the body and raises the breathing and heart rates, which have a systemic effect throughout the body. Jogging or fast walking works not only the leg muscles, but touches the heart, lungs, bones, and all other organs as well.

For weight control, exercising aerobically must be the number-one priority. Even though an aerobic exercise burns little fat during the exercise itself, it has tremendous effects on the metabolism of fat, including fat storage and the ability of muscles to burn fat. You may successfully lose pounds for a while on a low-calorie diet, but the diet will eventually cease to work because of lost muscle tissue and the need to cut calorie consumption to an unhealthy level for continued loss.

The word *aerobic* means "depending on oxygen." It is a term used by fitness specialists to describe exercises that increase breathing and pulse rates and produce predictable changes in the body (such as burning calories, strengthening the cardiovascular system, and toning the muscles). All aerobic exercises have one thing in common: As your muscles work hard, they demand and use more oxygen. The main objective of an aerobic exercise program, according to "the father of aerobics," Kenneth Cooper, is to increase the amount of oxygen the body can process within

253

Recommended Training Rates

Age	60%	70%	80%
20	120	140	160
30	114	133	152
40	108	126	144
50	102	119	136
60	96	112	128
70	90	105	120

a given time. Dr. Cooper calls this maximum amount *aerobic capacity*. It is dependent upon the ability to (1) rapidly breathe large amounts of air, (2) forcefully deliver large volumes of blood, and (3) effectively deliver oxygen to all parts of the body. Because it reflects the condition of the vital organs, aerobic capacity is often considered the best index of overall physical fitness.[5]

For your exercise workout to be aerobic, you must (1) engage in continuous activity (not stop-and-start) that works the muscles and the heart for a period of fifteen to thirty minutes, (2) exercise at a specified intensity, and (3) practice the exercise regularly—at least three times a week to maintain, five times to improve.

How hard you exercise is a personal decision that should be based on your heart rate. As intensity increases, oxygen demand goes up and your heart beats faster. The point is to keep within a specified range (your training rate) during the conditioning period.

It is important to determine the training rate that is right for you. You can do this by taking your pulse during the aerobic workout. If the exercise has truly been aerobic, your pulse will register between 60 and 80 percent of your maximum heart rate (MHR), which is around 220 beats a minute minus your age. The formula used to determine the training rate is based on your MHR and the percentage increase you want to achieve. The following example is for a person forty-five years old:

220 – 45 = 175 (maximum heart rate)

175 x .60 = 105 beats per minute

175 x .80 = 140 beats per minute

The training range is between 105 and 140 beats a minute.

The chart above will help you to select your target zone. As you can see, maximum heart rate drops with age, so you will need to make adjustments periodically.

Monitoring your pulse takes prior planning, especially if you train on your own—walking briskly, jogging, or riding a stationary bike, for example—and not in a class that includes pulse-taking as part of its program. First, you will need a watch with a second hand; second, you must know in advance what your training range is. After you have been exercising for about five minutes, slow down just enough to focus on the second hand of your watch and take your pulse. Do not stop exercising. Place your fingertips about an inch below your ear at the carotid artery and count the pulse beats for six seconds. (Do not use your thumb; it has a pulse of its own.) Add a zero to the number of beats you counted to get a per-minute rate. If you are over your range, slow your pace; if you are under, increase it; if you are right on, continue exercising for the full twenty to thirty minutes. Eventually, you will feel instinctively what it is like to be within your range and you won't have to bother with this ritual.

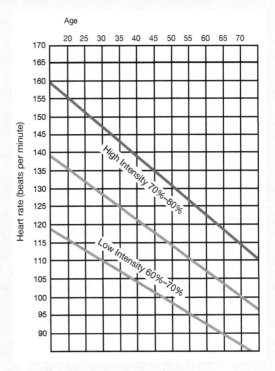

Figure 6. Determining Your Heart Rate

If you just can't be inconvenienced with such details, there is another reliable method for determining aerobic status, called the *perceived rate of exertion*. You can easily evaluate your own level of intensity by how heavily you are breathing. If you can't mumble a sound during your workout, chances are you have exceeded the 80 percent range. On the other hand, if you are not panting at all and can recite the Gettysburg Address without missing a beat, accelerate your stride.

There is a wide margin between the low-intensity training rate (60–70 percent) and the high-intensity training rate (70–80 percent); see Figure 6. What your rate should be depends on your fitness goals, age, and level of conditioning.

When you exercise within the low-intensity range, your heartbeat is slower and you are not burning as many calories. In some cases this is just the effect you want, because the calories you are burning are from fat only. Fat needs oxygen to burn, and at the lower rate more oxygen is taken in and is available for fat metabolism. As you increase the intensity of the exercise, it becomes more difficult to breathe deeply, so less oxygen is inhaled. Less fat is burned, and the balance is stored as glycogen; however, you are burning more calories. Each range has its own reward: At low intensity you burn fewer calories but more fat; at high intensity you burn less fat but more calories, which come first from the glycogen supply, then from the muscle.

If you are a beginner, your muscles have probably lost their ability to burn fat, and when you first start out, you will be primarily burning sugar.[6] When you go for a walk, your muscles will not yet be burning fat, even though you will be breathing heavily for twenty minutes. You may also tire easily and get discouraged when your results are less than you had anticipated. If you are overtired with your workout, cut back and start more slowly. Physical-fitness expert Covert Bailey recommends that the overweight beginning exerciser not limit her exercising to three times a week. Get out there every day—better yet, two or three times a day—for ten to fifteen minutes, to stimulate your body into initiating the fat-burning process.[7] The untrained body must be constantly introduced to exercise before it starts behaving the way it should. As you become fit, decrease the number of workout days and increase the duration to twenty to forty-five minutes.

If you have been exercising for a while and you feel your program is no longer working, you may need to give it a boost. Covert Bailey suggests adding intervals of greater intensity throughout your workout so your body can adjust to burning fat at higher levels. By including spurts of intensity in your program, your fat-burning potential goes up, and the body learns to be aerobic at levels of exercise that were once anaerobic. (Anaerobic exercise, which means "without oxygen," burns sugar and rapidly leads to exhaustion.) When you are out walking, for example, see if you can work in a few hills, not so difficult that you are gasping for air, but hard enough to make you slightly winded. If you live where there are no hills, you can create the same effect by walking faster for three to five minutes and then returning to your normal pace.

Exercise programs must be reevaluated periodically. Maybe we're not achieving the results we had hoped for, or maybe an injury forces us to alter our routine. Just because we've been doing something for many years, it doesn't mean that particular exercise will continue to be right for us forever. I hated having to give up jogging, but when my feet and knees started aching each time I hit the pavement, I knew my running days were numbered. Change is rarely welcome or fun, but once I adjusted to fast walking and hiking hills, I realized I'm much happier without the pain. What concerned me most was that I would be unable to get my heart rate up like I did with jogging, but I learned to accelerate my pace and to push up those hills, which more than compensated.

Your body may be providing signals that it's time to rethink your program. Be open to the possibility that a gentler form of exercise can also provide a healthy workout. Walking fast or walking with weights, low-impact dance classes, cycling, weight training, Pilates, tai chi, and yoga are alternatives worth considering. High-impact aerobics and marathons may be relegated to a past life, but that doesn't have to mean the end to new physical challenges.

⇒ Muscle Strengthening ⇐

Adding weight training to an aerobic program offers many benefits to the midlife woman. While strength training doesn't generally reduce body fat, it can help you reverse and rebuild the loss of muscle that comes with natural aging. Several studies suggest that fat mass increases with age, while both muscle mass and skeletal mass decline.[8] The reduction in muscle mass eventually leads to the decline in skeletal tissue. Research from the Midlife Center in Gainesville, Florida, found that postmenopausal women on hormonal therapy experienced an 8 percent increase in bone mass when they performed muscle-strengthening exercises, while a comparison group of women who took estrogen but didn't exercise neither gained nor lost bone mass.[9] Don't count on hormonal therapy alone to prevent osteoporosis; it is not an alternative to exercise.

Strong, toned muscles protect the joints and help prevent exercise-related injuries. They improve the way your clothes fit and the way you feel about yourself. Women who have not necessarily lost weight but notice definition in their muscles through exercise feel better about themselves.

There are several options for increasing your muscle strength. You can join a club that will introduce you to the proper use of free weights and weight machines like Cybex and Nautilus equipment, or if you prefer the privacy of your own home, you can purchase your own inexpensive equipment and any number of videos. (Some basic exercises are provided in Appendix D.) All you need are some three- to eight-pound dumbbells to build strength in your muscles and bones. Whatever you choose, be sure to get qualified instruction—proper form and technique are essential.

Some women still shy away from weight training and strange-looking machines. Lingering in some women's preconceptions are fears of bulking up or appearing "masculine." Most of us now know that this is a fallacy, because we lack high amounts of the male hormone, testosterone, that is primarily responsible for male musculature. Using light weights and high repetitions will just firm and strengthen muscles. Using heavier weights and fewer repetitions does build or add bulk, but not in the same way as it will for a man.

Sometimes, if a woman has a high percentage of body fat (about 28 percent) and starts a muscle-strengthening program before losing some of the fat, she may increase the muscle to a point where the additional muscle, along with her body fat, makes her look bulky. If you fall into this category, work first on losing some of your weight through reduced fat intake and aerobics, then add a weight-training program.

≋ Flexibility ≋

The third component of a well-rounded exercise program is flexibility. Muscles and connective tissue lose elasticity with disuse and age. Joints need to move through their full range of motion regularly to maintain flexibility. For many people, one simple form of exercise, stretching, will reduce joint pain and lower-back discomfort, improve posture, and minimize postexercise soreness.

There is a proper way to do everything—even stretching. Stretching should be slow and deliberate to be effective. Rapid or jerky movements, called *ballistic stretching*, are not beneficial and may even be harmful if there is too much tension placed on the muscle being stretched.

It is best to stretch your muscles when they are already warm, so before you start stretching, exercise slowly in the same way you will be using your muscle. For example, warm up for running by jogging slowly; warm up for tennis by swinging your racket. When you warm up, you raise the temperature of your muscles, enabling them to contract more. Stretching before a vigorous workout reduces your chances of being injured, and stretching after a hard workout reduces muscle soreness and enhances muscle relaxation. After exercise, your muscles gradually tighten, which reduces flexibility and increases your chances of injury. In summary, before each workout you should warm up and then stretch. After each workout, you should cool down and stretch again.

Stretching, in general, is the best way to increase flexibility and maintain a supple body. An excellent book on the subject is Bob Anderson's *Stretching*. He makes the point that any stretch must be slow and must be sustained for a minimum of twenty seconds to be effective.[10] Yoga, too, is excellent for improving flexibility and strength.

≋ The Bottom Line ≋

Optimal fitness requires more than one kind of exercise. Sheila Cluff from the Oaks at Ojai teaches that there are four major aspects to any fitness workout:

1. **A warm-up is very important.** You should not shock the body, especially at menopause, when it is already coping with many other changes. Move your body gradually from a sedentary mode to an exercise mode. The object is to increase the body temperature, the heart rate, and the muscle demand slowly. Stretching and low-impact exercises, in which the feet stay on the floor, are good warm-up exercises.

2. **Next comes the aerobic workout.** This doesn't have to be a class; it can be any kind of aerobic activity, but the social support and the music of a class may make it more enjoyable.

3. **After the aerobic session, when your muscles are warmed up, work on strengthening all the muscle groups.** Don't just concentrate on your "problem" areas; include every muscle from your shoulders to your ankles.

4. **Cooling down is as essential as warming up.** After a hard workout, you need to decrease your heart rate and body temperature gradually. Stretching will lengthen constricted muscles and help the body relieve itself of the toxins and lactic acid that have built up. Check your pulse rate again, making sure it is back to its normal resting rate.

As you become more physically fit, your resting pulse rate drops. Most women average around seventy-eight to eighty-four beats per minute, while men average seventy-two to seventy-eight. Athletes occasionally drop as low as thirty-five. My resting pulse rate was close to one hundred beats per minute before I started exercising; now it is consistently fifty-five. To get your true resting pulse rate, take it first thing in the morning, before you get out of bed. Activity, drugs, coffee—almost anything can cause it to fluctuate. Count the beats for an entire minute; a six-second count such as you take during aerobics is not sufficient. You can also find an average resting pulse by taking it several times during the day. If it stays within a few beats per minute, you are close enough to have an adequate reading.

As you begin your exercise program, proceed slowly and cautiously. Don't become discouraged; it takes time before results are noticeable. And don't try to keep up with women who have taken dance classes since they could walk. Go at your own pace. Excellent guides for beginning aerobic programs are Covert Bailey's *The Fit or Fat Woman*, Denise Austin's *Jump Start*, and Joanie Greggain's *Fit Happens*. Kathy Smith also offers a wonderful video called *Moving Through Menopause*, which includes twenty minutes of low-impact aerobics, twenty minutes of strength training, and twenty minutes of yoga, plus good information about menopause. You can find her products online at www.kathysmith.com.

NOTES

PART III

NUTRITION FOR LIFE
A WOMAN'S GUIDE

CHAPTER 14

FORMING NEW EATING HABITS

There is a definite tendency in our culture towards self-destructive behavior and living the "good life" despite dire consequences.

— KENNETH R. PELLETIER, *Holistic Medicine*

What we eat and drink every day plays a dynamic role in the way we look, act, and feel. Whether we feel and appear weary or energized, anxious or elated, sickly or fit is largely determined by our diet. Our future health, how quickly we age, and whether we will succumb to often fatal degenerative diseases have been proven to be directly related to our dietary lifestyle.

The ancients stressed the importance of good food in health. Some twenty-five hundred years ago, physician-teacher Hippocrates admonished his medical students, "Thy food shall be thy remedy." Today's variation on that axiom is "You are what you eat." Whatever the phrase, the point is that how you feed your body relates directly to your health.

Most of us don't think of nutrition as a separate, complete field of knowledge, but it is. It is a biochemical science based on the incontrovertible laws of nature. When these laws are broken, illness results. A great French physician, Henry Beiler, based his entire practice on the belief that improper foods cause disease and proper foods cure disease. In his famous book *Food Is Your Best Medicine*, he writes, "Health is not something bestowed on you by beneficent Nature at birth; it is achieved and maintained only by active participation in well-defined rules of healthful living—rules which you may be disregarding every day."[1] Food is not the only factor involved in healthy living, but it is a significant one.

⟫ **Diet Versus Disease** ⟪

It would appear that the American people are not conforming to the rules designed by nature. Despite the abundance of food in the United States, government studies, nutritional surveys, and medical evaluations reveal shocking statistics:

- ⊙ Lifestyle (meaning eating and exercise habits) may ultimately account for more than half of all deaths annually in the United States.[2]

- ⊙ Current dietary trends may lead to malnutrition through undernourishment.[3]

- ⊙ Only 15 percent of women between the ages of thirty and thirty-nine derive less than 30 percent of their calories from fat; only 2 percent get twenty-five grams of fiber a day.[4]

- ⊙ According to the US NHANES II survey, 41 percent of the population ate no fruit on the survey day; only 25 percent had a fruit or vegetable that contained vitamins A or C.[5]

- ⊙ The USDA National Food Consumption Survey showed that only 3 percent of the population eats a "balanced diet." Not a single person of the more than 21,500 surveyed obtained 100 percent of the RDA for all of ten nutrients listed.[6]

- ⊙ Iron deficiency is pervasive in three groups: preschoolers, adolescents, and women over eighteen.[7]

- ⊙ Of women aged eighteen to thirty years, 66 percent fail to meet the RDA for calcium; after age thirty-five, the proportion increases to 75 percent.[8]

The good news is that these statistics can be reversed by fairly simple changes in lifestyle. Many of the killer diseases we continually read and hear about (heart disease, arthritis, cancer, and diabetes) have been linked in one way or another to diet and daily habits. Interestingly, these often paralyzing and sometimes fatal conditions have been labeled "diseases of civilization" because of their prominence in rich, industrialized societies that have all the advantages of preserving and processing food.

It is well established that disease related to dietary deficiencies begins far in advance of symptoms. Subtle biochemical changes occur months—even years—before signs wake us up to a potential problem. In the early stages the individual feels nothing out of the ordinary, and medical tests reveal no malfunction. As the

disease progresses, there may be generalized symptoms such as fatigue, indigestion, or insomnia. At this point, the deficiency may still be difficult to determine, because the clues remain nebulous. Only when serious damage has occurred can a diagnosis be made. Consider the following likely symptoms of nutritional deficiencies. How many sound like menopausal complaints?

- low energy

- swollen glands

- digestive problems

- blood disorders

- irritability, nervousness

- mental problems

- insomnia

- poor concentration

- weight fluctuations

- frequent colds and infections

We need to change our frame of reference and concentrate on preventing disease and illness rather than just treating it. For so many life-threatening diseases—osteoporosis, heart disease, and cancer, to name a few—the best and possibly the only real cure is prevention. That voice crying out in the wilderness, out there beyond the "civilized" kingdom of the American Medical Association, is not a quack or an eccentric, but a responsible health professional, the holistic practitioner, saying, "Do something about it before it does something to you—before it kills you."

Whether or not you contract a disease depends on more than what you do or do not eat. Your genetic makeup may predispose you to certain illnesses. If your grandmother, mother, sister, or aunt had diabetes, your risk is heightened. Many findings, however, indicate that inherited characteristics exert less influence on our health than the way we live. Not only do genetic patterns occur within families; similar dietary habits may actually contribute more to the "familial weakness" than genetics. Does your family breakfast on croissants and coffee, lunch on hamburgers, fries, and cola, and dine on steak followed by dessert? You could be in trouble.

Breast cancer, the most common cause of cancer deaths among American women as well as women of other affluent Western countries, is one example of nurture taking precedence over nature. Several studies, including some conducted at the Tufts University School of Medicine and the New England Medical Center, in

Boston, support the theory that a major determinant for breast cancer in U.S. women appears to be the typical American diet.[9] Studies of disease in cultural populations and other cancer research over the past thirty years seem to confirm that women from Western countries suffer higher rates of breast cancer than women of most other nations because the Western diet is low in fiber and high in fat and sugar.

Poor daily habits make a person more susceptible to a variety of illnesses. We are all well informed now about the relationships between cigarette smoking and lung cancer, sugar intake and diabetes, stress and hypertension, cholesterol levels and heart disease, fiber intake and digestive disturbances. Whatever we do on a regular basis—whether it is smoking; drinking coffee, cola, or alcohol to excess; eating inordinate amounts of sugar; or working under stress—can promote and provoke very definite and predictable disease states in susceptible individuals.

Diet (and I use the term broadly, to encompass everything that enters the digestive tract, including drinks, drugs, and smoke) may not be the only factor for a healthy body, but it is an extremely vital one. All that you put into your mouth eventually reaches your body's cells, creating the environment in which they grow, replenish, and either thrive or struggle to survive.

What Do Healthy People Eat?

As part of a search to determine what we should do to become healthy, I have looked into societies and groups of people who have achieved a more optimal state of health. I found that the most robust people, living the longest number of years, eat foods as varied as the climates from which they come. Laplanders, who live in a bitterly cold climate, eat primarily reindeer meat and suffer none of the degenerative diseases afflicting more prosperous countries. The Polynesians thrive on poi, made from the root of the taro plant; raw or cooked fish; and an abundance of fresh tropical plants. The Hunzakuts of the Himalayas eat mainly whole grains, fresh fruits and vegetables, fresh milk and cheese, and, on occasion, meat, and they are known as the "healthiest people on Earth." In the United States, specific groups like the Seventh Day Adventists show lower rates of cancer and heart disease. Most of them are vegetarians, and they generally choose fresh organically grown grains and vegetables. In addition, they refrain from smoking as well as from drinking coffee and alcohol.

Even though the specific foods eaten by hearty people the world over are diverse, definite common denominators appear among their diets, and these can help us in determining what we should eat. Weston Price, author of *Nutrition and Physical Degeneration*, found that population groups who live on a natural, unadulterated diet display superb health and freedom from the "diseases of choice"

Figure 7. Revised Dietary Suggestions

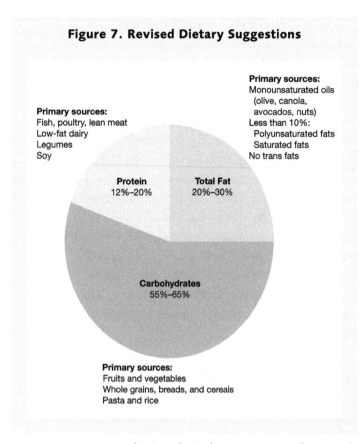

Primary sources:
Fish, poultry, lean meat
Low-fat dairy
Legumes
Soy

Primary sources:
Monounsaturated oils
(olive, canola,
avocados, nuts)
Less than 10%:
 Polyunsaturated fats
 Saturated fats
No trans fats

Protein
12%–20%

Total Fat
20%–30%

Carbohydrates
55%–65%

Primary sources:
Fruits and vegetables
Whole grains, breads, and cereals
Pasta and rice

mentioned earlier. When these more "primitive" people adopt modern eating habits, they contract the same degenerative diseases of "civilized" countries within a relatively short period of time (ten years on the average).[10]

The eating habits of healthy peoples, whether they come from the jungles of Africa, the mountains of Tibet, the beaches of the South Pacific, or midtown Manhattan, follow two general rules: Their food is of high nutritional value (what nutritionists call "nutrient dense") and is largely unadulterated (not highly processed).

The first component of a nutritious diet is nutrient density. Foods that healthy people consume are loaded with vitamins and minerals in their most natural state. These foods are fresh (locally grown and vine-ripened, and free from pesticides, herbicides, and additives) and raw or lightly cooked. Processed sugars and grains, packaged foods, and commercial additives are generally kept to a minimum.

The bottom line? Eat whole foods (foods that are as near to the way nature created them as possible), and reduce your intake of substitutes that originate in a test tube. This important rule becomes increasingly crucial to our health as we age. With the passing years, cells rebuild more slowly and deteriorate more rapidly. Some nutrients that are less efficiently absorbed may be required in greater amounts, even though calories need to be reduced as our metabolism slows with age. Obviously, we cannot afford to waste our caloric intake on foods that fail to feed the body properly.

The foods we consume most of the time must be high in nutrient density. We all have favorite recipes, snacks, and celebration delights, and I know you won't deny yourself Grandma's famous apple pie forever. As long as these foods are not a daily indulgence, a healthy body will be able to handle them.

For most of us in the United States, our priorities have become reversed over the past forty years. The balance of what we eat has swung more and more toward nonessential rather than essential foods. It is estimated that up to 80 percent of what the majority of Americans eat has no nutritive value whatsoever. No wonder, then, that the American way of life itself has been called a "high-risk

Figure 8. The Revised "Basic Four" Plan

High nutrient density	High fiber
Low fat	Low sugar

factor" in several diseases. The Senate Select Committee on Nutrition reports that the Standard American Diet (SAD) is high in fat, sugar, and calories and low in fiber and nutrients. To continue this way of eating when it is known to promote high blood pressure, heart disease, digestive disturbances, skin problems, obesity, blood-sugar imbalances, and accelerated aging is indeed SAD. Several leading nutritionists have proposed a variable scale for the major food groups based on the assumption that we are all unique and must tailor our food choices to individual needs. (For a summary of this guide, see Figure 7)

If you are at risk for any of the health problems listed above, it is important that you analyze exactly what you are eating. Consider your daily menus: Are the foods you normally eat high in nutrient density? High in fiber? Low in fat? Low in additives (sugar, salt, unnecessary chemicals)? When you choose your foods, keep these "revised basic four" nutrition goals in mind (see Figure 8).

DIFFERENT CULTURES, DIFFERENT DIETS

Do any cultures exist whose diets we can use as a model? Asian diets, particularly those high in soy-based products, have been shown to promote health, as this book discusses in several chapters. Soy is high in lignans and isoflavones, which have been shown to offer anticancer benefits and to aid in the management of menopausal symptoms. Adding liberal amounts of soy to a nutrient-dense, diverse diet based on unprocessed foods may be the best preventive medicine available.

Besides the traditional Asian diet, another demographic-specific diet has received a lot of press because of its supposed health benefits: the Mediterranean diet. Ancel Keys of the University of Minnesota began decades ago formally looking into the causes of heart disease. He studied the lifestyles of several thousand healthy, middle-aged men from seven countries. After ten years, the 655 subjects from the Greek island of Crete showed by far the best resistance to heart disease: Only 2 percent had developed heart disease, and none of them had died. Beginning with that research, guidelines for following the so-called Mediterranean diet have

emerged, including the development of a Mediterranean pyramid as an alternative to the USDA's Food Guide Pyramid (the one we frequently see on boxes of cereal and loaves of bread). The Mediterranean pyramid was developed by nutritionists and epidemiologists at the Harvard School of Public Health, the European office of the World Health Organization, and Oldways Preservation and Exchange Trust.

It is tempting to focus on the universally attractive elements of the Mediterranean diet because it allows liberal amounts of fat or oil in the diet (up to 40 percent of calories); limits but doesn't exclude red meat; recommends fish and poultry a few times a week; emphasizes fruits, vegetables, beans, pasta, and low-fat dairy products; and allows up to two glasses of alcohol per day. However, before we enthusiastically begin consuming high amounts of fat and daily alcohol, it's important to note, as always, that the *types* of these foods commonly eaten by the Cretans were very specific. Ancel Keys has noted that their diet was dominated by olive oil (we've already discussed the benefits of monounsaturated oils, such as olive oil and canola oil) and whole-grain breads. Together, these two elements accounted for 50 to 60 percent of their total calories. The diet also was rich in beans and fresh fruits and vegetables. Meat—even poultry—was rare, and so were sugar and most dairy products.

Cardiologist Stephen Sinatra, among others, believes that the Mediterranean diet reduces the risk of heart disease and sudden death more than any other program available. Indeed, new epidemiological (population) evidence and statistical evaluation confirm the protective effect of the Mediterranean diet when maintained for up to four years after the first myocardial infarction.[11]

Critics of the Mediterranean diet point out that a high-fat diet without sufficient exercise will add fat to the body, which is not good for the heart, and that two drinks a day may increase a woman's risk for breast cancer (remember, the Cretan study subjects were men). After reviewing all the evidence, it becomes clear that we cannot tout the miracles of the Mediterranean diet while ignoring the context of the total lifestyle enjoyed by the Cretan men of Keys' study, a lifestyle very different from that of most Americans today. The subjects from Crete got plenty of physical activity from their daily work (many were fishermen) and probably endured less stress as well—at least the kind of stress affiliated with our rush-around, get-ahead, achievement-obsessed society. Relaxing over a glass of wine at a leisurely lunch is not the same as a two-martini power lunch.

≋ Supplements? Yes! ≋

For decades I have espoused the necessity of taking vitamin and mineral supplements based on the probability that we are not eating all of the fruits and vegetables we require each day. I've presented governmental surveys indicating that few people in the United States are getting even the minimum daily allowances (RDAs). Moreover, I felt I built a solid case for the fact that nutritional research over the past two decades has shown that supplemental nutrients above the RDAs are critical in preventing and treating chronic diseases such as heart disease and cancer. But my presentation and passion, along with those of many other nutritionists, fell on deaf ears among the medically trained. Even in light of all the research supporting the benefits of supplementation, conventionally trained doctors on the whole maintained that a "balanced diet" was adequate to meet our dietary needs, and they collectively repeated the mantra over and over that vitamins only gave us expensive urine.

Nutritionists across America have been vindicated. In a landmark article published in June 2002 in the medical community's most prestigious periodical, *Journal of the American Medical Association*, researchers announced that pending strong evidence of effectiveness from randomized trials, it appears prudent that all adults should take vitamin supplements to help prevent chronic diseases.[12] Yippee!! Excuse my exuberance, but this has been a long time coming.

The authors of the study agree that most people fail to consume an optimal amount of all vitamins by diet alone. They point out that suboptimal levels of folic acid, vitamin B-6, and vitamin B-12 are a risk factor for heart disease, neural-tube defects, and colon and breast cancer; low levels of vitamin D contribute to bone fractures and osteopenia (lower than normal bone mass); and low levels of antioxidants (vitamins A, E, and C) may increase risk for several chronic diseases. And these are just the obvious nutrients. In another thirty years they will catch up with the rest of the scientific world and realize that other nutrients exist that contribute to optimum health.

Should you take vitamin/mineral supplements? Yes, your doctor says so.

WOMEN MAY BE NUTRIENT DEFICIENT

Human beings are not genetically uniform. They vary in body frame, weight, dietary preferences, the amount of exercise they take, their digestion and absorption of nutrients, and how they deal with stress. The nutritional requirements of healthy people can vary from "normal" by a factor of as much as thirty; those of sick people may vary by factors as high as one thousand.[13]

This diversity, both biochemical and nutritional, is even greater among women. Consider that some women have no children, some have one child, others have fourteen. There are women who nurse their babies for several months, women who are on the Pill, women who have undergone tubal ligations, women who have had partial or radical hysterectomies. Each of these situations usually

requires greater than "average" amounts of specific nutrients. When factors vary so dramatically, it is especially difficult if not impossible to formulate standard or average nutritional requirements.

Many people are born with or develop a need for larger quantities of some nutrients. Andrew Weil, M.D., author of *Health and Healing* and several other books on holistic health care, explains that our bodies have one or more weak points. Some people are prone to sore throats; others may have sensitive stomachs. Your diet may exacerbate this condition. Nowhere is this clearer than in the case of calcium and its relationship to osteoporosis. Many women inherit a predisposition to osteoporosis; others are at risk because of a lack of calcium in their diet or because of lifestyle habits that prevent calcium absorption. Whatever the case, increased calcium intake can significantly reduce bone loss in the midlife years.

What confuses many people about nutritional recommendations is the fact that there are always stories of individuals who beat the statistics. Why doesn't every smoker get lung cancer when the research so clearly shows a direct correlation between the two? Obviously, some fortunate individuals have strong constitutions or above-average respiratory systems.

The question you need to ask yourself is not "Am I average?" but "Do I have a weakness?" If so, you should design your diet to compensate for that weakness. And chances are, you have a weakness.

SHOULD YOU CONSIDER TAKING SUPPLEMENTS?

Nutritionists report that women are likely to be low in the following: vitamins A, D, C, and B-complex (especially B-6, B-12, and folic acid), and the minerals calcium, magnesium, zinc, selenium, and copper. Women who are menstruating can add iron to this list. The list expands with age, infection, disease, stress, smoking, and poor dietary habits, such as drinking in excess or eating primarily processed nonfoods.

At a minimum, you should consider taking supplements if you are

⊙ not eating two to three fruits and four to five vegetables a day;

⊙ drinking excess alcohol or caffeine, or eating sugar;

⊙ smoking or living with someone who does;

⊙ on a diet of fewer than one thousand calories per day;

⊙ on a fad diet that restricts a major food group;

⊙ pregnant, which usually indicates a need for additional iron and folic acid;

⊙ taking medications (diuretics and some hypertensive drugs deplete potassium; cholestyramine causes poor absorption of fat, vitamins A, B-12, and D, and the minerals iron and potassium; mineral oil and other laxatives cause a loss of vitamins A and D and the mineral calcium; and broad-spectrum antibiotics may decrease vitamin K and some of the B-complex vitamins);

⊙ diagnosed as having a disease in which diet is a recognized factor, including hypertension, heart disease, cancer, kidney disease, ulcers, alcoholism, adult-onset diabetes;

⊙ a burn patient, or suffering from a prolonged illness.

As strongly as I believe that most individuals require supplements to meet their nutritional needs, I want to make it very clear that pills are not a replacement for a nutritious diet. Researchers are continually identifying new substances in foods that promote health and protect against disease. Every day, scientists find more and more phytonutrients (nutrients in plants) that may be just as important to our health as well-known vitamins and nutrients. To rely too heavily on only the nutrients of which we are aware is a mistake. Also, don't think that you can eat all the junk food you want and pop a handful of pills as insurance. Who knows what nutritious substances we are missing because they are not found in a multivitamin pill?

CHOOSING OPTIMUM—NOT MINIMUM—NUTRITION

The recommended dietary allowances (RDAs), even though they were updated in the late 1990s and early 2000s, for the most part offer standards for minimum, rather than optimum, health. The RDAs were not designed to enhance health, to address people who are in less than perfect health, to include an aging population, or for anyone with specific nutritional needs, such as those who suffer from chronic disease or periodic infection or those who take medication. And in only a few cases do the RDAs consider the potential for optimal health and the relationship between nutrient intake and protection from disease.

Some progress was made when the RDAs were recently updated. For example, the National Institutes of Health found the previous RDAs for calcium to be inadequate across the board, but especially for postmenopausal women, and publicly recommended higher doses to help prevent and treat bone loss. In 1997, RDAs for calcium were increased for women to between 1,000 and 1,300 mg per day, depending on a woman's age and whether she is pregnant or lactating.

For another example, years of research have continued to confirm a strong association between vitamin E deficiency and heart disease. An individual's vitamin E status has been called a better predictor of heart disease than her or his blood cholesterol levels. Most of the research on vitamin E has found that people require supplemental doses in the range of 100 to 400 IU per day to prevent artery-clogging plaque, yet the RDA for women, updated in 2000, remains at a low 22 IU (15 mg) per day.

Instead of waiting for battling nutritionists to give us the official okay, we need to embrace current and ongoing knowledge that shows us ways to optimize our own health nutritionally.

ACCENTUATE THE POSITIVE

Life is a banquet, but most poor suckers are starving to death.

— AUNTIE MAME

Nutritionists rarely agree on what constitutes an optimum diet, usually for two reasons: First, much of nutrition is open to interpretation, and second, "optimum" is different for every individual. Nevertheless, certain principles can be applied when creating an individual program. An optimum diet should allow an individual to develop to his or her fullest potential, reach peak mental and physical performance, offer the greatest resistance to infection and disease, and not accelerate the aging process. These goals are widely accepted, so to start a program, let's fill in the dietary basics that also enjoy general acceptance.

First let's take a look at the so-called macronutrients: protein, carbohydrates, and fats. These are the nutrients that provide our bodies with energy. Besides alcohol, these three are the only substances that contain calories. (Because fiber is closely related to carbohydrate, although it contains no calories, it's also included in this first part of the chapter.)

⇒ Protein ⇐

Eating enough protein is not a problem for most American women, unless they are crash dieting on grapefruit and lettuce leaves. The average protein consumption in the United States substantially exceeds requirements.[1] Believing that a meal must center around meat, many people overdo it. The standard daily requirement of protein is 0.8 gram for every two pounds of ideal body weight. Thus, if you weigh 120 pounds, 48 grams of protein is the amount you need every day to build, repair, and maintain your cells. Women's average intake ranges between 40 and 60 grams per

day. The table titled "Are You Getting Adequate Protein?" translates the above formula into practical measurements (see the chart to the right).

We all know that protein is basic to life. Next to water, it is the most plentiful substance in the body, constituting 18 to 20 percent of body weight. Protein is the structural material that supports the cells, skin, hair, muscles, internal organs, and blood vessels. It builds cells during times of growth and repairs them in emergencies.

In the United States we have a rather empirical approach to diet. Because we are a relatively young country with a wide mix of national origins, we do not have a dominant "traditional" diet. So we tend to experiment a great deal, trying to sort out the good from the not-so-good. This also means that when something is proven to benefit our health, we have a strong tendency to go overboard. This certainly has happened with protein. For many years, a high-protein diet was the rage. Scores of people suffered dangerous side effects; some even sustained irreversible damage to their organs. As important as protein is to the maintenance of the body, an excess is not beneficial and may even cause serious problems.

For example, consider the following:

⊙ Some meats, especially red meats (beef, pork, lamb) are particularly high in saturated fat. A high-fat diet is known to promote obesity, hypertension, atherosclerosis, and cancer.

⊙ Red meats aggravate PMS and menstrual cramps.

⊙ Red meats are high in phosphates and acid, which increase the loss of calcium from the bones, creating a greater risk of osteoporosis.

⊙ Large amounts of protein put a strain on the kidneys, as they form and excrete organic compounds containing nitrogen waste.

⊙ Too much protein may deplete vitamins B-6 and B-3 (niacin), calcium, and magnesium.

⊙ Processed and smoked meats such as bacon, ham, salami, and luncheon meats contain nitrates and nitrites, which can lead to the formation of cancer-causing nitrosamines in the body.

Most cuts of meat contain nearly as much fat as protein and possibly even more. A slice of lean ham or a choice grade of slightly marbled sirloin is approximately 25 percent protein and 75 percent fat. Poultry is generally lower in fat and calories, providing, of course, that you remove the skin and don't fry the meat.

Much of the meat and poultry raised in the United States contains synthetic hormones, antibiotics, pesticide residues, and several other undesirable chemical additives. Fortunately, meat and poultry products that have been raised untreated are increasingly available. Ask about them at your local markets.

Fish is lower in fat than meat and chicken, yet still high in protein. Unless you fry the fish, bread it, or smother it in sauce, the fat content remains low. Of course, it is best to buy fresh fish, but even canned tuna (packed in water), shrimp, and crab are good sources of protein.

Meat, fish, eggs, and all dairy products provide what nutritionists call *complete proteins*. A complete protein contains all nine essential amino acids, or protein building blocks. Protein is also found in varying amounts in vegetables, grains, beans, peas, seeds, and nuts. Because these carbohydrate sources lack or are very low in one or more essential amino acids, they are considered incomplete; the one exception in the plant world is soy: It provides complete protein. Nutritionists used to think that one incomplete protein had to be combined with another incomplete protein at the same meal to get the complete benefit. This theory is no longer accepted, since the breakdown fragments of protein, the amino acids, circulate in the body long after a meal is eaten and are easily available for matching.

Though research on proteins and amino acids is fairly recent, cultures all over the world have been combining proteins since long before the word was coined. Latin Americans thrive on rice and beans. Corn tortillas and beans are a staple among Mexicans. Traditional dishes in the southeastern United States include corn bread and crowder peas or red beans and rice. In Chinese cuisine, tofu is added to vegetables and rice. Vegetarians have studied the art of food combining to achieve a healthier diet.

Dairy products are not only useful as accompaniments to grains; they are excellent by themselves as a protein source. Milk has been called "the perfect food" because its amino-acid balance matches that of meat, fish, and poultry. As with

Are You Getting Adequate Protein?

You need: Your body weight in pounds

_____ x 0.4 = _____ grams per day

Food	Protein (Grams)
Beef (8 oz)	64
Chicken (8 oz)	72
Fish (8 oz)	56
Tuna (3 oz)	24
Eggs (2)	14
Milk (1 cup)	9
Cottage cheese (1/2 cup)	14
Cheddar cheese (1 oz)	7
Beans (1/2 cup)	7
Beans with rice (1 cup)	17
Vegetarian lasagna (1 cup)	14
Rice pudding (1 cup)	17
Pasta (1 cup)	5
Wheat cereal with milk (1 cup)	28
Whole-wheat bread (1 slice)	3
Cornbread (4" x 3" slice)	4
Potato (1, medium)	5

other protein foods, those lowest in fat are preferred; these include nonfat milk, low-fat cottage cheese, low-fat yogurt, buttermilk, kefir, and cheeses such as mozzarella, baker's cheese, gammelost, krutt, pot, sapsago, and farmer's cheese. The most popular cheeses—Swiss, Cheddar, muenster, longhorn—are highest in fat. Since one ounce of these cheeses contains between 9 and 11 grams of fat, use these sparingly.

Cow's milk is not for everyone, however. Some people are allergic to milk products, and others may lack the enzyme needed to digest the lactose or milk sugar (a condition called *lactose intolerance*). If drinking cow's milk or eating processed cheese causes diarrhea, indigestion, or flatulence, try fermented milk alternatives (yogurt, kefir, buttermilk, or acidophilus milk). If digestive difficulties continue, drop dairy products from your diet. There are enough proteins available from other sources; if you are concerned about your calcium intake, take a supplement.

Seeds and nuts offer another alternative to meat and also double as a good source of fiber. They can be eaten raw and fresh and can be a convenient snack or combined in a meal for added nutrition, flavor, and texture. Still, power-packed as they are, it is best not to go overboard with these unless you can afford the calories. A half cup of peanuts or walnuts contains 36 grams of fat.

Tofu, made from soybean curd, is close in nutritional quality to meat protein and is an excellent complement to grains. Since tofu is easy to digest and low in saturated fats, cholesterol, and calories, it is recommended for those who cannot eat fat-rich meat and are sensitive to dairy foods.

⇒ Carbohydrates ⇐

The body runs on carbohydrates; they are the only true clean-burning fuel in the diet. Both protein and fat release toxic by-products as they are metabolized. Carbohydrates do not; in fact, they temper the toxins created by the processing of other nutrients. This is why a diet high in protein and fat and low in carbohydrates can overburden the organs and decrease energy. Athletes and exercise nuts know that carbohydrates are best for fueling the muscles before a workout to protect against muscular fatigue.

Since foods containing complex carbohydrates (such as whole grains, beans, rice, fruits, and vegetables) are rich in vitamins, minerals, antioxidants, and phytochemicals, are a great source of fiber, are low in fat, and can double as protein sources, they can potentially serve our total dietary needs. Vegetarians have long proven that fact. The bulk of our diet—55 to 65 percent of our total daily calories—should come from this important food group.

THE DOWNSIDE OF CARBS

Unfortunately, not all carbohydrates are healthy or good for us. With the advent of the fat-free revolution, when researchers linked dietary fat to obesity and coronary artery disease, women started eliminating fat from their diets and replacing it with concentrated carbohydrates. Sure these foods were devoid of fat, but the downside was that they were packed with sugar. And the end result wasn't weight loss. Unsuspectingly, women went overboard, consuming huge portions of nonfat ice cream, yogurt, salad dressing, cookies, and chips while thinking the fat would drip off their bodies. This didn't happen because the total caloric intake still exceeded the limit the body could use up. Obesity was not controlled; it climbed.

In some women, carbohydrates, even healthy ones, trigger overpowering food cravings. Foods affect all of us differently. One woman may be calmed and satisfied by her morning bagel, while another eating the same breakfast may be primed to hunt down anything remaining in the refrigerator or desk. Carbohydrates, especially those of the refined and sugarcoated variety, stimulate a rise in blood sugar and then in insulin levels, which eventually triggers the appetite and, in some people, uncontrollable cravings. (Read more about this phenomenon, called *insulin resistance*, in Chapter 4.) Women especially need to be aware of their particular sensitivity to carbohydrates and to work with reducing or eliminating offenders from their diet.

A tool called the *glycemic index* may help you make better choices about your carb-laden foods, especially if you are highly sensitive to sugars and starches. Food scientists have developed this system, which quantifies the rate at which a carbohydrate food enters the bloodstream and raises blood-sugar and insulin levels. Foods with a high glycemic index elevate blood sugar more rapidly than those with a moderate or lower score. That said, be aware that the chain of events is not exactly clearcut; for one thing, a particular food will impact individuals differently, and for another, when you eat a high-scoring carbohydrate with a low-scoring one, the effect is generally neutralized. For example, if you have cereal for breakfast but put milk on it, the spike in blood sugar is less immediate and doesn't go as high. Also, differences exist within the categories according to the amount of carbohydrate, fiber, or sugar content of the food. If you eat a carrot, which ranks high on the index list, it will not trigger a major spurt in your insulin level because it is low in both carbohydrate and sugar. I've read many diet books that stress eliminating carrots and potatoes from the diet because of their high glycemic-index score. I think we need to exercise some common sense and refrain from indiscriminately classifying all high-scoring carbs as evil. After all, a handful of baby carrots provides more than twice the RDA of pro-vitamin A, plus a decent amount of fiber.

Experiment with the following list and notice how you feel after eating some of these foods:

Glycemic Index of Selected Foods

High (Over 65)	Medium (45–65)	Low (Under 45)
Glucose, 100	Raisins, 65	All Bran, 43
Croissants, 96	Jelly, 63	Grapes, 43
Oatmeal (one minute), 93	Bananas (ripe), 62	Dried beans (cooked), 42
Carrots, 92	Sweet corn, 61	Pears, 41
Molasses, 87	Bran muffins, 60	Oranges, 40
Pancakes, 83	Table sugar, 59	Apples, 39
Cornflakes, 80	Apple juice, 58	Chocolate, 36
Baked potato, 73	Honey, 58	Wine, 35
White rice, 72	Oatmeal (cooked), 58	Beer, 35
Dark bread, 72	Kiwis, 58	Milk, 34
Watermelon, 72	Muesli cereal, 56	Yogurt, 33
Corn chips, 70	Oatmeal cookies, 55	Ice cream (full fat), 30
White bread, 69	Orange juice, 53	Strawberries, 25
Bagels, 69	Peas, 52	Cherries, 22
Corn meal, 68	Pasta, 50	Broccoli, 9
French fries, 67	Ice cream (low fat), 50	Spinach (cooked), 9
Brown rice, 66	Grapefruit juice, 48	Lettuce, 9

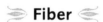

Fiber

The principal carbohydrates are sugars, starches, and fiber. Sugars and starches basically provide the body with energy, while dietary fiber serves several different functions.

Several varieties of fiber exist, and each participates differently in the body. Water-insoluble fiber, found in whole grains and the bran of wheat, rye, corn, and rice, and in some fruits and vegetables, keeps the gastrointestinal system running smoothly. It softens the stool, helps to prevent constipation, and exercises the muscles of the digestive system, keeping the intestines toned and more resistant to diverticulosis.

How Much Fiber Are You Getting?

Cereals   **Fiber**
(Grams)

All Bran with extra fiber (¹/₂ cup) . . . .
14.0
Wheat Bran (¹/₂ cup) . . . .
12.0
100% Bran (¹/₂ cup) . . . .
10.0
Bran Chex (²/₃ cup) . . . .
6.0
Fruit and Fiber (¹/₂ cup) . . . .
5.0
Oatmeal (³/₄ cup) . . . .
2.1
Cornflakes (³/₄ cup) . . . .
2.1
Oat granola (¹/₃ cup) . . . .
1.0

Bread

Pita bread, whole wheat (5" pocket) . . . . . .
4.4
100% whole wheat or rye (2 slices) . . . .
2.0
Bagel (1) . . . .
1.4
White bread, French, Italian (1 slice) . . . . .
0.6
Croissant (1) 0

Beans and Peas

Pinto or kidney beans (³/₄ cup, cooked) . .
14.0
Black-eyed peas (³/₄ cup, cooked) . . . . . .
12.3
Rice Krispies 0
Garbanzos (³/₄ cup, cooked) . . . .
7.0
Lentils (³/₄ cup, cooked) . . . .
5.6
Split peas (³/₄ cup, cooked) . . . .
4.0

Soluble fiber is found in high concentration in oat bran, dried peas and beans, barley, many fruits and vegetables, gums (guar, xanthan, locust bean), mucilages (psyllium), and pectin. A lot of current research proves soluble fiber to be effective in lowering both cholesterol and triglyceride levels in the blood and in aiding in the regulation of blood-sugar levels.

There is no question that dietary fiber is a major factor in achieving good health. Large-scale research throughout the world suggests that fiber may protect against some forms of cancer, reduce the risk of coronary heart disease, and help control obesity, constipation, diabetes, and a host of other maladies. Fibrous foods also contribute vitamins and minerals to the body. For example, whole-grain flours are rich in B vitamins and protein; fruits give us vitamin C and many minerals; and vegetables are high in vitamin A and minerals.

A quick digression: Let me reemphasize the superior nature of whole grains over processed cereals and breads. In the standard milling process, as much as 60 to 90 percent of vitamin B-6, folic acid, vitamin E, and many other nutrients are lost—as well as the fiber.[2]

Since we generally don't eat enough fruits and vegetables, and since a great deal of the fiber has been processed out of breads and

cereals, it is not surprising that fiber intake among Americans is abysmally low—less than half of what is considered healthy. Recommended dosage is approximately 30 to 40 grams of fiber per day; most Americans fall below 10 grams per day. Take a quick look at the table on page 279 and see how you score.

You may want to find ways to slowly introduce more fibrous foods into your diet. Adding too many too soon often causes discomfort, so go slowly and work up to at least 30 grams a day.

 Fat

About 40 percent of the calorie intake in the average American diet comes from fats and oils. This is equivalent to about three ounces of fat or three-quarters of a stick of butter per person per day. Surprised? Do you trim the fat off your meat and resist eating butter with your bread? Are you convinced that someone else—not you—makes up this "average"? The problem is that most of us are unaware of how many fats are camouflaged in our foods. How often do you eat fast foods, TV dinners, deli sand-

---

Suggestions for Increasing the Amount of Fiber in Your Diet

- Switch to a high-fiber bread, such as sprouted wheat, wheat berry, or 100 percent whole grain.
- Have a high-fiber cold cereal for breakfast three to four times a week. Try Bran Flakes, Bran Chex, Raisin Bran, or Cracklin' Oat Bran.
- Make a high-fiber soup once a week: bean soup, lentil soup, corn chowder, cabbage soup, or vegetable soup with beans.
- Use beans in your green salads: garbanzo beans, green beans, kidney beans, or peas.
- Make vegetable dishes that contain beans, such as three-bean salad, succotash, rice with peas, or broccoli with kidney beans.
- Eat high-fiber vegetables every day, including corn, broccoli, Brussels sprouts, spinach, peas, green beans, and potatoes.
- Serve fruit as often as possible, including blueberries, strawberries, pears, raisins, bananas, and apples.
- Use dark-green salad greens, such as spinach, romaine, and endive, instead of pale iceberg lettuce.
- Try bean dips served with chili, raw vegetables, or whole-wheat pita bread.
- Use unprocessed wheat bran and All Bran in regular recipes for pies, cakes, and cookies.
- Add unprocessed wheat and oat bran to meat loaf, casseroles, and vegetable dishes as an extender, or make crumb toppings for baked fruit desserts.
- Eat corn, bran, or oat muffins instead of cakes, doughnuts, and cookies.
- Add raisins to muffins, cereals, rice pudding, and cookies.
- Use part whole-wheat, soy, or oat flour in your standard recipes.
- Snack on whole-grain crackers and dried fruits.
- Use nuts and seeds on salads and in recipes.

wiches, hot dogs, luncheon meats, peanut butter, bread, crackers, nuts, potato chips, corn chips, avocados, cheese, quiche, salad dressing, pizza, rice pudding, potato salad, paté, pastries, mousse, croissants, dips, doughnuts, ice cream, cheesecake, cream soups, sauces, pie, cookies, or chocolate? These are all high in fat.

A high-fat diet contributes to obesity. Fat contains nine calories per gram, compared to four calories per gram for both protein and carbohydrates (alcohol contains seven calories per gram). A high-fat diet can contribute to the development of high blood pressure, heart disease, diabetes, and breast cancer. Reducing overall fat consumption to 25–30 percent of total calories should be your long-term goal.

Fats come in many forms, and some are worse for you than others. Two fats in particular, saturated fats and trans fatty acids, earn dishonorable mentions. So it's best to avoid them. It is also wise to avoid polyunsaturated fats, which are not much better. These fats are discussed in detail in Chapter 9.

Tips for Reducing Fat Content in Your Diet

- Cut down on red meats; use them as a side dish rather than as a main course.
- Buy leaner cuts of red meat, such as round steak, flank steak, and lean ground sirloin.
- Trim all visible fat from meat before cooking.
- Replace red meats with turkey and chicken—particularly the white meat parts.
- Skin poultry before cooking.
- Choose fish and seafood more often—especially scrod, flounder, cod, haddock, shrimp, lobster, red snapper, and tuna (packed in water).
- Bake, broil, or stir-fry rather than deep fry.
- Experiment with nonmeat dinners once or twice a week.
- Decrease use of oil and butter in cooking and baking.
- Minimize cheese, sauces, and dips, and use low-fat substitutes when you can (nonfat milk, low-fat plain yogurt, low-fat cottage cheese).
- Limit use of seeds, nuts, and avocados.
- Eliminate processed and packaged foods completely.
- Watch intake of desserts—especially pies, doughnuts, chocolate, ice cream, and other creamy, gooey concoctions. (Try substituting nonfat desserts instead.)

MONOUNSATURATED FATS

Monounsaturated fats are among the few that appear to heal rather than hurt. They include the oils canola, olive, peanut, and sesame and are your best bet for daily use in salads and cooking. In countries such as Greece and in southern Italy, where people take in relatively high amounts of these fats, the rates of heart disease are low.

ESSENTIAL FATTY ACIDS

A certain amount of dietary fat is vital to optimum health. Essential fatty acids (EFAs), the fats that we need daily for basic cellular function, are also being recognized for a variety of other therapeutic effects. EFAs have been found to lower cholesterol and blood pressure, to reduce the risk of heart disease and stroke, and, possibly, to be helpful for arthritis and some forms of cancer. They are particularly helpful to midlife women because low levels are partly responsible for drying of the tissues of the body, especially the vagina, skin, and hair.

The essential fatty acids, linoleic acid and linolenic acid, can be found in a variety of sources: raw nuts and seeds, vegetable oils, and fish oils. Getting essential oils through diet is not always easy, since few of us eat large enough amounts of sunflower or pumpkin seeds or mackerel, salmon, herring, and tuna. Supplementing the diet with EFAs is usually indicated for treatment of the conditions mentioned above and may be equally good for preventing problems generally. Recommended sources of EFAs are borage oil, black currant oil, evening primrose oil, and flaxseed oil. The latter is an excellent source of both EFAs, and it can be substituted for other, less nutritious oils in salad dressings and mayonnaise, or drizzled on vegetables. To take oils orally as a supplement, one to three tablespoons daily is adequate. Diabetics should avoid fish oil supplements, but can increase their consumption of fish.

The beneficial effects of EFAs do not mean that you can eat as much of these "healthful" oils as you like. All fats make you fat. Dietary fats are converted more efficiently into bodily fats than either protein or carbohydrates, and the body expends fewer calories to metabolize them than it does for the other two. If you are concerned about your weight, consume fewer total fats.

⬩ The Wonders of Soy ⬩

Soy is familiar to most Americans as a food staple for vegetarians. Soy is a protein powerhouse unique among plant foods: It is the only plant food that by itself provides complete protein. That means it houses all nine essential amino acids, which must be eaten within a few hours of each other to trigger the proper biochemical reactions in the human body. The only other foods that include complete protein are animal products: meat, eggs, dairy foods. That's why the Chinese call tofu (soybean curd) "meat without bones."

Soy is no longer relegated to the vegetarian's table. Following much research that has demonstrated its amazing health benefits, soy is enjoying a well-deserved boom in popularity. Containing estrogen-mimicking substances called *isoflavones* that appear to alleviate menopausal symptoms, reduce the risk of breast cancer, protect bones from osteoporosis, and help prevent heart disease, soy is being touted as a veritable wonder food.

Even with the flood of information about soy's benefits, habits often prove slow—and difficult—to change. How do we Americans begin on a daily basis to include a food in our diet that most of us have hardly been exposed to? This section aims to help you do just that—but first, a little more overview about the amazing soybean.

CHECK THE LABELS

Even the often slow-to-respond Food and Drug Administration has pronounced that eating soy-based foods can help fight heart disease. In 1999, the FDA authorized the use of health claims on food labels promoting the association of soy protein and the reduced risk of coronary heart disease. The two must-haves on the labels include: (1) a statement that 25 grams of soy protein a day, as part of a diet low in saturated fat and cholesterol, may reduce the risk of heart disease; (2) a statement about the amount of soy protein per serving contained in that particular food product.

To claim the health benefits of soy, a food product must contain

⊙ at least 6.25 grams of soy protein per serving;

⊙ low fat (less than 3 grams per serving);

⊙ low saturated fat (less than 1 gram per serving);

⊙ low cholesterol (less than 20 mg per serving).

Foods made with the whole soybean may also qualify for the health claim if they contain no fat in addition to that present in the whole soybean. These would include products such as tofu, soy milk, soy-based burgers, tempeh, and soy nuts.

A partial list of food companies whose products meet these criteria appears on the website of the U.S. Soyfoods Directory (www.soyfoods.com). According to the FDA, foods that may be eligible for the health claim include soy beverages, tempeh, tofu, soy-based meat alternatives such as soy patties, soy nuts, and maybe some baked goods. Soy sauce fails to meet minimum requirements.

SOY'S NUTRITIONAL CONTENT

Soy is what nutritionists call a nutrient-dense food. It is packed with nutrition. Besides being a complete protein, it is rich in complex carbohydrates and fiber. While some soy foods might be high in fat (sometimes containing up to 40 percent of calories from fat), soy itself is low in saturated fat. Soy's predominant fat is the essential fatty acid linoleic acid, an omega-6 fatty acid. It also contains some

of the super-healthy omega-3 fatty acids. And not all soy products are high in fat: Texturized soy protein (TSP) has no fat, and many products are manufactured with the fat content reduced. Finally, soy is a good source for B vitamins and for the estrogen-like isoflavones that appear to be so beneficial in treating menopausal symptoms and preventing breast cancer and osteoporosis.

THE DIVERSITY OF SOY

Soybeans, used in China for thousands of years, belong to the legume family. The plant produces pods that contain two to three seeds each; these are the soybeans themselves, sometimes called *soya beans*, or, in China, *wang tul*, "yellow bean." Raw, the soybean is totally indigestible and even contains some chemicals that deactivate vital enzymes in the body. The cooking process neutralizes those unfavorable chemicals.

Soy can be eaten in many forms, some of which are listed below.

Soybeans

Soybeans can be purchased dried, like other legumes, or fresh, as green soybeans. Either way they are a good source of all the health-promoting nutrients. They can be hard to find, and many people find the flavor on the strong side, so you may find other soy foods more to your liking.

Dried soybeans can be boiled for several hours (like other dried beans) and served as a side dish or added to salads and casseroles. Fresh green soybeans look like fuzzy green pods. Steamed until tender, when they are known as *edamame*, they are sweet and crunchy and make a nice addition to salads or by themselves. Restaurants in Japan serve them as finger food before the meal. Canned soybeans can also be found in some stores, fully cooked and ready to eat.

Soy Beverages

Soy milk is a liquid prepared from ground soybeans and water. Since it is lactose-free, people who cannot tolerate cow's milk often drink soy milk as a substitute. It does not contain as much calcium as cow's milk, but like regular milk it can be fortified with calcium, vitamin D, and sometimes vitamin B-12.

No longer is soy milk the gritty, unpalatable product of the past. It is light and smooth and, besides plain, comes in flavors such as chocolate, almond, and vanilla. It also is offered in low-fat or nonfat varieties. You can find it in the dairy section or packaged in aseptic cartons that don't need refrigeration (until after being opened).

Drink soy milk as a beverage, pour it over cereal, or substitute it for milk in cooking. Consider using it in your favorite decaf latte.

Soy Nuts

With the same nutrient quality as plain soybeans, piquantly seasoned deep-fried or dry-roasted soybeans are now easy to find in the bulk-foods section of most natural foods stores. They make a quick, crunchy snack, but they're high in fat and calories. Use them sparingly, in breads and other baked goods.

Miso

A fermented soybean paste made from soybeans, salt, water, and a cultured grain (usually rice or barley), miso is sold in Asian groceries. A tablespoon contains virtually no fat; however, it is high in sodium. Use sparingly.

Miso can be used like bouillon to flavor soups; it can be added to salad dressings and sauces for vegetables; it can be used to marinate meat for barbecue. Several types of miso exist; they vary in taste and usage depending on their color. Darker ones tend to be stronger tasting than the lighter varieties.

Tofu

Chinese for "soybean curd," tofu is made from soy milk. Dried soybeans are crushed and boiled, and a curdling agent is added to separate the curds from the whey. The pieces of the curd are then poured into square molds, where they become firm.

Tofu is loaded with nutrients: protein, essential fats, zinc, iron, B vitamins, and calcium (if it is made with calcium sulfate). It is bland, so it takes on the flavor of any food it is cooked with. It must be refrigerated.

Several forms of tofu are generally available in the refrigerated section of the grocery store:

Silken or soft tofu has a creamy consistency and is best for soups, desserts, sauces, and as a substitute for scrambled eggs. Blend it into drinks, puddings, and pureed vegetables, or make a tofu scramble with your favorite chopped vegetables and seasonings.

Firm tofu is easily cut. It is a great alternative to meat in most dishes: stir-fries, casseroles, chili, stews, and tacos.

Hard or extra-firm tofu can be deep-fried, marinated for barbecuing, crumbled into salads, or used as a topping for pasta.

Tofu desserts, mayonnaise, "cream cheese," yogurt, "ice cream," and *dips* are some of the newer soy products available, some of which are excellent substitutes for the traditional products. Check the labels for fat content and other added ingredients.

Tempeh

Made from fermented soybeans and usually including a grain such as rice or millet, tempeh has a meatlike texture and tastes somewhat nutty. It can be marinated for grilling or barbecuing, cubed to add to chili or spaghetti sauce, stir-fried with vegetables, grated and made into vegetarian burgers, or diced into salads. Tempeh is rich in protein, fiber, isoflavones, iron, potassium, calcium, and B vitamins.

Nutritional Content of Soy Foods

	Soy Protein (grams)	Fat (grams)	Calories
Miso (1 tablespoon)	2	1	35
Soy flour (3^1/$_2$ ounces)			
regular	35	22	441
defatted	47	1.2	329
Soy milk (1 cup)			
regular	10	4	140
reduced fat	4	2	100
Soy nuts (1 ounce)	13.3	5.5	127
Soy oil (1 tablespoon)	0	13.6	120
Soy sprouts (^{1}/$_2$ cup)	4.6	2.5	45
Soybeans, dried (^{1}/$_2$ cup, cooked)	14.3	7.7	149
Soybeans, green, without pods (^{1}/$_2$ cup, cooked)	6	2	60
Tofu (^{1}/$_2$ cup)			
firm	13	6	120
soft	9	5	80
silken	9.6	2.4	72
Tempeh (^{1}/$_2$ cup)	17	8	204
TVP (1 cup, reconstituted)	22	0.2	120

Soy Flour

Soy flour is made from the dehulled soybean, which is milled, toasted, and ground. Look for defatted soy flour, in which the oil has been extracted during processing, as the full-fat soy flour is very high in fat.

Defatted soy flour is lower in calories and fat than wheat flour and higher in protein. It is heavier and creamy in color, with a distinctly "beany" smell that usually translates into a rather nutty flavor after cooking. Baked goods can be made from soy flour, but it must be used in combination with a lighter flour. Try substituting it for between 20 and 50 percent of the regular flour in your recipes. Add more moisture if the dough seems too dry, and experiment by doing things such as reducing the baking temperature by 25°F.

Soy flour contains no gluten, so it can't be substituted entirely for wheat flour in yeast breads. Because it is gluten-free, it is a good alternative for individuals with a gluten intolerance.

Soybean Sprouts

Not to be confused with mung bean sprouts, which are easy to find fresh in most supermarkets, soybean sprouts can be bought in packages from Asian groceries and some specialty stores. With slightly stringy roots and broad yellow seed leaves, they take longer to cook than mung bean sprouts. The seed leaves (cotyledons) contain the most nutrients and lend the sprouts a nutty taste. Like the mung bean sprout, the soybean sprout is a good source of vitamin C. And the phytoestrogen content is about fourteen times greater than that in alfalfa sprouts, and seventy times greater than that in frozen green or string beans.

Lecithin

Lecithin is a by-product of soybean oil. It is a natural emulsifier found in many products, such as candy, baked goods, chocolate coatings, and margarine. It offers antioxidant properties and a potential cholesterol-lowering effect. Lecithin is available in powdered and granular forms—which can be added to shakes, smoothies, and soups or sprinkled over breakfast cereals and salads—and in tablets, often combined with other vitamins and minerals.

Soybean Oil

Oil extracted from the soybean has a light, bland flavor and a high smoking point, both of which qualities make it attractive for cooking or stir-frying vegetables, a process requiring a high heat. Although soybean oil contains no isoflavones or soy proteins, it is rich in omega-3 and omega-6 fatty acids, as well as linolenic and linoleic acid, both thought to help prevent bowel and breast cancers. Many commercially baked goods are prepared with soybean oil.

Soy Grits

Soy grits are made by removing the skin from soybeans, then lightly steaming and grinding them. They have a taste and nutritional value similar to that of soybeans. With a texture comparable to ground meat, they make a good substitute in chili, meat loaf, casseroles, and spaghetti sauce.

Texturized Soy Protein (TSP)

TSP (also known as *texturized vegetable protein* or *TVP*) is used to extend ground-meat dishes, such as chili, meat loaf, and hamburgers. An excellent source of soy protein and isoflavones, and containing almost no fat, TSP must be rehydrated before use. It keeps for several days in the refrigerator once it is made.

Nutritional Content of Brand-Name Soy Drinks and Foods

Drinks (1 cup unless indicated; each cup has approximately 300 milligrams of calcium)	Soy Protein (grams)	Fat (grams)	Calories
Edensoy Extra Original Soy Milk	10	4	130
Pacific Lite Plain	4	2.5	100
Pacific Lite Cocoa	4	2	160
Revival Soy Meal-Replacement Drink	20	2.5	240
Solair Vanilla Bean	3	2	98
Trader Joe's Soy-Um	4	3	100
VitaSoy Enriched Original	6	3	110
VitaSoy Enriched Vanilla	6	3	140
West Soy Dessert Drink (6 fl. oz)	6	4	160

Foods

	Soy Protein (grams)	Fat (grams)	Calories
Boca Burger (original; 1)	12	0	84
BodyLogic Super Bumble Crumble (¹/₂ cup)	14	15	310
Fantastic Foods Mandarin Chow Mein with Tofu (1 package)	22	5	330
Hickory Baked Tofu (3 ounces)	18	3.5	140
Light Life Smart Dogs (1)	9	0	45
Morningstar Breakfast Links (2)	n/a	5	90
Nancy's Soy Yogurt (8 oz)	7	4	200
Trader Joe's Eggless Salad (¹/₂ cup)	7	8	120
TofuRella Tofu Cheese (1 oz)	6	5	80
Wildwood Tofu Cutlets (3 oz)	13	12	180
Wildwood Veggie Burger (1)	11	10	150
Yamato Boiled Soybeans (¹/₂ cup)	9	5	103
Yves Veggie Cuisine Tofu Wieners (1)	9	0	45

Soy Snacks

- soy nuts
- soy milk, flavored or plain
- fresh, steamed soybeans
- soy yogurt
- soy cheese on pita bread, tortillas, or crackers
- smoothie made with soy protein or pureed tofu and fruits
- soy trail mix
- soy flour substituted (20 percent) in a muffin or pancake recipe

Breakfast
- tofu crumbled in a skillet and cooked like scrambled eggs
- soy milk poured over high-fiber cereal
- soy yogurt mixed into high-fiber cereal
- isolated soy protein (ISP) sprinkled on cereal or fruit
- ISP added to baked goods
- ISP blended into juice

Lunch and Dinner
- steamed fresh soybeans added to salads
- soy milk substituted for white sauce or pudding or used as a base for a cream soup
- blended tofu as a base for a cream soup
- firm tofu cubed and added to soups, stews, casseroles, or chili
- takeout miso soup, also suitable as a base for your favorite homemade soups
- creamed tofu substituted for cheese in lasagna and enchiladas
- firm tofu marinated and grilled or made into kebabs
- tempeh grilled like a burger
- tofu or tempeh added to vegetable soup
- firm tofu stir-fried with vegetables
- tofu chili on a baked potato
- soy dogs with vegetarian chili, topped with soy cheese
- sliced soy hot dogs added to bean or pea soups
- tofu tacos or burritos made from crumbled firm tofu and taco spices
- soy burgers—store-bought or homemade—on whole-wheat bun with condiments and vegetables

Soy Sauce

Although a tasty condiment, soy sauce offers virtually none of the nutritional benefits of other soy foods, especially since it is used in such minuscule quantities. Made from salted, roasted soybeans that have been fermented for several months in huge vats, it is high in sodium and therefore should be used only sparingly. Low-salt versions are available.

Other Soy Products

More and more soy products are taking up residence in supermarkets. Soy cheeses in a variety of flavors are now found next to regular cheeses. They look and act like cheese and usually include small amounts of milk solids to aid in melting. Try them on sandwiches, pizzas, quiches, and lasagna, or as a snack with crackers.

Soy-based hot dogs, sausages, and hamburgers are usually lower in fat than the real thing, but they are often a poor source of isoflavones and, unless fortified, do not have the same nutritional content as other, purer soy products. Soy cookies, breads, yogurts, mayonnaise, and smoothies might also merit a try, but here, as elsewhere, it's a good idea to get into the habit of reading labels for nutritional information. Don't assume that all products with the word *soy* in the name are created equal.

SOY—QUICK AND EASY

Because it can be hard to start a new dietary program, listed on the previous page are some handy recommendations for incorporating soy foods into your diet. After you've made small changes, you may be ready to try some additional ideas. Who knows? In a few weeks or months you may find yourself buying an entire book of soy recipes.

≈ Water ≈

Water is an often overlooked ingredient in the good health and energy equation. Next to oxygen, it is the most important nutrient we can give our bodies. A healthy adult can survive for weeks without food, but only days without water. A loss of even 10 percent of total body fluid is serious.

Water is essential to all living organisms. It is the major constituent of body fluid, making up about half of the body weight in an average adult female and about 60 percent in an adult male. This percentage varies inversely with the fat content of the body: When less fat is present, water is a greater percentage of the body weight.

Water is absolutely essential to blood building and internal cleansing, to the proper functioning of the kidneys and sweat glands, and to the entire digestive process. It facilitates the transportation of nutrients and hormones to the cells and flushes toxic wastes from the body. People who drink a lot of water seldom have elimination problems.

In addition to transporting molecules of oxygen and hydrogen to the cells, water is also, in itself, a source of minerals that are particularly important to the blood, bones, and heart. Several studies in both the United States and the United Kingdom have found that rates of death from heart disease are generally lower in regions where people drink mineralized "hard" water. Soft water may be great for laundry, but its lack of calcium and magnesium, in addition to its high sodium content, make it a poor choice for drinking.

Many people mistakenly feel they are consuming their quota of liquid because they continually drink coffee, tea, soft drinks, and diet drinks. Even though these beverages are water-based, the pure water has been corrupted with syrup, caffeine, and chemical additives. Instead of hydrating the system, these draw the water out; instead of cleansing, they pollute and burden the dried-out organs; instead of quenching, they cause thirst.

As we age, we naturally lose about 10 to 15 percent of our body fluid. If we compound this loss by continually dehydrating our bodies with coffee, sugar, and alcohol, we are likely to wrinkle and age prematurely. For moist mucous membranes on the inside, and plump-looking, wrinkle-free skin on the outside, we must drink a lot of fresh water.

Certain foods contain a great deal of water and are refreshing, cleansing, and energizing. More than 90 percent of juicy fruits and vegetables such as tomatoes, lettuce, cauliflower, eggplant, watermelon, and strawberries are water. Whole milk is 87 percent water; avocados, bananas, and sweet potatoes contain 75 percent water; and, strangely enough, many kinds of low-fat fish are a fair source of water.

However, we cannot depend on foods to fill our need for fluid. Persons of average build should drink six to eight 8-ounce glasses of pure spring or bottled water each day—more if it is hot, if they are exercising, if they are having hot flushes, and (believe it or not) if they are bloated or retaining water.

The foods we eat and the fluids we drink all work together in creating good health. High-quality proteins, fibrous carbohydrates low in saturated fat, and essential fatty acids provide the raw materials necessary for a healthy body.

CHAPTER 16

ELIMINATE
THE NEGATIVE

*Every day you do one of two things: build health
or produce disease in yourself.*

— ADELLE DAVIS

≽ Nonfood Additives ≼

To choose healthful foods, look for those that are as close as possible to their original, whole state. This means avoiding foods whose natural integrity has been violated. Foods created in a laboratory cannot match the nutritional quality of a natural product. Even if they have been carefully designed to incorporate several vitamins and minerals, they do not contain the mysterious micronutrients—enzymes and trace minerals—that have yet to be discovered and duplicated. For these elusive elements, we need "real" food. This is why most nutritionists prefer foods to pills as the source of nutrients.

Almost all reports and research indicate that the health and longevity of a population are related to the naturalness and wholesomeness of the foods its members eat. In cultures where the diet consists totally of fresh, whole, unprocessed, and unrefined foods, people (if they get enough to eat) enjoy good health, long life, and a relative absence of disease. Once their diet changes to include denatured, refined, human-made foods, disease creeps in and people lose their mysterious secret of life and good health.

Virtually all supermarket food today contains chemicals that were added either in the growing stage or during processing. Long before most foods reach manufacturers, they are treated with fertilizers, herbicides, and pesticides; injected with hormones, tranquilizers, and antibiotics; or exposed to the chemical wastes of industrial society. In a survey released in April 1994, the USDA found residues of forty-nine different chemicals in 61.2 percent of the apples, bananas, carrots, celery, grapes, grapefruit, oranges, peaches, lettuce, and potatoes sampled. Of these, about 1 percent had residues above the legal limits set by the Environmental Protection Agency.[1] Apples had the highest pesticide findings, with 88.5 percent of those sampled containing at least one residue.

As a food is prepared and packaged, it may be treated with a number of additional chemicals, some of which may be harmful. For example, a group of acknowledged carcinogens—sodium nitrate and sodium nitrite—are routinely used to preserve luncheon meats, hot dogs, smoked fish, bacon, and ham. There is no question that these additives produce a cancer-causing substance, yet they continue to be used—supposedly in quantities small enough to be harmless.

To list all the pollutants and poisons found in processed foods would take a book in itself. There are literally thousands, disguised as stabilizers, imitation flavors, thickeners, softeners, emulsifiers, sweeteners, bleaches, enhancers, conditioners, ripeners, waxes, acidifiers—and the list goes on. Yet many research studies show that when taken together and given the chance to interact, they may not be harmless at all, and that we—or the food manufacturers—may be playing Russian roulette with our lives and health. It may shock you to know that each of us supposedly consumes about five pounds of these additives per year. The long-term effects of many of them are still unknown, as are the cumulative consequences of a lifetime of ingesting these substances.

The food industry determined long ago that these substances are necessary to maintain the shelf life, to preserve the appearance, or to enhance the appeal of a product. There appears little chance that the industry will stop using them anytime soon in the interest of better nutrition. Large-scale production has always been motivated more by profits than by health. As consumers, we have two choices: We can vow never to eat a food that has been "adulterated" (eliminating just about everything at the grocery store), or we can be prudent in our selection of products, taking the time to read and compare labels. In time, if enough consumers select foods with fewer additives, the food industry will respond and start reducing, perhaps even eliminating, the additives. One more safeguard is to eat a variety of foods, reducing the risk of getting too much of a particular additive.

Whenever possible, look for produce, meat, and processed foods (including eggs and dairy products) that are organically cultivated, that is, grown without the aid of pesticides, herbicides, and hormones. Many states have adopted laws governing organic food and farming practices, and in early 2000, the USDA adopted national organic standards, after some hard lobbying by consumers and organic farmers to ensure that the national standards were rigorous enough. Organic

products are widely available in specialty markets, natural-food stores, and local farmers' markets and are beginning to infiltrate major market chains. If everyone began asking his or her local grocery manager about incorporating more organically grown foods into the inventory, we would enjoy a greater selection, ultimately leading to lower prices for these products. If you have no choice in the matter and are forced to purchase conventionally grown produce, wash it well in a mild soap free of additives, or peel off the skin and remove the outer layers.

⮞ Sugar ⮜

Two food additives, sugar and salt, deserve special mention because they are so terribly overused in the Western diet. Since both are relatively inexpensive, they are used extensively to preserve, flavor, and extend the shelf life of many products. If you think your diet is relatively low in sugar, go into your pantry and read the labels. Sugar, disguised in its many different forms as dextrose, sucrose, fructose, maltose, corn syrup, beet sugar, honey, and molasses, probably appears on all your product labels: canned fruits and vegetables, yogurt, salad dressing, pickles, catsup, antacids, and cough medicine. Many items contain more than one form of sugar, so be assured you are getting better than your fair share. Believe it or not, most Americans individually consume 140 pounds of sugar per year.

As we approach menopause, we require fewer calories but the same amount of nutrients. We need to minimize foods that not only lack nutritive value but also destroy the nutrients we have consumed. Sugar is at the top of the list. How bad is it? So bad that not even a lowly microbe can survive in it.

As sugar is metabolized, it drains the body of many vitamins. Unlike complex carbohydrates—such as those contained in apples, oranges, and whole grains—refined white sugar enters the body unaccompanied by the team of nutrients needed to facilitate its digestion and assimilation. These nutrients are leached out of the body's resources. Over time, this creates multiple deficiencies, especially within the B-complex family. As a result, most women with a sweet tooth are deficient in B vitamins. Initial signs of such deficiency are relatively minor: fatigue, water retention, anxiety, irritability, and depression. Long-term deficiencies, however, may have serious consequences. Studies at McGill Medical School have determined that there is a direct correlation between B-vitamin deficiency and estrogen-based cancers.[2] In the absence of adequate B vitamins, estrogen builds up and is subsequently stored in the estrogen receptors of the breast and uterus. A vicious cycle results: As the production of estrogen increases, the deficiency becomes more pronounced; the greater the deficiency, the more estrogen is secreted.

Sugar significantly alters the levels of several hormones as they attempt to maintain a chemical balance within the body. The pancreas, liver, and adrenal glands are all overstimulated by fluctuation in blood-sugar levels. While our bodies can handle blood-sugar highs and lows in our youthful years, the day of reckoning comes when our systems lose their resilience.

For menopausal women, symptoms of this change may be related to the inability of the worn-out adrenal glands to take over estrogen production as the ovaries decline. When the glands are strong and healthy, they are much more capable of secreting the amounts of estrogen needed to prevent dramatic hormonal fluctuations, which are related to menopausal symptoms.

Probably the most critical problem women face, both before and during menopause, is getting and absorbing enough calcium to prevent osteoporosis. Eaters of sweets beware! Sugar inhibits calcium absorption. To guard against the most devastating of all menopausal problems—brittle bones—watch your sugar intake starting *now.*

A sweet tooth, like any bad habit or addiction, can be brought under control if one is truly motivated. For some women, conscious awareness is enough to make the change. Women who have become physically addicted to sugar may actually experience withdrawal symptoms when it is eliminated. Approach the change with care, planning, self-love, and patience. Retraining your taste buds will take time and effort. Don't try to reverse thirty years of indiscriminate eating in two days, or two weeks.

Everyone asks for advice on how to handle sugar cravings. I recommend that you concentrate on the specific micronutrients affected by eating sugar: the B vitamins, magnesium, chromium, zinc, and manganese. Foods rich in these substances include certain fruits and vegetables, whole grains, and wheat germ. But don't wait until you have given in to the desire for a double hot-fudge sundae to start suddenly eating greens. Prepare your body in advance by keeping it well nourished and well supplied.

Why Women Must Control Their Cravings for Sweets

- Sugars are nonnutritive.
- They deplete vitamin and mineral stores, especially vitamins B and C and the minerals magnesium and chromium.
- They create hormonal fluctuations and imbalances, aggravating menstrual problems.
- They cause extremes in blood-sugar levels.
- They create severe stress in the endocrine glands (adrenals and pancreas).
- They trigger hot flashes.
- They inhibit calcium absorption and thus can contribute to osteoporosis.
- They are addictive.
- They have been linked to obesity, digestive disturbances, tooth decay, diabetes, increased blood cholesterol and triglyceride levels, and urinary tract infections.

Artificial sweeteners are not the best alternative to sugar, although they may be temporarily useful. Saccharine, cyclamates, and aspartame have all been linked to cancer and have various side effects. To replace one potential enemy with another is hardly satisfactory. What we ultimately must do is to retrain the expectation of our taste buds for sweetness.

You are probably wondering about the value of raw sugar, molasses, carob, and honey—the so-called natural sugars. Bad news: All forms of sugar, in the amounts we normally eat them, deplete the nutrient supply and cause a sudden elevation in the blood sugar. Unlike table sugar or sucrose, however, these more natural sweeteners do have some nutritional value: Carob is rich in B vitamins and minerals; honey contains small amounts of trace minerals and traces of the vitamins B, C, D, and E; molasses is high in iron, calcium, copper, magnesium, phosphorus, and vitamins B and E. If you must use a sweetener for baking or on your cereals, the natural ones are slightly better. Just use them sparingly.

⇒ Salt ⇐

Table salt, or sodium chloride, has been used for a long time to preserve food. Unlike simple sugar, however, sodium is an essential nutrient. It is required for the maintenance of blood volume, the regulation of fluid balance, the transport of molecules across cell walls, and the transmission of impulses along nerve fibers.

Recent government studies indicate that most Americans consume far more table salt than they need. Even when no salt is added during cooking or at the table, the sodium quickly adds up. We take in daily, on the average, between 6 and 20 grams of sodium chloride; we need no more than 1 to 3 grams per day, which is no more than is found in the foods we normally eat.

Eating too much salt can raise the blood pressure and increase the risk of heart and kidney disease. Salt stimulates water retention, which is uncomfortable, adds unwanted pounds to the body, and prevents the loss of fat. In the menopausal woman, salt may trigger annoying hot flashes and promote loss of calcium from the bones. The exact amount of calcium loss and bone breakdown caused by high salt intake is not known, but any loss is significant for high-risk women in their middle years.

Sodium can also aggravate premenstrual syndrome. Niels Lauersen writes that eliminating salt from their diet alone has helped many PMS sufferers reduce their bloatedness, premenstrual irritability, and headaches.[3] He indicates that it is especially important for women with PMS to reduce their salt intake during the two weeks preceding their periods, when PMS symptoms can be the worst.

To reduce salt in your diet, start with the obvious offenders: chips, crackers, ham, bacon, other smoked or cured meats, processed cheese, and table salt. Then look for the hidden salt in processed foods. In checking labels, look for anything with the word *sodium* in it, such as monosodium glutamate and sodium nitrate, and watch for the abbreviated chemical symbol for sodium, Na.

Commonly available salt substitutes contain potassium in place of all or part of the sodium. People under medical supervision, particularly for kidney problems, should check with their physicians before using salt substitutes. Alternatives that contain mixtures of spices and herbs, such as Veg-It, may be better choices. You can also substitute mixed herbs, fresh spices, garlic, lemon juice, and unsalted salad dressing. Be creative, find new tastes you like, and experiment with them. Once you do, you will find it difficult to eat something that is highly salted. Many good books have also been written with excellent recipes for a low-salt diet. My favorite is *The American Heart Association Cookbook*.

You should also be cautious of what you drink. Soft water, carbonated soda, and some bottled waters contain sodium. Ordinary club soda has 241 mg; Perrier water, 14 mg; and Poland Spring water, 4 mg. This may be more important to notice if you are prone to PMS, water retention, or high blood pressure.

Sodium Content of Common Foods

Food	Sodium
Eggs (2, medium)	108 mg
Ground beef ($^1/_4$ lb)	76
Hamburger (1 commercial)	950
Hot dog	627
Haddock (4 oz)	201
Whole-wheat bread (1 slice)	148
Cornflakes ($^1/_2$ cup)	126
Waffle	356
Chocolate cake (1 piece)	233
Fresh peas ($^1/_2$ cup)	2
Canned peas ($^1/_2$ cup)	200
Potato (1 medium)	6
Hash brown potatoes ($^1/_2$ cup)	223
Milk (1 cup)	128
Low-fat cottage cheese (1 cup)	918
Cheddar cheese (1 oz)	176
Roquefort cheese (1 oz)	513
Dill pickle	928
Commercial salad dressing (1 tbsp)	219
Canned minestrone soup (1 cup)	2,033

Caffeine

Coffee is the most widely used stimulant in the United States. Hidden behind the friendly color and delicious aroma of brewing coffee is the stimulant drug caffeine. This white crystalline alkaloid produces strong physiological effects, some of which we know and desire, and others about which we are uninformed. Caffeine stimulates the central nervous system, warding off fatigue and temporarily giving us the feeling of mental alertness. In some individuals it may create a general sense of well-being, improve reaction time, enhance accuracy, and even enhance endurance. But that is only half the story.

Determining Caffeine Levels

Source	Milligrams
Coffee (1 cup)	
drip	110–150
percolated	64–124
instant	40–108
Tea (1 cup)	
black, brewed 5 min	20–50
black, brewed 1 min	9–33
green	30–50
instant	12–28
iced	22–36
Soft drinks (12 oz)	
Coke	46
Pepsi	41
Mountain Dew	54
Diet Coke	46
Chocolate	
milk chocolate (1 oz)	20–35
hot chocolate (1 cup)	5–10
Medications	
Excedrin (Excedrin P.M. has no caffeine)	65
Anacin	32
Midol	32
Cope	32
Dexatrim	200
No Doz	100
Darvon	32
Vivarin	100
Aspirin	0

When caffeine is taken in excess—and that limit is a function of individual tolerance—the entire central nervous system is overstimulated. Nervous reactions that result may include shakiness, heart palpitations, chronic anxiety, and dizziness. Menopausal women report that caffeine often triggers hot flashes, sweating, and insomnia.

Caffeine promotes the release of insulin from the pancreas and of adrenaline from the adrenal cortex, raising the blood-sugar level initially to an unnatural high, which soon drops to an unhealthy low. Contrary to the hopes and dreams of dieters, the insulin response initiated by the stimulant winds up increasing the appetite, enhancing the craving for sweets, and encouraging the storage of fat.

An effective diuretic, coffee forces the excretion of more than normal amounts of water, vitamins, and minerals. The water-soluble vitamins B and C are particularly susceptible to forced water loss. Calcium can also be lost by drinking too much coffee.

Caffeine has been implicated in the development of fibrocystic breast disease. Eliminating caffeine completely has been shown to reduce both the size and painfulness of the cysts in two to six months.[4] As both a coffee lover and a woman with fibrocystic breast pain, I can confirm the results of this research. Only one small latte will give me pains within the hour, and forget espresso.

Caffeine affects the gastrointestinal, cardiovascular, and circulatory systems as well. Shortly after you drink a cappuccino, your stomach temperature rises, your hydrochloric acid output increases, your heart beats faster, and the blood vessels constrict (narrow) around your brain, yet dilate (widen) around your heart. Your metabolic rate increases, the uric acid in your blood increases, the blood flow to your extremities is reduced, and your eyeball pressure is raised. Anyone suffering from glaucoma should be warned against drinking coffee.

The effects of caffeine are systemwide, touching every organ, tissue, and cell in the body. Caffeine has also been linked to the incidence of several cancers; however, more studies are needed to confirm these reports.

A "moderate" dose of caffeine is 2 mg per pound of body weight; thus, if you weigh 130 pounds, it is considered "safe" for you to take in 260 mg of caffeine per day. This isn't very much when you consider that a single cup of coffee contains between 100 and 150 mg of caffeine. Remember, too, that coffee is not the only common source of caffeine, which is also a major ingredient in many over-the-counter diet pills and in prescription drugs for pain, menstrual cramps, allergies, and headaches. Use the table titled "Determining Caffeine Levels" to the left to determine how much caffeine you may be taking into your body.

Changing any lifelong pattern can be stressful. Most experts suggest a gradual process for weaning yourself off of coffee, rather than stopping cold turkey. Because caffeine is a drug, when you stop abruptly, you may experience withdrawal symptoms: headaches, drowsiness, nausea, nervousness, depression, indigestion, edema, constipation, cramps, and, strangely, even a runny nose. Give yourself time to make this transition. Taper off by eliminating a few cups a day if you are a heavy coffee drinker. Substitute with decaffeinated coffee some of the time, or try tea or, better yet, herb tea, Postum, juice, mineral water, or plain water with a twist of lemon. Once you have kicked the coffee habit, you will have more natural energy than you did after your four-cup fix.

⇒ Alcohol ⇐

Alcohol provides little or no nutrition, depletes vital nutrients, and places a heavy burden on the hormonal system, the digestive system, and the kidneys. Taken to extremes, alcohol consumption actively damages organs such as the pancreas and the liver and can disrupt the entire nervous system permanently. It increases the risk of diabetes, heart disease, and cancer, and its addictive qualities are, for some people, a nightmare.

Certain women are hypersensitive to alcohol. PMS sufferers have a lowered alcohol tolerance during the days preceding their periods. Even one glass of wine may be enough to cause intoxication.

The potential long-term effects of alcohol consumption are even more frightening. One British study indicates that women who drink regularly sustain a one and one-half to two times higher rate of breast cancer than those who never drink.[5] Women who both smoke and drink are at even greater risk, suggesting that there may be multiple adverse factors in effect when both habits are involved.

One explanation for why alcohol may increase the risk of breast cancer is proposed by nutritional biochemist Jeffrey Bland. He believes that the phenomenon is related to the adverse effect of alcohol on the liver. One function of the liver is to break down estrogen so that it can be excreted safely from the body. Bland writes,

"The inability to properly metabolize estrogen can lead to the buildup of certain estrogenic substances within the body that can overly stimulate receptors in the breast, ovary, or uterine wall and initiate a cancer process."[6] As was noted previously, B-vitamin deficiencies can also cause estrogen oversecretion, and alcohol depletes B vitamins.

Over half of the problems associated with excessive long-term alcohol consumption stem from the malnutrition that results from continual use. Alcohol, a derivative of sugar, is metabolized in the body in a similar way. It requires substantial nutrients from other sources or from the body's reserves before it can be metabolized, or converted into energy. Thus, it creates deficiencies of the B vitamins, vitamin C, calcium, magnesium, potassium, and zinc.

Any woman at risk for osteoporosis should carefully monitor her alcohol intake. Alcohol impairs calcium absorption and may affect the ability of the liver to activate vitamin D. It is not known how much alcohol it takes to effect significant bone loss; what has been established, though, is the fact that alcoholics are at much greater risk for developing osteoporosis.

Alcohol has also been reported to aggravate the common menopausal symptoms of hot flashes, insomnia, and depression. Since it is high in calories, it easily adds unwanted pounds around the midsection. And as a dehydrant, alcohol, in excess, can result in premature wrinkling and loss of skin tone.

Individuals who eat healthy diets and are in good physical condition can take the occasional drink without serious detrimental effects; it may even have some health benefits. Alcohol in moderation is a social lubricant. It can relieve tension, stimulate the appetite (aperitif), and aid digestion (digestif). As I have said, it is not what you eat or drink *occasionally* that will harm you; it's what you put into your body on a regular basis.

Recent reports have indicated that one or two ounces of alcohol a day may slightly decrease the risk of heart disease by increasing high-density lipoproteins—the type of cholesterol that seems to protect against atherosclerosis. I do not advocate drinking alcohol in order to raise your HDLs, however; exercise is every bit as effective and has only positive side effects.

To a large degree, alcohol tolerance is an individual—or family—matter. If you are hypoglycemic; have a history of breast cancer in your family; are prone to osteoporosis; suffer from hot flashes, depression, insomnia, or PMS; or have a problem with moderate drinking, you probably need to refrain from alcohol completely.

⪜ Cigarettes ⪛

Smoking is the largest single cause of premature death and ill health for women and men in America. A woman who smokes runs twice the risk of dying from stroke, and eight to twelve times the risk of dying from lung cancer. Because women are now smoking as much as men, they have caught up with men in incidence of lung cancer, which is now the number-one cancer killer of women, exceeding even breast cancer.

The risks of smoking increase with age and the number of years one has smoked. They include osteoporosis, glaucoma, cardiovascular disease, and several kinds of cancer. An increased risk of heart disease occurs among women who both take oral contraceptives and smoke, and an increased risk of cancer of the mouth, pharynx, larynx, and esophagus occurs among people who both smoke and drink.

A wonderful book that addresses the reasons women smoke and the unique difficulties—physiologically and psychologically—they have quitting is *How Women Can* Finally *Stop Smoking,* by Dr. Robert Klesges and Margaret DeBon.

CHAPTER 17

PUTTING YOUR DIET INTO ACTION

Knowing is not enough; we must apply.
Willing is not enough; we must do.

— GOETHE

What we eat and how we live in our younger years directly determine the quality of our future health. For this reason, we need to analyze our eating habits and see if we are adequately prepared.

As we get older, it becomes increasingly important to monitor the quality of food we eat. Physical problems increase because the body cannot produce hormones, enzymes, and antibodies at the same rate and in the same amounts as before. Nutrients are absorbed and used less efficiently. To maintain health, we must provide the body with a steady supply of high-grade nutrients and avoid foods and substances that strain the system.

For some, this may mean embarking on a major program to take charge of their health. The first steps are determining where you are and what you want to accomplish. Awareness of the need to change always precedes action, and you should take some time now to understand your individualized needs. Before you make any specific dietary alterations or go out and spend a fortune on supplements, first analyze your eating habits, your lifestyle, and your present symptoms.

⋙ Charting for Health ⋘

Prior to taking action, check any and every unusual symptom with your family doctor. Even something as seemingly innocuous as fatigue could indicate a serious problem. When you have a clean bill of health, then proceed.

Dietary and Lifestyle Analysis

1. Do you frequently (more than four times a week) eat
   - ☐ fast foods
   - ☐ canned fruits, canned vegetables, or canned soups
   - ☐ fried, breaded, or deep-fried meats or vegetables
   - ☐ desserts, doughnuts, cupcakes, cookies, pie, ice cream
   - ☐ packaged or frozen foods, instant products
   - ☐ white bread, white rice
   - ☐ hot dogs, bacon, luncheon meats
   - ☐ chips and crackers
   - ☐ condiments (catsup, mustard, syrups, jam, mayonnaise)
   - ☐ candy?

2. Do you frequently drink
   - ☐ coffee, more than two cups a day
   - ☐ soft drinks, diet drinks, tea, decaffeinated coffee, daily
   - ☐ alcohol, more than five times a week?

3. Do you often skip one or more meals? . . . .

4. Are you on a diet of fewer than 1,000 calories per day? . . . .

5. Do you smoke? . . . .

6. Do you take medication? . . . .

7. Are you continually under stress? . . . .

8. Are you inactive, having no regular exercise program? . . . .

9. Do you have several annoying symptoms (gas, fatigue,
   headaches, hemorrhoids, insomnia)? . . . .

Any new program must begin with the basics, and that is precisely where we will start, with the most basic substance our body needs: good, wholesome, nutritious food. The first step is to review everything that enters your mouth. The most effective way to do this is by charting—writing down every day, for several weeks, exactly what you eat and drink.

You could use a very large calendar, such as a desk calendar, or buy some poster paper and make your own chart. This will also reinforce your serious intent to change your habits. Next, write down your eating patterns for three weeks. Why so long? For several reasons: It is important to record and review different eating situations, such as weekend parties, family get-togethers, lunches out, office meals, and days alone. It is especially important to analyze the week before, during, and after your menstrual period.

The same kind of dieting chart illustrated in Chapter 12 and suggested for use in gaining control of your weight is excellent for helping you gain control of your nutrition. Make three columns: a narrow one for the times of day you eat or snack; a wider one for the type, preparation method, and quantity of food; and another narrow one for recurring feelings or symptoms. Be specific when you fill it in—for example, write down the *kind* of cereal (oatmeal, cornflakes, or bran flakes), the *kind* of bread (white, rye, whole-grain wheat), *how* the food was prepared (fried, broiled, steamed, raw), and *how much* you ate. Don't forget condiments: catsup, mustard, mayonnaise, pickles, and so on. In the symptom column, record how you feel; you can use your own system of abbreviations or symbols. Fill in this column as and when your symptoms occur—midmorning, after lunch, and so on.

After a very interesting—and revealing—three weeks, you will be ready for the dietary and lifestyle test on the previous page. It might be easier if you go through your chart and circle specific categories with different-colored pens (e.g., sugar foods with red, fatty foods with green, and processed foods with blue). After three weeks have gone by, you will definitely be in touch with your eating habits. Not only will you know the types of foods you eat regularly, but you will also see how often you eat (or don't eat) and how frequently you experience symptoms.

As a cross-check or a quick self-test, you can get a general idea of your dietary habits right now. In the questionnaire, put a check next to each item for which your answer is yes.

If you checked fewer than five items, your diet is probably healthful. If you checked close to half, you need to make some adjustments in your diet or lifestyle. If you checked most of the items, you should get a physical and reevaluate your lifestyle. You definitely need both a drastic change of diet and nutritional reinforcement.

Are You Depriving Your Body of Nutrients?

Your next step is to determine whether your daily habits are diminishing your vitamin and mineral supply. Many people do not realize the serious consequences environmental forces, drugs, and their own daily habits can have in terms of nutritional deficiencies. Some factors, such as the air we breathe, are unavoidable; some, such as medications and stress, can be controlled somewhat; and many, such as sugar, salt, and fat consumption, are completely within our power to change. The ideal is to avoid as many of these poor habits as possible. If you are not ready to give up your favorite vice, the least you can do is to fortify the body so your overall health will not be compromised.

Review the chart titled "Vitamin and Mineral Depleters" to the right. How many of these items are a part of your life? Circle them. What nutrients might you be compromising? Do they appear more than once? Twice? Refer to your daily food-intake chart. Are you eating foods that supply these nutrients? For example, if you smoke, eat a lot of cooked and frozen foods, lunch meats, and bacon (high in nitrates), and take medications such as aspirin or Indocin, you may require additional vitamin C. Keeping this in mind, check your food-intake chart again. How many foods do you eat that are high in vitamin C? (See Appendix C for a list of nutrients and some of the foods that contain them.) If you are not eating fresh fruits and vegetables every day, you need to add them to your diet. Supplementing with vitamin C also is probably called for, but remember, no pill is a substitute for good nutrition.

Vitamin and Mineral Depleters

Depleter	Nutrient Depleted
Caffeine	B-complex, especially thiamine (B-1); inositol, potassium, zinc
Alcohol	B-complex, C, A, magnesium, zinc
Sugar	B-complex, chromium, zinc, manganese
High-fat/high-protein diet	calcium
Refining process	B-complex, many minerals
Crash dieting	A, B-complex, C, D, E, calcium, zinc, potassium
Chlorinated water	E
Inorganic iron	E
Cigarettes	A, C, E, calcium, selenium
Pollution	A, C, E, selenium
Stress	B-complex, C, zinc, all nutrients
Infection	A, B-complex, C, E, zinc
Cooking	A, B-complex, C
Freezing	C, E
Nitrites	A, C, E
ERT	E, zinc, magnesium
Aspirin	C, folic acid, pyridoxine (B-6)
Antibiotics	B-complex, C, K, potassium
Antacids	thiamine (B-1), phosphorus
Antihistamines	C
Barbiturates	A, C, D, folic acid
Cortisone	A, pyridoxine (B-6), C, D, zinc, potassium
Indocin	thiamine (B-1), C
Laxatives/diuretics	A, D, E, K, potassium

Once you have analyzed your dietary habits, you are ready to make some changes. Whatever you do, don't try to tackle all your problems in the first week. You will just give up in frustration. Choose one area that you want to work on; when you feel it is under control, go for another.

You may not feel immediate improvement, but after a few months you should notice subtle changes: an increase in energy, less stomach distress, a clearer mind, more radiant skin and hair, stronger nails, easier and shorter menstrual periods, a sense of well-being, and a feeling of calmly energetic good health. I have experienced it, and I have seen it happen to many others. A healthier diet and lifestyle will reward you in ways you cannot imagine.

Reading Your Body

Don't trash your food-intake chart yet, even if you feel you know all about your eating patterns. There is a third column, remember? Symptoms. What are yours? Do you have a lot of those "normal" complaints? Are you run down? Do you have the Monday-morning droops? The afternoon slump? The blahs? Are you tired? Listless? Have "female problems"? Cramps? The premenstrual crazies? Read on.

Many people suffer from marginal nutrient deficiencies. These individuals are not what you would call "sick"—that is, they don't have anything with a Latin-sounding name. A marginal deficiency is "a condition of gradual vitamin or mineral depletion in which there is evidence of lack of personal well-being associated with impaired physiological function."[1] Roughly translated, that means you can feel that something is out of sync, but tests don't reveal any major functional problem.

The body operates on a fresh and continuing supply of nutrients. When these are missing for an extended period of time, functions deteriorate, setting off a series of reactions that begin subtly at the cellular level and gradually move up to the tissue and organ level. Initially, the body compensates for deficiencies by using stored nutrients. Some nutrients, however, cannot be stored for more than one day, and in time the stores of others get seriously low. Examples of these are the B vitamins and vitamin C.

Myron Brin, Ph.D., a nutrition researcher at Hoffman–La Roche (a pharmaceutical firm) and one of the pioneers in this area, has identified consecutive phases of marginal deficiencies in the body. In the preliminary stage, nutrients stored in the body's tissues are gradually depleted, because of low intake, poor absorption, or abnormal metabolism. At this point there are no symptoms or detectable physical signs. As deficiencies progress to the biochemical stage (the stage at which changes can be detected through chemical tests), tissue stores are depleted. There are still no obvious clues, but silent destruction is occurring beneath the sur-

face of the skin. Even though nothing can be detected on the outside, the tissue damage can have a significant effect on functions such as the body's ability to handle drugs, alcohol, or exposure to environmental chemicals, and its immunity to disease.[2]

Clues start appearing only in the final stage, where they show up as behavioral and psychological manifestations. Nonspecific symptoms such as loss of appetite, depression, anxiety, or insomnia may be among the first signals that you are undernourished. If you notice yourself writing these symptoms in several entries on your daily chart, consider it a warning of marginal nutrient deficiencies.

> **Your Plan of Action**
>
> ◎ Chart your dietary and lifestyle habits.
> ◎ Check for nutrients taken in.
> ◎ Check for nutrients depleted.
> ◎ Determine your symptoms and signs.
> ◎ Determine whether you have special needs (for example, high blood pressure).
> ◎ Compare your diet to the proposed diet plan on page 308.

In the final stages, definite clinical signs appear and, if left untreated, eventually result in disease. Of course, this is what we want to avoid, and we can to a certain degree, by heeding our bodies' subtle, nonspecific signals before they reach a critical point.

Most bodily reactions involve several biochemical pathways or steps. Several nutrients, enzymes, and hormones may be required for one particular organ system to function. A shortage of just one vitamin can result in a collection of different symptoms involving the skin, hair, eyes, mouth, or teeth, or the digestive, muscular, nervous, or reproductive systems. Adding to the confusion is the fact that the initial indications of many deficiencies are alarmingly similar: fatigue, weakness, minor aches and pains, headache, and so on.

Most researchers and practitioners in nutritional medicine agree, however, that certain physical clues point to specific nutrient deficiencies. For example, spoon-shaped fingernails with white spots, loss of the sense of smell or taste, and stretch marks are clinical signs of a zinc deficiency. These clues may be telling you that you are not taking in enough zinc, that you have an increased need for the mineral, or that you are not absorbing it.

Check Appendix B for a list of common physical symptoms and the associated nutrient deficiencies. While this list should not be used to try to make an exact diagnosis of your nutrient needs (because other vitamins and minerals may also be involved), it gives the most common relationships and is a guide to help you establish which nutrients you may need to supplement. If some of the signs apply to you, circle the nutrients that correspond to the symptoms. Certain nutrients may appear more than once, indicating a likely deficiency. Before you run out and buy

Proposed Diet Plan

Daily caloric intake

Inactive women . . . . Ideal weight x 11
Moderately active
  women . . . . Ideal weight x 14
Active women . . . . Ideal weight x 18
Men . . . . Ideal weight x 18

Protein
(12–15 percent of total calories)

Women . . . . 40–60 g/day
Men . . . . 45–75 g/day

Low-fat sources of protein
(1 g or less of fat/serving)

Chicken breast, skinless (4 oz) . . . . 35 g
Shellfish: shrimp, scallops,
  lobster (4 oz) . . . . 23–35 g
Fish: cod, flounder, sole,
  halibut, trout (4 oz) . . . . 21–30 g
Tuna, packed in water (2 oz) . . . . 14 g
Cooked beans, peas, lentils
  (1 cup) . . . . 9–18 g
Tofu (4 oz) . . . . 10 g
Milk, nonfat (1 cup) . . . . 8 g
Yogurt, nonfat (1 cup) . . . . 8 g
Pasta (1 cup) . . . . 7 g
Bulgur (1 cup) . . . . 6 g
Oatmeal (1 cup) . . . . 6 g
Macaroni (1 cup) . . . . 5 g
Bread, whole wheat (2 slices) . . . . 5 g
Rice, brown (1 cup) . . . . 5 g
Rice, white (1 cup) . . . . 4 g
Tortilla, flour (1 medium) . . . . 4 g

Medium-fat sources of protein
(1.5–3 g of fat/serving)

Beef, sirloin, choice or select (4 oz) . . . . 34 g
Beef, bottom round, choice
  or select (4 oz) . . . . 33 g
Chicken, dark meat (4 oz) . . . . 29–31 g
Salmon (4 oz) . . . . 31 g

Eggs (2, large) . . . . 13 g
Cheese, reduced fat (1 oz) . . . . 8 g
Milk, 1 or 2 percent (1 cup) . . . . 8 g

High-fat sources of protein
(4–7 g of fat/serving)

Beef, chuck blade roast, choice
  or select (4 oz) . . . . 35 g
Ground beef, regular, lean,
  or extra-lean (4 oz) . . . . 28 g
Mackerel (4 oz) . . . . 28 g
Corned beef brisket (4 oz) . . . . 21 g
Milk, whole (1 cup) . . . . 8 g
Peanut butter (2 tbsps) . . . . 8 g
Cheddar cheese (1 oz) . . . . 7 g
Hot dog, beef or pork (2 oz) . . . . 7 g

Carbohydrates
(65–80 percent of total calories)

Increase complex carbohydrates
  (aim for 25–40 g/day of fiber)

Fruits (2–4 servings/day)
  1 serving = 1 medium fruit,
  $1/2$ cup diced fruit, $3/4$ cup juice

Vegetables (4–5 servings/day)
  1 serving = 1 cup raw or $1/2$ cup cooked

Breads, cereals, rice, pasta
  (6–11 servings/day)
  1 serving = 1 slice bread; $1/2$ cup cooked
    cereal, pasta, or rice

Fats (20–30 percent of total calories)

Reduce saturated fats and trans fatty acids (red
meats, butter, high-fat dairy products, margarine,
tropical oils, hydrogenated fats)

Increase monounsaturated oils (olive, canola,
peanut)

Include essential fatty acids and omega-3 fatty
acids (fish oils, salmon, trout, tuna, flaxseed oil)

several bottles of vitamins, however, look at your diet. Are you eating foods that supply these nutrients? Are you engaging in habits that flush them out? Start here first to make needed changes.

Fine-tuning your diet is a continuous exercise, because your needs vary from day to day, month to month, and season to season. As we move to a new stage of development, or into unusual circumstances (undergoing an operation, going on the Pill, fighting illness), we need to reevaluate and rebalance. What is correct for your body this month may not work in five years. Being tuned in to the workings of our bodies becomes a constant challenge and, as our bodies respond to our care and attention, a constant reward.

⇒ Eating for Life ⇐

Use the following diet-plan outline for comparison; it can help you to determine the areas in your diet that need improvement. Remember, it is a balanced food plan in itself, but it does not take into account special needs and biochemical differences.

Many women have no idea how many calories they should be eating in one day. Many charts are available, and most of them conflict in the number and range of calories. I have found the following formula fairly accurate for a wide range of women. Keep in mind that it is an approximate number and is only a guide for redesigning your daily intake.

CHAPTER 18

DESIGNING YOUR SUPPLEMENT PROGRAM

Preparing for menopause by eating the right foods and exercising is a great place to start, but it may not be enough to prevent menopausal symptoms or guard against bone loss. Women should consider the advantages of supplementation. The effectiveness of vitamin supplements and nutritional remedies in treating a variety of symptoms has been proven. Controlled scientific studies and epidemiological surveys have validated many of the theories of nutrition researchers in the last few years.

Providing the body with a complete supply of vitamins, minerals, enzymes, amino acids, fatty acids, trace elements, and fluids is the surest safeguard against poorly functioning glands, hormonal disturbances, and physiological imbalances. It is simple logic: When the restorative and regenerative cycles in the body are supplied with the raw materials they need, the body has a better chance to maintain optimum functioning.

One thing cannot be emphasized enough: Supplements, even food-based vitamins and minerals, cannot replace healthful eating. Continuing to eat junk food while taking megadoses of vitamins is ridiculous—and probably dangerous. In fact, most supplements will not work in the context of an improper diet.

Supplements are best taken with food and with other nutrients. Vitamins and minerals rarely function independently. Whether any one nutrient is digested, absorbed, and properly utilized usually depends on the amount and availability of one or several others. If even one nutrient is missing, or in short supply, entire metabolic processes slow down or stop. Some of the interdependent nutrients you should remember from this book are calcium and magnesium, iron and vitamin C, and calcium and vitamin D.

How much of each vitamin and mineral do you personally need? No book can tell you; it depends on your diet history, your family history, and clinical symp-

toms. The best that nutritionists and researchers can do is to provide guidelines and indicate the different nutrients that have benefited most individuals under specific, monitored circumstances. It is up to you to determine how closely your condition matches these standards, to judge when you might need more or less, and to decide when you need to revise your program. You know your body better than anyone else. Using the information in this book, you can analyze the data and work out your own program. If you are ever in doubt, or feel uneasy about the effects of your program, seek the guidance of a qualified nutritionist or consult your family doctor.

So, let us begin.

The nucleus of any supplement program is generally the multivitamin and mineral formula, and many women will find that it meets most of their needs. Appendix A lists vitamins and minerals and the dosage ranges generally recommended by nutritionists and clinicians. Though some of the amounts go beyond RDA requirements, they are not unreasonable or excessive. When megadoses are called for, however, it is important to work with a physician; in large doses, any vitamin or mineral or other supplement acts as a drug and must be carefully monitored. If you have any doubts or questions about vitamin and mineral safety, I recommend consulting Patricia Hausman's *The Right Dose.*[1]

In addition to the basic formula outlined in Appendix A, further supplementation may be beneficial. If the multiple supplement you are taking doesn't contain an adequate amount of any nutrient (this is often true of calcium), or if you need a larger amount because of a specific problem (for example, vitamin E for breast pain), or if your daily habits are not going to change immediately (long-term smokers, drinkers, or coffee addicts), it would be wise to add single nutrients.

⋙ Supplement Safety ⋘

Supplement skeptics spend a good deal of time worrying about the alleged toxicity of vitamins and minerals. I think this needs to be addressed and put into perspective. According to the American Association of Poison Control Centers, the total number of accidental fatalities from legal FDA-approved prescription and over-the-counter drugs was 1,132 from 1983 to 1987. During this same time period, the total number of fatalities from vitamin supplements was zero. The incidence and likelihood of adverse reactions from supplemental use are miniscule. The very few cases recorded in medical journals usually involved massive doses taken over long periods of time. That is not to say that overdose is impossible; it's just highly improbable. Extremely large doses of vitamins A and D can cause problems, but staying within the recommended doses is quite safe.

⪘ Buyer Beware ⪗

Americans are spending more than fourteen billion dollars a year on supplements, according to a Washington-based market-research firm.[2] With so many people realizing they need additional vitamins and minerals, the supplement industry is producing more and more products. The question is, are we getting what we pay for? Does the capsule, powder, or pill deliver the amount that is stated on the label—an especially pertinent question since the supplement industry is largely unregulated. ConsumerLab, a private company founded by a physician and former natural-products chemist for the FDA, tests nutritional supplements and offers a "seal of approval" if they measure up to certain criteria. ConsumerLab operates a website (www.consumerlab.com) where visitors can see if their vitamin or herbal supplement has been examined and meets the organization's standards. Their most recent findings on ginkgo biloba, for example, showed that only three of the four samples tested contained the actual amount of the herb specified on the label. Of the twenty-six vitamin C preparations examined, four failed to pass and others contained less of the vitamin than claimed.[3] (ConsumerLab has not tested all supplements, and only one sample per brand is selected.) Unfortunately, the website does not reveal which supplements failed the test, which is what I would love to know. Still, it's a way to check up on some of the companies that manufacture the nutrients and herbs we're consuming. To give you a head start, I'll mention some of the better-scoring companies that I'm familiar with; remember, this is not an inclusive list: Shaklee, Solgar, Twin Labs, Nature Made, USANA, K-Mart, GNC, Puritan's Pride, Walgreen Co., and Bayer.

⪘ Natural Versus Synthetic ⪗

There is much confusion concerning the relative virtues of natural versus synthetic supplements. The naturalists claim that their products, derived chiefly from plant sources, contain still unidentified "associated cofactors"; for example, natural vitamin C contains the entire C complex, which makes it that much more effective, whereas synthetic C is just ascorbic acid, nothing more. Many clinicians I admire have found that natural vitamins are much less toxic when given in large amounts and yield better results than the artificially produced varieties. On the other side of the debate are researchers with equally impressive degrees and experience. Those favoring synthetic products deny that there is any chemical difference, because in the test tube they all possess the same molecular properties. They also observe that, for people suffering from food allergies, the nonfood supplements are safer.

I don't predict any agreement between these two camps; however, there is a consensus on two nutrients. Vitamin E is better when taken from natural sources. Natural vitamin E (d-alpha tocopherol) is absorbed better than the synthetic (dl-alpha tocopherol). Don't be misled by labels that say the supplement contains vitamin E with d-alpha tocopherol; chances are the "with" greatly dilutes the active amount. As for folic acid, synthetic is the way to go, since it is more biologically available than the natural form.

≳ Brand Name or Generic? ≲

This issue is continually debated by the experts and manufacturers, and, of course, they are not in agreement. The advice of Sheldon Hendler, author of *The Doctor's Vitamin and Mineral Encyclopedia*, is that all vitamins are essentially the same, so buy the least expensive.[4] "Only about a half-dozen drug companies actually make vitamins," says Hendler. They supply the basic raw materials, and the manufacturer mixes the blend, adding ingredients like sugar, coloring, bindings, and preservatives. However, many supplements list as many additives as they do nutrients, and, personally, I think these should be avoided. When I hear that people have a difficult time digesting supplements, I often wonder if they might be allergic to one of the ingredients. If a supplement causes you distress, try another brand.

≳ Dissolution Statement ≲

Supplement manufacturers use a scientific procedure called a *disintegration test*, which mimics the action of the digestive tract, to test their products for dissolution and disintegration time. In January 1993, the U.S. Pharmacopoeia (USP) adopted a voluntary supplement dissolution standard: Water-soluble vitamins (B and C) should disintegrate in the digestive tract within forty-five minutes. Look for information on the label about the supplier's testing procedures.

≳ Expiration Dates ≲

Not all supplements list a date, and even when they do, it does not guarantee freshness. Nevertheless, a date does suggest that the manufacturer is aware that nutrients have a finite shelf life and is trying to offer a good product. If properly stored (covered, cool, and away from direct light), supplements retain their potency for two to three years from date of manufacturing. After opening, supplements keep for up to one year.

⇒ Proceed Slowly ⇐

When you first begin your program, start slowly, adding one supplement at a time. That way, if you have an allergic reaction to a particular ingredient, you will be able to determine the cause of the allergy more easily.

After a few months of a change in diet or supplementing, you should begin to notice subtle changes in your hair, eyes, fingernails, energy level, and sense of well-being. It is exciting to know that you can control to such a large extent how you feel and look by how well you nourish yourself and take care of your body.

Once you start your program to revamp your life and promote health and well-being, don't expect miracles. Nutrients don't work like drugs; they act slowly to rebuild tissue and reestablish homeostasis. If it has taken your body years to create a hormonal imbalance, don't expect it to reverse in a few days. It may actually take a few months. Be patient. Let the body mend in its own time. I must also mention that, as your body changes, you may actually feel worse for a few days before you feel better. This is normal, and you will find that the results are well worth the temporary transition.

The program you are designing now is not set in stone. Your needs, like your life, are constantly changing. Some changes are short-term (for example, pregnancy); others stay with us for the rest of our lives. I continually readjust and fine-tune my program as my lifestyle changes and my eating habits improve. In the process I become more and more aware that the "purer" my daily intake—the less junk I put into my body—the less I need to supplement.

The real key to preparing for a healthy menopause—menopause without medicine—and a healthy second half of life is all-around good health: a nutritive diet, wise supplementation, regular physical exercise, and a positive mental attitude. Don't wait until you are going through the change to start thinking about your health. If you have prepared for the excitement and challenge of menopause far in advance of the midlife years, you will be ahead of the game, and your life will be the celebration it was meant to be. Think about it, and start now.

APPENDIXES

ENDNOTES

GLOSSARY

RESOURCES

INDEX

NOTES

A BASIC NUTRIENT FORMULA FOR WOMEN

The following dosages are recommended for the average healthy woman. Some of the dosages suggested in various chapters of the book for the treatment of specific problems may exceed these amounts. Whenever using higher dosages, consult your health-care professional.

Nutrient	Recommended Range*	Toxicity Level
Fat-soluble vitamins		
Vitamin A	5,000–20,000 IU	100,000 IU
Beta-carotene	5,000–25,000 IU	10,000 IU
Vitamin D	400–800 IU	1,000 IU
Vitamin E (d-alpha)	25–800 IU	1,500 IU
Vitamin K	70–100 mcg	n/a
Water-soluble vitamins (and vitamin-like substances)		
Vitamin B-1 (thiamine)	25–100 mg	n/a
Vitamin B-2 (riboflavin)	25–100 mg	n/a
Vitamin B-3 (niacin/niacinamide)	19–100 mg	2,000 mg
Vitamin B-5 (panthothenic acid)	25–100 mg	n/a
Vitamin B-6 (pyridoxine)	25–100 mg	200 mg
Vitamin B-12 (cobalamine)	100–200 mcg	n/a
Vitamin C	60–200 mg	2,000 mg
Bioflavonoids	500–2,000 mg	n/a
Biotin	150–300 mcg	n/a
Choline	25–100 mg	n/a
Folic acid	400–800 mcg	1,000 mcg
Inositol	25–100 mg	n/a
PABA (para-aminobenzoic acid)	25–50 mg	n/a

Nutrient	Recommended Range*	Toxicity Level
Minerals		
Boron	3 mg	20 mg
Calcium	800–2,000 mg	3,000 mg
Chromium	200–300 mcg	n/a
Copper	2–3 mg	n/a
Iodine (kelp)	150 mcg	1,000 mcg
Iron		
Premenopause	18 mg	45 mg
Postmenopause	8–10 mg	n/a
Magnesium	300–800 mg	8,000 mg
Manganese	3 mg	11 mg
Molybdenum	45 mcg	1,000 mcg
Potassium	100–300 mg	n/a
Selenium	70–400 mcg	1,000 mcg
Sodium	1,100–2,400 mg	n/a
Zinc	15–50 mg	40 mg
Other nutrients		
omega-3 fatty acids (DHA and EPA)	300 mg	n/a

* Individual recommendations in various chapters of this book may be specific to a symptom or problem. The ranges given here are general to therapeutic.

CLINICAL SYMPTOMS OF NUTRIENT DEFICIENCIES

Ca–calcium
Cr–chromium
Cu–copper
EFA–essential fatty acids
Fe–iron
I–iodine

K–potassium
Mg–magnesium
PABA–para-aminobenzoic acid
Se–selenium
Zn–zinc

Body Area	Symptom	Possible Deficiency
Skin	dry, flaky	A, B, E, EFA
	oily	B-complex (especially B-6, choline, inositol)
	bruise easily	C, K
	wounds heal slowly	C, Zn
	yellow color	B-6, choline, Mg
	brown pigmentation	B, C, E
	prominent veins	C, bioflavonoids, Zn
	pale, white	B, C, Fe
	stretch marks on hips, thighs, breasts	B, E, Zn
	backs of arms rough	A
Nails	brittle	Fe, Ca, protein, EFA
	white spots	Zn, Ca
	spoon-shaped	Fe, Zn
Eyes	dark circles underneath	B, K
	small yellow lumps on white part	A, E, Zn
	night blindness, dry eyes	A
	red blood vessels around corners	general poor health
Hair	dull, dry	protein
	oily	choline, inositol
	hair splits and grows poorly	protein, Zn

Body Area	Symptom	Possible Deficiency
Hair (continued)	dermatitis	B, Zn, EFA
	hair thins out	B, protein, EFA
	dandruff	B
Mouth	canker sores	A, B-complex, Zn
	bad breath	B-complex (especially B-3)
	cracks on corner of lips	B-1, B-2, B-3
Tongue	magenta coating	B-complex (especially B-12), K
	green cast	B-complex (especially B-6, choline)
	white	B-complex (especially choline), C
	thick white spots	A, B-complex
	scalloped sides	B-6, B-12, folic acid
Teeth	bleeding and spongy gums	C, B-complex
	cavities	B-complex, Ca, Zn
	grinding teeth	Ca, Mg
	periodontal disease	Ca
Gastrointestinal system	enlarged liver	B-complex (especially choline, inositol), protein, lecithin
	nausea	A, B-3, B-6, Mg
	hemorrhoids	B-6, C, bioflavonoids, Mg
	bloating (gas)	B-complex, Zn
	hard bowel movements (infrequent)	Fe, fiber
Respiratory system	prone to infections	A, B-complex, C
	sinus	A, B-complex, C, K, Zn
	loss of sense of smell	A, B-complex, Zn
	dry membranes	A, D, E, Zn
Cardiovascular system	increased heart rate	B-complex, C, E, Ca, Mg
	slow, irregular heartbeat	B-complex, K
	elevated blood pressure	Choline, Ca, K, Se, Cr

Body Area	Symptom	Possible Deficiency
Muscular/ skeletal	muscle weakness	B-complex, K
	muscle cramps	D, B-5 (panthothenic acid), Ca, Mg
	stiff joints	B-complex, Ca, Mg
General	cold hands and feet	I
	loss of sense of taste	Zn
	insomnia	D, Ca, Mg
	varicose veins	C, E, Fe, Cu
	nervousness	B-complex (especially PABA), Ca, Mg
	low energy	B-complex, I, Fe
	poor memory	B-complex (especially inositol, choline), I, Mg
	inability to recall dreams	B-6
	frequent ear wax	B-complex (especially choline, inositol)

Sources: Jeffrey Bland, Ph.D., *Nutraerobics* (New York: Harper and Row, 1983); Richard A. Kunin, M.D., *Mega-Nutrition for Women* (New York: McGraw-Hill, 1983).

MAJOR NUTRIENT GUIDE

Source	Amount
VITAMIN A	

Beef liver (3 oz) . . . . 45,400 IU
Carrot (1, medium) 7,900
Sweet potato, cooked (1/2 cup) 7,850
Pumpkin, cooked (1/2 cup) 7,840
Spinach, cooked (1/2 cup) 7,300
Cantaloupe (1/2) 5,400
Tomato juice (3/4 cup) 1,460

Other sources: squash, red peppers, eggs, peaches, Swiss chard, endive, beet greens, broccoli, papaya, crab

Depleters: ERT, heat, coffee, processed foods, low-fat diet

Source	Amount
VITAMIN B-1: THIAMINE	

Brewer's yeast (2 tbsps) . . . . 3.00 mg
Sunflower seeds (1 cup) 2.84
Split peas, cooked (1 cup) 1.48
Black beans (1 cup) 1.10
Pecans (1 cup) 0.96
Wheat germ, toasted (1/4 cup) 0.44
Asparagus (1 cup) 0.24

Other sources: oatmeal, peanuts, liver, brown rice, fish

Depleters: heat, ERT, stress, sulfa drugs, sugar, processed foods, cigarettes, alcohol, dieting, surgery, illness, coffee, tea

Source	Amount
VITAMIN B-2: RIBOFLAVIN	

Beef liver (3 oz) . . . . 3.65 mg
Brussels sprouts (1 cup) 2.00
Almonds (1 cup) 1.31
Brewer's yeast (3 tbsps) 1.00
Split peas, cooked (1 cup) 0.58
Milk (1 cup) 0.34
Broccoli, cooked (1 cup) 0.31

Other sources: organ meats, wheat cereals, red meats, yogurt, eggs, poultry, wheat germ, nuts, sesame seeds

Depleters: alcohol, antibiotics, ERT, light, stress, junk foods, sulfa drugs, coffee, tea

Source	Amount
VITAMIN B-3: NIACIN/NIACINAMIDE	

Tuna, in water (1 cup) . . . . 47.3 mg
Chicken, light meat (3 oz) 10.0
Broccoli (1 cup) 9.7
Sunflower seeds (1 cup) 9.0
Mushrooms (1 cup) 5.7
Haddock (6 oz) 5.4
Peanut butter (2 tbsps) 2.4

Other sources: pumpkin and squash seeds, cashews, uncreamed cottage cheese, split peas, beans, avocado, brewer's yeast

Depleters: sugar, antibiotics, alcohol, coffee, stress, ERT, sulfa drugs, sleeping pills

Source	Amount

VITAMIN B-5: PANTOTHENIC ACID

Beef liver (3 oz). . . . . 7.7 mg
Mushrooms (1 cup) 2.7
Sunflower seeds (1 cup). 2.0
Wheat bran (1 cup). 1.6
Egg (1) 1.6
Cabbage, raw (1 cup) 1.3

Other sources: cashews, whole grains, wheat germ, salmon, beans, broccoli, peas, avocado, milk, chicken, peanut butter, bananas, potatoes

Depleters: heat, stress, methyl bromide, alcohol, sugar, coffee, cigarettes

VITAMIN B-6: PYRIDOXINE

Brown rice (1 cup) . . . . 1.00 mg
Tuna, in water (1 cup). 0.85
Beef liver (3 oz). 0.84
Chicken, white meat (3 oz). 0.68
Banana (1, medium) 0.76
Fresh chestnuts (1 cup) 0.53

Other sources: sunflower seeds, alfalfa sprouts, wheat germ, fish, prunes, avocado, cabbage, grapes, green peas

Depleters: ERT, cortisone, penicillin, heat, light, high-protein diet, sugar, alcohol, stress, coffee

VITAMIN C

Kiwi fruit (1) . . . . 108 mg
Orange juice (6 oz). 87
Orange (1) 85
Broccoli, cooked (1/2 cup) 70
Brussels sprouts, cooked (1/2 cup) 65
Grapefruit juice (6 oz) 57
Strawberries (1/2 cup) 48
Tomato, raw (1) 46
Potato (1) 29

Source	Amount

Other sources: raw green peppers, cantaloupe, grapes, watermelon

Depleters: stress, cigarettes, pollution

VITAMIN D

Canned tuna/salmon (1/4 lb). . . . . 400 IU
Whole milk (1 cup) 100
Beef liver (1/4 lb). 40
Butter (1 oz) 28
Egg yolk (1) 27

Other sources: fatty fish, organ meats, shrimp, fish liver oils, sun

Depleters: smog, mineral oil, cortisone, anticonvulsants

VITAMIN E

Sunflower seeds (1/4 cup) . . . . 27.1 IU
Raw filberts (1 cup). 13.5
Almonds (1 cup) 12.7
Cucumber, raw (1 cup). 12.6
Kale, raw (1 cup). 12.0
Coleslaw (1 cup). 10.5
Crab (6 oz) 9.0

Other sources: vegetable oils, asparagus, whole-wheat breads, eggs, liver, collards, peanuts, wheat germ

Depleters: ERT, mineral oil, chlorine, freezing temperatures, heat, oxygen, thyroid hormone, excess polyunsaturated oil

VITAMIN K

Spinach (1/2 cup) . . . . 360 mcg
Brussels sprouts (1/2 cup) 235
Broccoli (1/2 cup) 113
Cabbage (1/2 cup) 75
Green apple (1/2 cup). 60

Depleters: large doses of vitamin E impair absorption

Source	Amount

FOLIC ACID

Brewer's yeast (1 tbsp)	313 mcg
Black-eyed peas (1/2 cup)	230
Orange juice (1 cup)	136
Beef liver (3 oz)	123
Romaine lettuce (1 cup).	98
Cantaloupe (1/2)	82

Other sources: spinach, broccoli, beets, Brussels sprouts, potatoes, almonds

Depleters: alcohol, stress, ERT, heat, light, oxygen, sulfa drugs, sugar, caffeine

CALCIUM

Sardines (4 oz).	496 mg
Almonds (1 cup)	333
Whole milk (1 cup)	298
Yogurt, skim milk (1 cup)	294
Salmon, with bones (3 oz)	275
Tofu (4 oz)	154
Broccoli (1 cup)	136

Other sources: cheese, corn tortillas, pinto beans, blackstrap molasses, sunflower seeds, chickpeas, kale

Depleters: antibiotics, cigarettes, high-protein diet, sugar, fat, oxalic acid in spinach, inactivity

IRON

Beef liver (3 oz).	7.5 mg
Wheat bran (1/2 cup).	7.2
Pistachios (1 cup)	7.2
Sunflower seeds (1/2 cup)	5.1
Dried apricots (1/2 cup).	3.6
Blackstrap molasses (1 tbsp)	3.2
Almonds (1/2 cup)	2.7
Raisins (1/2 cup).	2.5
Tofu (4 oz)	2.5

Source	Amount

Other sources: turkey, haddock, spinach, pumpkin seeds, cashews, lima beans, soybeans, peanuts, sprouts, peas, brewer's yeast

Depleters: ERT, blood loss, high altitude, coffee, tea

MAGNESIUM

Peanuts (1/4 cup)	247 mg
Lentils, cooked (1/2 cup)	134
Tofu (4 oz)	126
Wheat germ (1/4 cup).	97
Almonds (1/4 cup)	96
Shredded wheat (1 cup)	67
Banana (1, medium).	58
Oatmeal (1 cup)	50

Other sources: split peas, kidney beans, potatoes, raw spinach, brown rice, salmon, milk, most nuts

Depleters: diuretics, alcohol, ERT, phytic acid in whole grains, large amounts of zinc or fluoride

POTASSIUM

Fish (6 oz).	760 mg
Papaya (1 medium)	710
Cantaloupe (1/2)	682
Butternut squash, cooked (1/2 cup)	600
Lima beans (1/2 cup).	600
Blackstrap molasses (1 tbsp)	585
Prunes (1/2 cup)	559
Orange juice (1 cup)	496

Other sources: spinach, pinto beans, halibut, banana, potato, sweet potato, green pepper, peach, apricot, tomato, soybeans, watermelon

Depleters: diuretics, laxatives, malnutrition, fasting, surgery, ERT, sugar, stress, coffee, alcohol

Source	Amount	Source	Amount

SELENIUM

Lobster (6 oz) . . . . 132 mcg
Tuna (6 oz) 120
Shrimp (6 oz) 108
Ham (6 oz) 58
Egg (1) 37

Other sources: chicken, whole-wheat breads, whole grain cereals

Depleters: It is not known what depletes selenium. Some parts of the country have selenium-depleted soils; produce from those areas will not contain the selenium content of produce from other areas.

ZINC

Pacific oysters (100 g) . . . . 9.0 mg
Brazil nuts, raw (1 cup) 7.1
Cashews (1 cup) 6.1
Turkey, dark meat (3 oz) 4.0
Turkey, light meat (3 oz) 2.0
White fish (6 oz) 2.0
Wheat germ (1 tbsp) 1.0

Other sources: red meat, almonds, lobster, whole grains, eggs, bran flakes, lentils, soybean sprouts

Depleters: infection, pernicious anemia, overactive thyroid, excessive sweating, alcohol, diabetes, large amounts of vitamins B and C

STRENGTHENING EXERCISES
FOR WOMEN

The muscle-strengthening exercises presented here have been specially designed to be of maximum benefit for menopausal women. Before you begin any exercise regimen, see your doctor for a complete physical, and review the exercises with him or her. If specific exercises, or a high level of exertion, are contraindicated, do not proceed except under supervision. Always stop if you experience ongoing pain or joint soreness. Remember, no amount of exercise is healthful if it is harming any part of your body.

The exercises are illustrated in two positions: A, the starting position, and B, the finishing position. Read the complete exercise before attempting it. Pay particular attention to the "don'ts" that are shown next to the figures in the illustrations.

Repetitions for all dumbbell movements: Two sets of 15 repetitions with five-pound weights. Fewer repetitions are required for heavier weights, more for lighter.

Cautions for all standing exercises: Keep back straight and knees slightly bent. Hold stomach muscles in. Keep breathing, and control the movement.

Cautions for floor stomach exercises: Do not arch your back. Check with your hand to make sure your lower back touches the floor. When pulling up, use your stomach muscles and not your neck. Control the movement at all times.

EXERCISE 1—ALTERNATING DUMBBELL CURL

Benefit: *Tones the biceps and forearms.*

Stand with torso straight and knees slightly bent. Hold a dumbbell in each hand, with arms bent at the waist and palms facing upward. Keeping elbows close to the sides, raise one weight while the other arm remains bent at the waist. Repeat this motion with the other arm and continue to alternate. Repeat 12 times for each arm, then rest and repeat 12 more times.

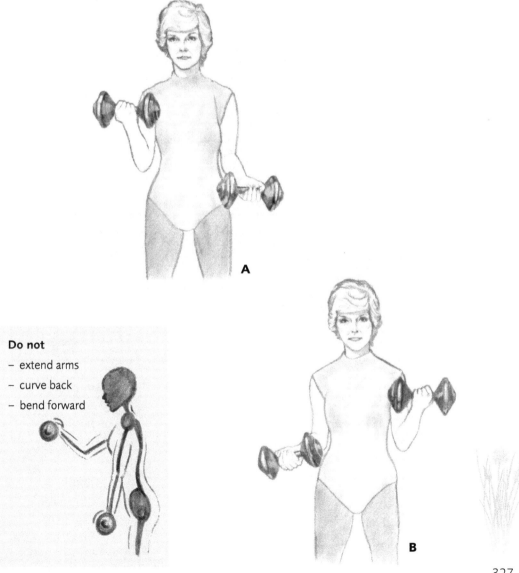

A

Do not

– extend arms
– curve back
– bend forward

B

327

EXERCISE 2—DUMBBELL PRESS

Benefit: *Works all three sections of the shoulder muscles (deltoids), triceps, and upper chest.*

Stand or sit erect. Hold one dumbbell in each hand at shoulder level. Weights should be parallel to the floor, with palms facing forward. Press dumbbell slowly overhead as you exhale. Inhale and slowly lower dumbbell back to shoulder level. Repetitions are the same as for Exercise 1.

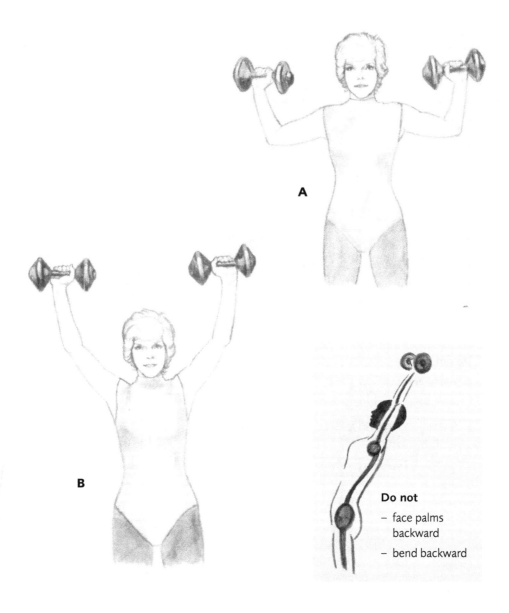

A

B

Do not
- face palms backward
- bend backward

EXERCISE 3—TWO-ARM DUMBBELL EXTENSION

Benefit: *An all-around triceps developer.*

Stand or sit, clasping one dumbbell with both hands, palms facing upward. Raise dumbbell above the head. Arms should be pulled all the way up so that the elbows are close to the ears. Inhale as you lower the dumbbell behind your head. Exhale as you raise the dumbbell over your head until elbows are nearly straight. Repetitions are the same as for Exercise 1.

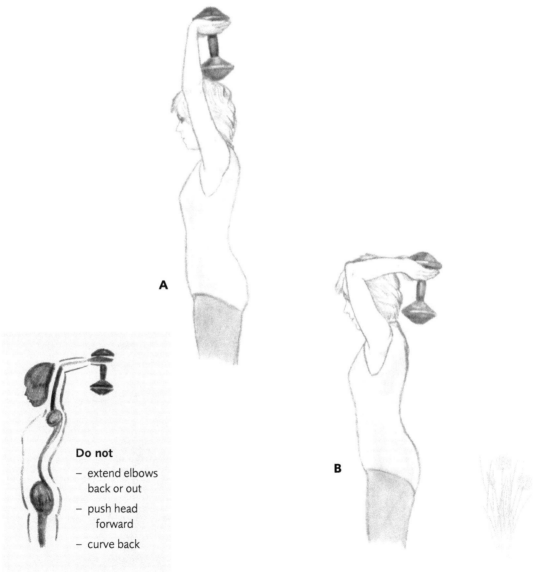

Do not

– extend elbows
   back or out
– push head
   forward
– curve back

EXERCISE 4—ARM PULL

Benefit: *An all-around shoulder and arm developer.*

Stand with knees slightly bent; lean over a bit from the hips, not the waist, with stomach and buttock muscles held firm. Hold arms directly in front of you. Pull arms back to the waist and then push them out straight. Extend and pull as many times as you can until your arms get tired. Wearing or holding weights makes the exercise more effective.

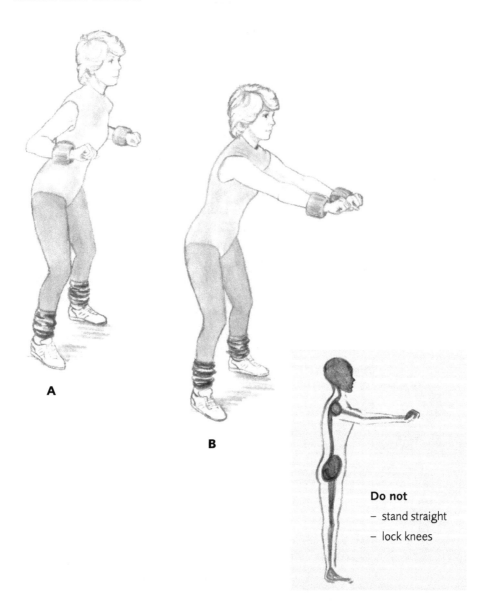

A

B

Do not
– stand straight
– lock knees

EXERCISE 5—SIT-UP CRUNCH

Benefit: *Strengthens abdominal muscles directly and back muscles indirectly.*

Lie on the floor on your back, with knees bent. With arms extended above chest, point hands toward the ceiling and look directly up. Raise upper torso, keeping stomach muscles tight and lower back pressed to the floor at all times. Be careful not to arch back. Exhale as you curl up, inhale as you release. Stay in control at all times. Go for 20 repetitions to start, and add more as you are able.

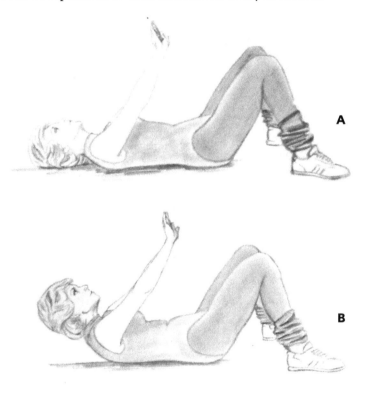

Do not
- look at your knees
- use your neck
- arch your back

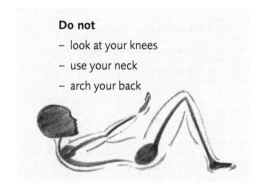

EXERCISE 6—SIDE SIT-UP

Benefit: *Strengthens the obliques (side abdominal muscles).*

Lie on the floor on your back, with legs bent and dropped to one side. Fold arms and place them behind the head to support neck. Looking up at the ceiling, exhale and lift up. Inhale as you lower both legs to the other side. Start with 20 repetitions, and work up to 50 on each side.

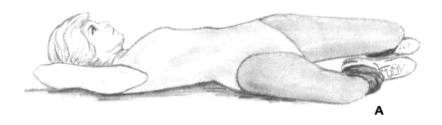

A

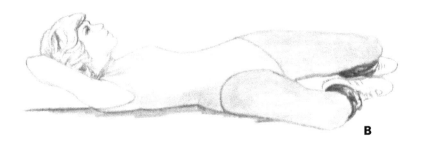

B

Do not

- push up with arms and neck
- roll to the side
- straighten legs

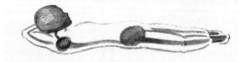

EXERCISE 7—BICYCLE TWIST

Benefit: *Works the abdominals, waist, shoulders, and upper thighs.*

Lie on the floor on your back, with arms clasped behind the head and legs straight. Lift both the left shoulder and the right knee off the floor simultaneously. Bring them as close together as is comfortably possible—without pulling on your neck. Reverse arm and leg and continue cycling motion until tired.

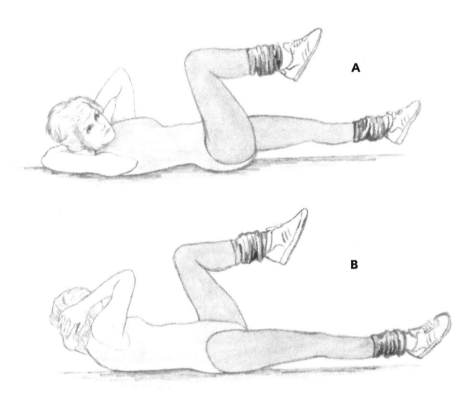

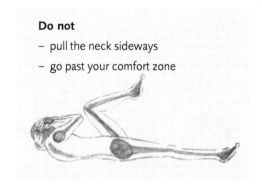

Do not
- pull the neck sideways
- go past your comfort zone

EXERCISE 8—PELVIC TILT

Benefit: *Strengthens and tones the abdominals, buttocks, lower back, and internal organs. Also reverses the flow of blood and stimulates circulation.*

Lie on the floor on your back, with knees bent. Raise the lower trunk, keeping upper back on the floor. Raise four to five inches, hold, and then lower. Keep the buttocks tight at all times. Remember, do not raise too high. Do as many as you can.

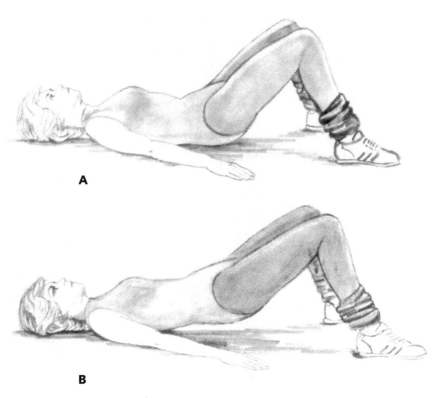

A

B

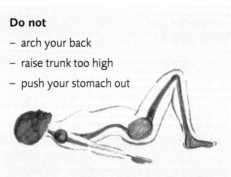

Do not

– arch your back
– raise trunk too high
– push your stomach out

ENDNOTES

CHAPTER 1

1. Robert A. Wilson, *Feminine Forever* (New York: M. Evans, 1966).

2. David R. Reuben, M.D., *Everything You Always Wanted to Know about Sex, but Were Afraid to Ask* (New York: Hawthorne Books, 1977), 292.

3. Wulf H. Utian and Pamela P. Boggs, "The North American Menopause Society 1998 Menopause Survey. Part I: Postmenopausal Women's Perceptions about Menopause and Midlife," *Menopause: The Journal of the North American Menopause Society* 6 (1999): 122–28.

4. Ibid.

5. Sheldon H. Cherry, M.D., *For Women of All Ages: A Gynecologist's Guide to Modern Female Health Care* (New York: Macmillan, 1979), 205.

6. M. C. Martin, J. E. Block, S. D. Sanchez, et al., "Menopause Without Symptoms: The Endocrinology of Menopause among Rural Mayan Indians," *American Journal of Obstetrics and Gynecology* 168 (1993): 1839–45.

7. Cathy Perlmutter, Toby Hanlon, and Maureen Sangiorgio, "Triumph over Menopause: Results from Our Exclusive Woman-to-Woman Survey with the Center for Women's Health at Columbia-Presbyterian Medical Center, New York," *Prevention* (August 1994).

8. Cherry, *For Women of All Ages*, 205.

9. Barbara Evans, M.D., *Life Change: A Guide to the Menopause: Its Effects and Treatment* (London: Pan Books, 1979), 92.

10. Letty Cottin Pogrebin, *Getting over Getting Older* (New York: Berkley Books, 1996), 13.

11. Howard J. Osofsky, M.D., and Robert Seidenburg, M.D., "Is Female Menopausal Depression Inevitable?" *Obstetrics/Gynecology* 36 (October 1970): 611–14.

12. Juanita Williams, *Psychology of Women* (New York: W. W. Norton, 1977), 360.

13. Maxwell Maltz, *Psycho-Cybernetics* (Englewood Cliffs, NJ: Prentice-Hall, 1960).

14. R. J. Beard, ed., *The Menopause: A Guide to Current Research and Practice* (Lancaster, England: MTP Press, 1976), 30; Edmund R. Novak, M.D., Robert B. Greenblatt, M.D., and Herbert S. Kupperman, M.D., "Treating Menopausal Women—and Climacteric Men," *Medical World News* (28 July 1974): 32–44.

15. Beard, *The Menopause*, 27.

16. Hershel Jick, Jane Porter, and Alan S. Morrison, "Relation Between Smoking and Age of Natural Menopause," Report from the Boston Collaborative Drug Surveillance Program, Boston University Medical Center, *Lancet* 1 (25 June 1977): 1354–55.

17. Louisa Rose, ed., *The Menopause Book* (New York: Hawthorne Books, Inc., 1977), 22.

18. Lila Nachtigall, M.D., with Joan Heilman, *The Lila Nachtigall Report* (New York: G. P. Putnam, 1977), 165.

19. Elizabeth Plourde, C.L.S., M.A., *Hysterectomy and Ovary Removal* (Irvine, CA: New Voice Publications, 2002).

20. Evans, *Life Change*, 92.

21. Rosetta Reitz, *Menopause: A Positive Approach* (Radnor, PA: Chilton, 1977), 19.

22. Louis Parish, M.D., *No Pause At All* (New York: Reader's Digest Press, 1977), 30.

23. Winnifred Berg Cutler, Ph.D., Celso-Ramon Garcia, M.D., and David A. Edwards, Ph.D., *Menopause: A Guide for Women and the Men Who Love Them* (New York: W. W. Norton, 1983), 66.

24. Penny Wise Budoff, M.D., *No More Hot Flashes and Other Good News* (New York: G. P. Putnam, 1983), 19.

25. Beard, *The Menopause*, 46.

26. Howard L. Judd, M.D., "Menopause and Postmenopause," in Ralph C. Benson, M.D., *Current Obstetric and Gynecologic Diagnosis and Treatment*, 4th ed. (Los Altos, CA: Lange Medical Publications, 1982), 550.

CHAPTER 2

1. N. Keating, P. Cleary, A. Aossi, et al., "Use of Hormone Replacement Therapy by Postmenopausal Women in the United States," *Annals of Internal Medicine* 130 (1999): 545–53.

2. S. Fletcher and G. Colditz, "Failure of Estrogen plus Progestin Therapy for Prevention," *Journal of the American Medical Association* 288 (2002): 366–67.

3. Gina Kolata, "Risk of Breast Cancer Halts Hormone Replacement Study," *San Francisco Chronicle* (9 July 2002): D1.

4. Writing Group for the Women's Health Initiative Investigators, "Risks and Benefits of Estrogen plus Progestin in Healthy Postmenopausal Women," *Journal of the American Medical Association* 288 (2002): 321–33.

5. John R. Lee, M.D., "Getting off HRT and onto Natural Hormones," *The John R. Lee, M.D., Medical Letter* (July 2002): 2.

6. Jonathan Wright, M.D., and John Morgenthaler, *Hormone Replacement for Women over 45* (Petaluma, CA.: Smart Publications, 1997), 24.

7. Jonathan Wright, M.D., and John Morgenthaler, "Don't Let Your Doctor Give You Horse Urine," *Smart Publications Update*, no.101 (www.smart-publications.com), 2.

8. Kathleen A. Head, "Estriol: Safety and Efficacy," *Alternative Medicine Review* 3 (1998): 101–13.

9. K. Takahashi, M. Okada, T. Ozaki, et al., "Safety and Efficacy of Oestriol for Symptoms of Natural or Surgically Induced Menopause," *Human Reproduction* 15 (2000): 1028–36.

10. H. Itoi, H. Minakami, R. Iwaski, and I. Santo, "Comparison of the Long-Term Effects of Oral Estriol with the Effects of Conjugated Estrogen on Serum Lipid Profile in Early Menopausal Women," *Maturitas* 36 (2000): 217–22.

11. A. Tzingounis, M. Aksu, and R. Greenblatt, "Estriol in the Management of the Menopause," *Journal of the American Medical Association* 239 (1978): 1638–41.

12. Henry M. Lemon, et al., "Reduced Estriol Excretion in Patients with Breast Cancer Prior to Endocrine Therapy, " *Journal of the American Medical Association* 196 (1966): 1128–34.

13. Alvin H. Follingstad, M.D., "Estriol: The Forgotton Estrogen?" *Journal of the American Medical Association* 239 (1978): 293.

14. Jonathan V. Wright, M.D., and John Morgenthaler, *Natural Hormone Replacement* (Petaluma, CA: Smart Publications, 1997), 104.

15. Barbara S. Hulka, M.D., Lloyd E. Chambles, Ph.D., David Kaufman, M.D., et al., "Protection Against Endometrial Carcinoma by Combination-Product Oral Contraceptives," *Journal of the American Medical Association* 247 (1982): 475–77.

16. Catherine Schairer, Jay Lubin, Rebecca Troisi, et al., "Menopausal Estrogen and Estrogen-Progestin Replacement Therapy and Breast Cancer Risk," *Journal of the American Medical Association* 283 (2000): 485–91.

17. R. K. Ross, A. Paganini-Hill, P. C. Wan, and M. C. Pike, "Effect of Hormone Replacement Therapy on Breast Cancer Risk: Estrogen Versus Estrogen plus Progestin," *Journal of the National Cancer Institute* 92 (2000): 328–32.

18. E. Barrett-Connor, S. Slone, G. Greendale, et al., "The Postmenopausal Estrogen/Progestin Intervention Study," *Maturitas* 27 (1997): 261–74.

19. United States Pharmacopeia, *The Complete Drug Reference* (Yonkers, New York: Consumer Reports Books, 1992), 1069.

20. J. Hargrove, W. Maxson, et al., "Menopausal Hormone Replacement Therapy with Continuous Daily Oral Micronized Estradiol and Progesterone," *Obstetrics and Gynecology* 73 (1989): 606–12.

21. B. de Lignieres, "Oral Micronized Progesterone," *Clinical Therapeutics* 21 (1999): 41–59.

22. J. Hargrove, W. Maxson, A. Wentz, and L. Burnett, "Menopausal Hormone Replacement Therapy with Continuous Daily Oral Micronized Estradiol and Progesterone," *Obstetrics and Gynecology* 73 (1989): 606.

23. John Lee, M.D., "Osteoporosis Reversal with Transdermal Progesterone," *Lancet* 336 (1990): 1327.

24. Cowan, A.D., et al., "Breast Cancer Incidence in Women with a History of Progesterone Deficiency," *American Journal of Epidemiology* 114 (1966): 209.

25. D. de Ziegler, R. Ferriani, L. A. M. Moreales, and C. Bulletti, "Vaginal Progesterone in Menopause: Crinone 4% in Cyclical and Constant Combined Regimens," *Human Reproduction* 15 (2000): 149–58.

26. N. Watts, M. Notelvitz, M. C. Timmons, et al., "Comparison of Oral Estrogens and Estrogens plus Androgen on Bone Mineral Density, Menopausal Symptoms, and Lipid-Liproprotein Profiles in Surgical Menopause," *Obstetrics Gynecology* 85 (1995): 529–37.

27. B. B. Sherwin, and M. M. Gelfand, "Differential Symptom Response to Parenteral Estrogen and/or Androgen Administration in the Surgical Menopause," *American Journal of Obstetrics and Gynecology* 151 (1987): 153–60.

28. D. C. Bauer, D. Grady, A. Pressman, et al., "Long-Term Effects of the Menopause and Sex Hormones on Skin Thickness," *British Journal of Obstetrics and Gynecology* 92 (1985): 256–59.

29. Eugene Shippen, M.D., and William Fryer, *The Testosterone Syndrome* (New York: M. Evans and Company, Inc., 1998), 152.

30. F. Labrie, P. Diamond, L. Cusan, et al., "Effect of 12-Month Dehydroepiandrosterone Replacement Therapy on Bone, Vagina, and Endometrium in Postmenopausal Women," *Journal of Clinical Endocrinology and Metabolism* 82 (1997): 3498–505.

31. P. Diamond, L. Cusan, J. Gomez, et al., "Metabolic Effects of 12-Month Percutaneous DHEA Replacement Therapy in Postmenopausal Women," *Journal of Endocrinology* 150 (1996): S43–S50.

32. John R. Lee, M.D., David Zava, Ph.D., and Virginia Hopkins, *What Your Doctor May Not Tell You about Breast Cancer* (New York: Warner Books, Inc., 2002), 162.

33. Marla Ahlgrimm, R.P.H., and John Kells, *The HRT Solution: Optimizing Your Hormone Potential* (Garden City Park, NY: Avery Publishing Group, 1999), 64.

34. Christiane Northrup, M.D., "The Latest News about HRT—and What You Can Do about It," *Christiane Northrup's Health Wisdom for Women* 9, 9 (2002), 2.

CHAPTER 3

1. Margaret Locke, "Contested Meanings of the Menopause," *Lancet* 337 (1991): 1270–72.

2. M. C. Martin, J. E. Block, S. D. Sanchez, et al., "Menopause Without Symptoms: The Endocrinology of Menopause among Rural Mayan Indians," *American Journal of Obstetrics and Gynecology* 168 (1993): 1839–45.

3. H. Aldercreutz, E. Hamalainen, S. Gorbach, and B. Goldin, "Dietary Phyto-oestrogens and the Menopause in Japan," *Lancet* 339 (1992): 1233.

4. Niels H. Lauersen, M.D., and Eileen Stukane, *Listen to Your Body: A Gynecologist Answers Women's Most Intimate Questions* (New York: Berkley Books, 1983), 377.

5. Mats Hammar, Goran Berg, and Richard Lindgren, "Does Physical Exercise Influence the Frequency of Postmenopausal Hot Flashes?" *Acta Obstet Gynecol Scand* 69 (1990): 409–12.

6. Robert Freedman and Suzanne Woodward, "Behavioral Treatment of Menopausal Hot Flushes: Evaluation by Ambulatory Monitoring," *American Journal of Obstetrics and Gynecology* 167 (1992): 436–39.

7. John Yudkin, M.D., *Sweet and Dangerous* (New York: Bantam Books, 1973), 164.

8. Federation of Feminist Women's Health Centers, *A New View of a Woman's Body* (New York: Simon and Schuster, 1981), 96.

9. G. Wilcox, M. L. Wahlquist, H. G. Burger, and G. Medley, "Oestrogenic Effects of Plant Foods in Postmenopausal Women," *British Medical Journal* 301 (1990): 905–6.

10. Mark Messina and Stephan Barnes, "Commentary: The Role of Soy Products in Reducing the Risk of Cancer," *Journal of the National Cancer Institute* 83 (1991): 541–46.

11. The Second International Symposium on the Role of Soy in Preventing and Treating Chronic Disease, Brussels, Belgium, 15–18 Sept. 1996. Guest scientific editors: Mark Messina, Ph.D., and John Erdman. Website www.soyfoods.com.

12. Alice L. Murkies, Catherine Lombard, Boyd Strauss, et al., "Postmenopausal Hot Flushes Decreased by Dietary Flour Supplementation: Effects of Soy and Wheat," *American Journal of Clinical Nutrition* 68, supplement (1998): 1532S–33S.

13. Paola Albertazzi, et al., "The Effect of Dietary Soy Supplementation on Hot Flushes," *Obstetrics and Gynecology* 91 (1998): 6–11.

14. H. Aldercreutz, H. Markkanen, and S. Watanabe, "Plasma Concentration of Phyto-oestrogens in Japanese Men," *Lancet* 342 (1993): 1209–10

15. J. J. B. Anderson, H. Aldercreutz, S. Barnes, et al., "Appropiate Isoflavone Food Fortification Levels: Results of a Consensus Conference," *Experimental Biology* (San Diego CA, 15–18 April 2000).

16. P. Albertazzi, F. Pansini, G. Bonaccorsi, et al., "The Effect of Dietary Soy Supplements on Hot Flushes," *Obstetrics and Gynecology* 91 (1998): 6–11.

17. G. J. Christy, "Vitamin E in Menopause: Preliminary Reports of Experimental and Clinical Study," *American Journal of Obstetrics and Gynecology* 50 (1945): 84.

18. Michael Lesser, M.D., *Nutrition and Vitamin Therapy* (New York: Grove Press, 1980), 98.

19. Barbara Seaman and Gideon Seaman, M.D., *Women and the Crisis in Sex Hormones* (New York: Bantam Books, 1979), 445.

20. *Physician's Desk Reference for Herbal Medicines*, 1st ed. (1998), 746–47.

21. Sarah Harriman, *The Book of Ginseng* (New York: Jove, 1973), 25.

22. Tzay-Shing Yang, Shun-Hwa Tsan, Sheng-Ping Chang, and Heung-Tat Ng, "Efficacy and Safety of Estriol Replacement Therapy for Climacteric Women," *Chinese Medical Journal* (Taipei) 55 (1995): 386–91.

23. H. B. Leonetti, S. Longo, and J. Anasti, "Transdermal Progesterone Cream for Vasomotor Symptoms and Postmenopausal Bone Loss," *Obstetrics and Gynecology* 94 (1999): 225–28.

24. Robert C. Atkins, *Dr. Atkins' Nutrition Breakthrough: How to Treat Your Medical Condition Without Drugs* (New York: William Morrow, 1981), 131.

CHAPTER 4

1. Barbara Edelstein, M.D., *The Woman Doctor's Medical Guide for Women* (New York: William Morrow, 1982), 82.

2. R. O. Brennan, M.D., with William C. Mulligan, *Nutrigenetics: New Concepts for Relieving Hypoglycemia* (New York: Signet Books, 1977), 9.

3. William Dufty, *Sugar Blues* (New York: Warner Books, 1975), 43.

4. Kathleen DesMaisons, Ph.D., *The Sugar Addict's Total Recovery Program* (New York: Ballantine Books, 2000), 14.

5. Clement G. Martin, M.D., *Low Blood Sugar: The Hidden Menace of Hypoglycemia* (New York: Arco Publishing, 1981), 41.

6. Earl Mindell, *Earl Mindell's Vitamin Bible* (New York: Rawson, Wade, 1979), 176.

7. G. Collier and K. O'Dea, "Effect of Physical Form of Carbohydrate on the Postprandial Glucose, Insulin, and Gastric Inhibitory Polypeptide in Type-2 Diabetes," *American Journal of Clinical Nutrition* 36 (1982): 10.

8. T. Poynard and G. Tchobroutsky, "Pectin Efficacy in Insulin-Treated Diabetes," *Lancet* (18 January 1980): 158.

9. Jeffrey Bland and Scott Rigden, *A Physician and Patient Survival Guide: Resource Guide to Treating the Burnout Syndrome* (Gig Harbor, WA: Health Communication, 1987), 87.

10. Julian Whitaker, M.D., "99 Medical Secrets Your Doctor Won't Tell You," *Health and Healing* (Potomac, MD: Phillips Publishing, 1993).

11. R. A. Anderson, M. Polansky, N. Bryden, et al., "Urinary Chromium Excretion of Human Subjects: Effects of Chromium Supplementation and Glucose Loading," *American Journal of Clinical Nutrition* 36 (1982): 118–24.

12. Brennan, *Nutrigenetics*, 160.

13. Richard A. Kunin, M.D., *Mega-Nutrition* (New York: McGraw-Hill, 1981), 125.

14. Stephen Sinatra, M.D., "Too Little Thyroid Hormone Can Make You Old Before Your Time," *HeartSense* 6.9 (September 2000): 1.

15. Richard L. Shames, M.D., and Karilee H. Shames, R.N., Ph.D., *Thyroid Power* (New York: Harper Collins Publishers, Inc., 2002), 14.

16. A. E. Hak, et al., "Subclinical Hypothyroidism Is an Independent Risk Factor for Atherosclerosis and Myocardial Infarction in Elderly Women: The Rotterdam Study," *Annals of Internal Medicine* 132 (2000): 270–78.

17. Baha M. Arafah, "Increased Need for Thyroxine in Women with Hypothyroidism During Estrogen Therapy," *New England Journal of Medicine* 344 (2001): 1743–49.

18. John R. Lee, M.D., *The John R. Lee Medical Letter* (July 2000): 1.

19. Broda Barnes, M.D., and Charlotte Barnes, *Hope for Hypoglycemia* (Fort Collins, CO: Robinson Press, 1978), 11.

20. Susan S. Weed, *New Menopausal Years* (Woodstock, New York: Ash Tree Publishing, 2002), 55.

21. "Essential Trace Elements and Thyroid Hormones," *Lancet* 339 (1992): 1575–76, editorial.

22. John R. Lee, M.D., "Interview with James Kwako, M.D., How to Recognize and Treat Tired Adrenals," *The John R. Lee Medical Letter* (July 1998), 5.

23. Ann Louise Gittleman, M.S., with Melissa Diane Smith, *Why Am I Always So Tired?* (San Francisco: Harper Collins Publishers, 1999).

24. J. Kleijnen and P. Knipschild, "Drug Profiles—Ginkgo Biloba," *Lancet* 340 (1993): 1136–39.

25. Georgia Witkin-Lanoil, Ph.D., *The Female Stress Syndrome: How to Recognize and Live with It* (New York: Newmarket Press, 1984).

CHAPTER 5

1. Shere Hite, *The Hite Report: A Nationwide Study of Female Sexuality* (New York: Dell, 1981), 508.

2. Kaylan Pickford, *Always a Woman* (New York: Bantam Books, Inc., 1982).

3. Linda Madaras, Jane Patterson, and Peter Schlick, *Womancare: Gynecological Guide to Your Body* (New York: Avon, 1981), 611.

4. Norma McCoy, Winnifred Cutler, and Julian Davidson, "Relationships among Sexual Behavior, Hot Flashes, and Hormone Levels in Perimenopausal Women," *Archives of Sexual Behavior* 14 (1985): 385–88.

5. Niels H. Lauersen, M.D., and Eileen Stukane, *Listen to Your Body: A Gynecologist Answers Women's Most Intimate Questions* (New York: Berkley Books, 1983), 386.

6. Susan R. Davis, "The Clinical Use of Androgens in Female Sexual Disorders," *Journal of Sex and Marital Therapy* 24 (1998): 153–63.

7. Christiane Northrup, M.D., *The Wisdom of Menopause* (New York: Bantam Books, 2001), 259.

8. John R. Lee, M.D., with Virginia Hopkins, *What Your Doctor May Not Tell You about Menopause* (New York: Warner Books, Inc., 1996), 76.

9. Susan Rako, M.D., *The Hormone of Desire* (New York: Three Rivers Press, 1999), 14.

10. Salender Bhasin and William J. Bremner, "Emerging Issues in Androgen Replacement Therapy," *Journal of Clinical Endocrinology and Metabolism* 82 (1996): 3–7.

11. P. R. Casson, et al., "Effect of Postmenopausal Estrogen Replacement of Circulating Androgens," *American College of Obstetrics and Gynecology* 90 (1997): 995–98.

12. R. M. J. Rosenberg, T. D. N. King, and M. C. Timmons, "Estrogen-Angrogen for Hormone Replacement: A Review," *Journal of Reproductive Medicine* 42 (1997): 394–404.

13. H. Adlercreutz, et al., "Urinary Excretion of Lignans and Isoflavenoids, Phytoestrogens in Japanese Men and Women Consuming a Traditional Japanese Diet," *American Journal of Clinical Nutrition* 54 (1991): 1093–1100.

14. J. T. Dwyer, B. R. Goldin, N. Saul, et al., "Tofu and Soy Drinks Contain Phytoestrogens," *Journal of the American Dietetic Association* 94 (1994): 739–43.

15. John Lee, M.D., *Natural Progesterone: The Multiple Roles of a Remarkable Hormone* (Sebastopol, CA: BLL Publishing, 1993), 58.

16. J. Ofek, et al., "Anti-*Escherichia Coli* Adhesion Activity of Cranberry and Blueberry Juice," *New England Journal of Medicine* 324 (1991): 1599.

17. Vidal S. Clay, *Women: Menopause and Middle Age* (Pittsburgh, PA: Know, 1977), 92.

18. Baha M. Arafah, "Increased Need for Thyroxine in Women with Hypothyroidism During Estrogen Therapy," *New England Journal of Medicine* 344 (2001): 1743–49.

19. Richard L. Shames, M.D., and Karilee Halo Shames, R.N., Ph.D., *Thyroid Power* (New York: HarperCollins Publisher, 2002), 118.

20. Jeffrey Bland, Ph.D., *Nutraerobics* (New York: Harper and Row, 1983), 17.

21. Durk Pearson and Sandy Shaw, *Life Extension: A Practical Scientific Approach* (New York: Warner Books, 1982), 205.

CHAPTER 6

1. J. B. McKinlay, S. M. McKinlay, and D. Bramvilla, "The Relative Contributions of Endocrine Changes and Social Circumstances to Depression in Middle-Aged Women," *Journal of Health and Social Behavior* 28 (1987): 345–63.

2. Sadja Greenwood, M.D., *Menopause Naturally: Preparing for the Second Half of Life* (San Francisco, CA: Volcano Press, 1984), 73.

3. Lonnie Barbach, Ph.D., *The Pause: Positive Approaches to Menopause* (New York: Penguin Books, 1993), 41.

4. P. J. Schmidt, L. Nieman, M. A. Danaceau, et al., "Estrogen Replacement in Perimenopause-Related Depression: A Preliminary Report," *American Journal of Obstetrics and Gynecology* 183 (2000): 414–20.

5. M. Rosenberg, T. King, and M. Chrystie Timmons, "Estrogen-Androgen for Hormone Replacement: A Review," *Journal of Reproductive Medicine* 41 (1997): 394–404.

6. R. A. Mulnard, et al., "Estrogen Replacement Therapy for Treatment of Mild to Moderate Alzheimer Disease: A Randomized Controlled Trial," *Journal of the American Medical Association* 283 (2000): 1007–15.

7. M. J. Engelhart, M. I. Geerlings, and A. Ruitenberg, "Dietary Intake of Antioxidants and Risk of Alzheimer Disease," *Journal of the American Medical Association* 287 (2002): 3223–29.

8. Deborah Sichel, M.D., and Jeanne Watson Driscoll, M.S., R.N., *Women's Moods* (New York: William Morrow and Company, Inc., 1999), 6.

9. Margaret Lock, "Contested Meanings of Menopause," *Lancet* 337 (1991): 1270–72.

10. Allan Chinen, M.D., *Once upon a Midlife* (New York: Jeremy P. Tarcher/Perigee, 1993), 211.

11. Alice Miller, *The Truth Will Set You Free* (New York: Basic Books, 2001), 45.

12. Ibid., 124.

13. William Bridges, *Transitions* (Reading, MA: Addison-Wesley Publishing Company, 1980), 14.

14. Gloria Steinem, *Revolution from Within: A Book of Self-Esteem* (Boston: Little, Brown and Company, 1992), 3.

15. Lillian B. Rubin, *Women of a Certain Age: The Midlife Search for Self* (New York: Harper and Row, 1979), 54.

16. Pauline Bart, "Depression in Middle-Aged Women," in Vivian Gornick and Barbara K. Moran, eds., *Woman in Sexist Society: Studies in Power and Powerlessness* (New York: Basic Books, 1971), 110.

17. Judith Wurtman, *Managing Your Mind and Mood Through Food* (New York: Harper and Row, 1988), 5.

18. Debra Waterhouse, "The Brain-Body Connection: Hormones, Diet and Behavior," seminar, Corte Madera, CA: Institute for Natural Resources, 1993.

19. Mona M. Shangold, "Exercise in the Menopausal Woman," *Obstetrics and Gynecology* 75 (1990): 53S.

20. *American Health* (March/April 1984): 28.

21. E. Cheraskin, M.D., and W. M. Ringdorf, Jr., with Arline Brecher, *Psychodietetics: Food as Key to Emotional Health* (New York: Bantam Books, 1981), 72.

22. Susan Lark, M.D., "The Serotonin-Depression Connection," *The Lark Letter* (October 2000), 5.

23. Michael Lesser, M.D., *The Brain Chemistry Diet* (New York: G.P. Putnam's Sons, 2002), 91.

24. Ibid., 93.

25. Christiane Northrup, M.D., "Why SAMe Helps Depression, Arthritis, and Overall Brain Function," *Dr. Christiane Northrup's Health Wisdom for Women* 9.1 (January 2002), 7.

26. Roger J. Williams, Ph.D., *Nutrition in a Nutshell* (Garden City, NY: Doubleday, 1962), 94.

27. *Women's Health Advocate* (September 1999), 6.

28. *Women's Health Advocate* (July 1999), 6.

29. *Prevention* (March 2000), 103.

30. Lawrence C. Katz, Ph.D., and Manning Rubin, *Keep Your Brain Alive* (New York: Workman Publishing Company, 1999).

31. Jos Kleijnen and Paul Knipschild, "Ginkgo Biloba," *Lancet* 340 (1993): 1136–39.

32. K. Linde, G. Ramirez, C. D. Mulrow, et al., "St. John's Wort for Depression: An Overview and Meta-Analysis of Randomized Clinical Trials," *British Medical Journal* 313 (1996): 253–58.

33. *Physician's Desk Reference for Herbal Medicines*, 1st ed. (1998).

CHAPTER 7

1. Lois McBean, Tab Forgac, and Susan Calvert Finn, "Osteoporosis: Visions for Care and Prevention—A Conference Report," *Journal of the American Diabetic Association* 94 (1994): 668–71.

2. Morris Notelovitz, M.D., and Marsha Ware, *Stand Tall! The Informed Woman's Guide to Preventing Osteoporosis* (Gainesville, FL: Triad Publishing, 1982), 40.

3. Howard L. Judd, M.D., "Menopause and Postmenopause," in Ralph C. Benson, M.D., *Current Obstetric and Gynecologic Diagnosis and Treatment*, 4th ed. (Los Altos, CA: Lange Medical Publications, 1982), 554.

4. Thomas J. Silber, "Osteoporosis in Anorexia Nervosa," *New England Journal of Medicine* 312 (1985): 990–91.

5. *American Journal of Clinical Nutrition* (June 1986): 910.

6. C. Rosen, M. Holick, and P. Millard, "Premature Graying of Hair Is a Risk Maker for Osteopenia," *Journal of Clinical Endocrinology and Metabolism* 79 (1994): 854–57.

7. Notelovitz and Ware, *Stand Tall!*, 72.

8. D. E. Sellmeyer, K. L. Stone, A. Sebastian, and S. R. Cummings, "A High Ratio of Dietary Animal to Vegetable Protein Increases the Rate of Bone Loss and the Risk of Fracture in Postmenopausal Women," *American Journal of Clinical Nutrition* 73 (2001): 118–22.

9. B. Arjmandi, et al., "Flaxseed Supplementation Positively Influences Bone Metabolism in Postmenopausal Women," *Journal of the American Neutraceutical Association* (Summer 2001). Retrieved online <www.americanutra.com/janav1n2.html>.

10. E. Barret-Connor, J. C. Chang, and S. L. Edelson, "Coffee-Associated Osteoporosis Offset by Daily Milk Consumption," *Journal of the American Medical Association* 271 (1994): 280–83.

11. T. L. Holbrook, "A Prospective Study of Alcohol Consumption and Bone Mineral Density," *British Medical Journal* 306 (1993): 1506–9.

12. Morris Notelovitz, M.D., and Diana Tonnessen, *Menopause and Midlife Health* (New York: St. Martin's Press, 1993), 102.

13. M. A. Fiatarone, et al., "High-Intensity Strength Training in Nonagenarians," *Journal of the American Medical Association* 263 (1990): 3029–34.

14. John F. Aloia, M.D., et al., "Prevention of Involutional Bone Loss by Exercise," *Annals of Internal Medicine* 89 (1978): 356–58.

15. Richard Prince, et al., "Prevention of Premenopausal Osteoporosis," *New England Journal of Medicine* 325 (1991): 1189.

16. "High-Impact Aerobics Are Not for Everyone," *Tufts University Health and Nutrition Letter* 19.2 (April 2001): 3.

17. D. Schneider, E. Barrett-Connor, and D. Morton, "Timing of Postmenopausal Estrogen for Optimal Bone Mineral Density," *Journal of the American Medical Association* 277 (1997): 543–47.

18. G. Colditz, "Relationship Between Estrogen Levels, Use of Hormone Replacement Therapy, and Breast Cancer," *Journal of the National Cancer Institute* 90 (1998): 814–23.

19. H. Minaguchi, et al., "Effect of Estriol on Bone Loss in Postmenopausal Japanese Women: A Multicenter Prospective Open Study," *Journal of Obstetrics and Gynecology Research* 3 (1996): 259–65.

20. J. C. Prior, "Progesterone as a Bone-Tropic Hormone," *Endocrine Review* 2 (1990): 386–98.

21. John Lee, M.D., "Osteoporosis Reversal with Transdermal Progesterone," *Lancet* 336 (1990): 1327.

22. N. B. Watts, et al., "Comparison of Oral Estrogens and Estrogens plus Androgen on Bone Mineral Density, Menopausal Symptoms, and Lipid-Lipoprotein Profiles in Surgical Menopause," *Obstetrics and Gynecology* 85 (1995): 529–37.

23. Gill Sanson, "The Osteoporosis 'Epidemic': Well Women and the Marketing of Fear," *Dr. Christiane Northrup's Health Wisdom for Women* 9 (November 2002): 3.

24. B. J. Abelow, T. R. Holford, and K. L. Insogna, "Cross-Cultural Association Between Dietary Animal Protein and Hip Fracture: A Hypothesis," *Calcif Tissue* 50 (1992): 1448.

25. D. W. Dempster and R. Lindsay, "Pathogenesis of Osteoporosis," *Lancet* 341 (1993): 797–805.

26. Robert Recker, M.D., "Calcium Absorption and Achlorhydria," *New England Journal of Medicine* 313 (1985): 70.

27. Susan Whiting, "Safety of Some Calcium Supplements Questioned," *Nutrition Reviews* 52 (1994): 95–97.

28. N. A. Breslau, L. Brinkley, K. D. Hill, and C. C. Kak, "Relationship of Animal Protein–Rich Diet to Kidney Stone Formation and Calcium Metabolism," *Journal of Clinical Endocrinology and Metabolism* 66 (1988): 140–46.

29. M. L. Brandi, "Flavenoids: Biochemical Effects on Therapeutic Applications," *Bone and Mineral* 19, suppl. (1992): S3–S14.

30. C. R. Draper, et al., "Phytoestrogens Reduce Bone Loss and Bone Resorption in Oophorectomized Rats," *Journal of Nutrition* 127 (1997): 1795–99.

31. Susan M. Potter, "Overview of Proposed Mechanisms for the Hypocholesterolemic Effect of Soy," *Journal of Nutrition* 125 (1995): 606S.

32. J. J. B. Anderson and S. C. Garner, "The Effects of Phytoestrogens on Bone," *Nutrition Research* 17 (1997): 1617–32.

33. P. Alexandersen, et al., "Ipriflavone in the Treatment of Postmenopausal Osteoporosis: A Randomized Controlled Trial," *Journal of the American Medical Association* 285 (2001): 1482–88.

34. R. W. Smith, W. R. Eyler, and R. C. Mellinger, "On the Incidence of Senile Osteoporosis," *Annals of Internal Medicine* 52 (1960): 773–76.

35. M. Chapuy, et al., "Vitamin D-3 and Calcium to Prevent Hip Fractures in Elderly Women," *New England Journal of Medicine* 327 (1992): 1637–42.

36. L. Bitensky, et al., "Circulating Vitamin K Levels in Patients with Fractures," *Journal of Bone and Joint Surgery* 70-B (1988): 663–64.

37. Diane Feskanich, et al., "Vitamin K Intake and Hip Fractures in Women: A Prospective Study," *American Journal of Clinical Nutrition* 69 (1999): 74–79.

38. F. H. Nielson, C. D. Hunt, L. M. Mullen, and J. R. Hunt, "Effect of Dietary Boron on Mineral, Estrogen, and Testosterone Metabolism in Postmenopausal Women," *FASEB Journal* 1 (1987): 394–97.

CHAPTER 8

1. M. L. Taymor, S. H. Sturgis, and C. Yahia, "The Etiological Role of Chronic Iron Deficiency in Production of Menorrhagia," *Journal of the American Medical Association* 187 (1964): 323–27.

2. M. S. Biskind and G. R. Biskind, "Effects of Vitamin B Complex Deficiency on Inactivated Estrone in the Liver," *Endocrinology* 31 (1942): 109.

3. H. L. Newbold, *Mega-Nutrients for Your Nerves* (New York: Berkley Publishing Co., 1975), 213.

4. Katharina Dalton, M.D., *Once a Month* (Alameda, CA: Hunter House Publishers, 1994), 18.

5. Richard Passwater, *Evening Primrose Oil* (New Canaan, CT: Keats Publishing, 1981), 22.

6. Richard M. Kunin, M.D., and Richard A. Kunin, *Mega-Nutrition for Women* (New York: McGraw-Hill, 1981), 76.

7. R. Schellenberg for the study group, "Treatment for the Premenstrual Sundrome with Agnus Castus Fruit Extract: Prospective, Randomised, Placebo-Controlled Study," *British Medical Journal* 322 (2001): 134–37.

8. J. Minton, et al., "Response of Fibrocystic Breast Disease to Caffeine Withdrawal and Correlation of Cyclic Nucleotides with Breast Disease," *American Journal of Obstetrics and Gynecology* 135 (1979): 157.

9. Penny Wise Budoff, M.D., *No More Menstrual Cramps and Other Good News* (New York: G. P. Putnam, 1981), 73.

10. P. M. Farrell and J. G. Bieri, "Megavitamin E Supplementation in Man," *American Journal of Clinical Nutrition* 28 (1975): 1381.

11. M. S. Biskind, "Nutritional Deficiency in the Etiology of Menorrhagia, Cystic Mastitis and Premenstrual Tension, Treatment with Vitamin B Complex," *Journal of Clinical Endocrinology and Metabolism* 3 (1943): 227.

12. R. A. Anderson, et al., "Urinary Chromium Excretion of Human Subjects: Effects of Chromium Supplementation and Glucose Loading," *American Journal of Clinical Nutrition* 36 (1982): 1184–93.

13. P. D. Leathwood and F. Chauffard, "Aqueous Extract of Valerian Reduces Latency to Fall Asleep in Man," *Planta Medica* (1985): 144–48.

14. Susan E. Hankinson, R.N., Sc.D., Graham A. Colditz, M.D., JoAnn E. Manson, M.D., and Frank E. Speizer, M.D., eds., *Healthy Women, Healthy Lives: A Guide to Preventing Disease, from the Landmark Nurses' Health Study* (New York: Simon and Schuster, 2001), 260.

15. Susan Lark, M.D., "Heal Arthritis Naturally," *The Lark Letter* (July 2000), 5.

16. Andrew Weil, M.D., "Gentle Relief for Rheumatoid Arthritis," *Dr. Andrew Weil's Self Healing* (February, 2001), 3.

17. J. M. Smyth, A. A. Stone, A. Hurewitz, and A. Kaell, "Effects of Writing about Stressful Experiences on Symptom Reduction in Patients with Asthma or Rheumatoid Arthritis: A Randomized Trial," *Journal of the American Medical Association* 281 (1999): 1304–9.

18. M. X. Sullivan and W. C. Hess, "Cysteine Content of Fingernails in Arthritis," *Journal of Bone and Joint Surgery* 16 (1935): 185–88.

19. J. M. Kraemer, et al., "Effects of Manipulation of Dietary Fatty Acids on Clinical Manifestations of Rheumatoid Arthritis," *Lancet* 1 (1985): 184–87.

20. Norman Childers, *A Diet to Stop Arthritis* (Somerville, NJ: Somerset Press, 1991).

21. L. G. Darlington, N. W. Ramsey, and J. C. Mansfield, "Placebo-Controlled, Blind Study of Dietary Manipulation Therapy in Rheumatoid Arthritis," *Lancet* (1 Feb. 1986): 236.

22. E. R. Schwartz, "The Modulation of Osteoarthritis Development by Vitamin C and E," *International Journal of Vitamin and Nutrition Research* 26, suppl. (1984): 141–46.

23. I. Machtey and L. Ouaknine, "Tocopherol in Osteoarthritis: A Controlled Pilot Study," *Journal of the American Geriatric Society* 26 (1978): 328–30.

24. E. C. Barton-Wright and W. A. Elliot, "The Pantothenic Acid Metabolism of Rheumatoid Arthritis," *Lancet* 2 (1963): 862–63.

25. J. C. Arnand, "Osteoarthritis and Pantothenic Acid," *Lancet* 2 (1963): 1168.

26. Peter Simpkin, "Oral Zinc Sulphate in Rheumatoid Arthritis," *Lancet* ii (1976): 539.

27. Antoniohopes Vaz, "Double-Blind Clinical Evaluation of the Related Efficacy of Ibuprofen and Glucosamine Sulfate in the Management of the Knee In-Out Patients," *Current Medical Research and Opinion* 8 (1982): 145–49.

28. P. M. Brooks, S. R. Potter, and W. W. Buchanan, "NSAID and Osteoarthritis—Help or Hindrance," *Journal of Rheumatology* 9 (1982): 35.

29. Jason Theodosakis, M.D., Brenda Adderly, M.H.A., and Barry Fox, Ph.D., *Maximizing the Arthritis Cure* (New York: St. Martin's Press, 1998), xvii.

30. Ibid., 188.

CHAPTER 9

1. Marianne Legato, M.D., and Carol Colman, *The Female Heart: The Truth about Women and Coronary Artery Disease* (New York: Simon and Schuster, 1992), xii.

2. Margie Patlak, "Women and Heart Disease," *FDA Consumer* 28.9 (Nov. 1994): 710.

3. Legato, *The Female Heart*, 16.

4. S. Hully, et al., "Randomized Trial of Estrogen plus Progestin for Secondary Prevention of Coronary Heart Disease in Postmenopausal Women," *Journal of the American Medical Association* 280 (1998): 605–13.

5. D. Grady, et al., "Cardiovascular Disease Outcomes During 6.8 Years of Hormone Therapy: Heart and Estrogen/Progestin Replacement Study Follow-Up (HERS II)," *Journal of the American Medical Association* 288 (2002): 49–57.

6. Andrew Stern, "Hormone Treatment Gives No Heart Benefit—U.S. Study," *Reuters*, (2 July 2002), 1. Retrieved on-line at <www.ivillagehealth.com/news/women/>.

7. Writing Group for the Women's Health Initiative Investigators, "Risks and Benefits of Estrogen plus Progestin in Healthy Postmenopausal Women: Principal Results from the Women's Health Initiative Randomized Controlled Trial," *Journal of the American Medical Association* 288 (2002): 321–33.

8. K. Ten, H. Boman, and S. P. Darger, "Increased Frequency of Coronary Heart Disease in Relatives of Wives of Myocardial Infarct Survivors: Assortive Mating for Lifestyle and Risk Factors," *American Journal of Cardiology* 53 (1984): 399–403.

9. Susan E. Hankinson, R.N., Graham A. Colditz, M.D., JoAnn E. Manson, M.D., and Frank E. Speizer, M.D., *Healthy Women, Healthy Lives: A Guide to Preventing Disease from the Landmark Nurses' Study* (New York: Simon and Schuster, 2001), 39.

10. Jeff Down, "Doctors Err More on Blacks, Women," *The Orange County Register* (20 April 2002), 22.

11. Marian Sandmaker, *The Healthy Heart Handbook* (National Institutes of Health Pub. No. 922720: 1992), 11.

12. Richard Helfant, M.D., *Women Take Heart* (New York: G. P. Putnams Sons, 1993), 18.

13. Morris Notelovitz, M.D., and Diana Tonnessen, *Menopause and Midlife Health* (New York: St. Martin's Press, 1993), 327.

14. Helfant, *Women Take Heart*, 17.

15. Hankinson, 56.

16. E. N. Frankel, et al., "Inhibition of Oxidation of Human Low-Density Lipoprotein by Phenolic Substances in Red Wine," *Lancet* 341 (1993): 454–57.

17. J. L. Abramson, S. A. Williams, H. M. Krumholz, and V. Vaccarino, "Moderate Alcohol Consumption and Risk of Heart Failure among Older Persons," *Journal of the American Medical Association* 285 (2001): 1971–77.

18. Elizabeth Barret-Connor, et al., "Why Is Diabetes Mellitus a Stronger Risk Factor for Ischemic Heart Disease in Women?" *Journal of the American Medical Association* 265 (1991): 627–31.

19. J. E. Manson, et al., "A Prospective Study of Obesity and Risk in Coronary Heart Disease in Women," *New England Journal of Medicine* 322 (1990): 882–89.

20. K. E. Powell, P. D. Thompson, I. J. Caspersen, and J. S. Kendrick, "Physical Activity and the Incidence of Coronary Heart Disease," *Annual Review of Public Health* 8 (1987): 253–87.

21. S. N. Blair, et al., "Physical Fitness and All-Cause Mortality: A Prospective Study of Healthy Men and Women," *Journal of the American Medical Association* 262 (1987): 2395–2401.

22. J. S. House, K. R. Landis, and D. Umberson, "Social Relationships and Health," *Science* 241 (1988): 540–45.

23. L. Schervitz, L. E. Graham, G. Grandits, and J. Billings, "Speech Characteristics and Behavior-Type Assessment in the Multiple Risk Factor Intervention Trial (MRFIT)," *Journal of Behavioral Medicine* 10.2 (1987): 173–95.

24. Herbert Benson, M.D., *The Mind/Body Effect: How Behavioral Medicine Can Show You the Way to Better Health* (New York: Berkley Books, 1981), 98.

25. National Heart and Lung Institute, "What Every Woman Should Know about High Blood Pressure."

26. Boston Women's Health Book Collective, *The New Our Bodies, Ourselves* (New York: Simon and Schuster, 1984), 541.

27. R. Stamler, et al., "Nutrition Therapy for High Blood Pressure: Final Report of a Four-Year Randomized Controlled Trial—The Hypertension Control Program," *Journal of the American Medical Association* 257 (1987): 1484.

28. Peter Wilson, "High-Density Lipoprotein, Low-Density Lipoprotein and Coronary Artery Disease," *The American Journal of Cardiology* 66 (1990): 7A–10A.

29. *Arteriol Thrombosis* 12 (1992): 529.

30. Bruce Kinosian, Henry Glick, and Gonzalo Garland, "Cholesterol and Coronary Heart Disease: Predicting Risks by Levels and Ratios," *Annals of Internal Medicine* 121 (1994): 641–47.

31. Stephen Sinatra, M.D., "Hormone Replacement and Women's Hearts: The Evolving Truth," *The Sinatra Health Report* (November 2001): 5.

32. Jean Carper, *Stop Aging Now* (New York: HarperCollins Publishers, 1995), 5.

33. Daniel Q. Haney, "Inflammation Worse for Health than Cholesterol," *San Francisco Chronicle* (4 August 2002), A9.

34. P. M. Ridker, C. H. Hennekens, J. E. Buring, and N. Rifai, "C-Reactive Protein and Other Markers of Inflammation in the Prediction of Cardiovascular Disease in Women," *New England Journal of Medicine* 342 (2000): 836–43.

35. "C-Reactive Protein, Coronary Risk, and Statins," *Harvard Women's Health Watch* 9.1 (September 2001): 2.

36. D. Ornish, et al., "Can Lifestyle Changes Reverse Coronary Heart Disease?" *Lancet* 336 (1990): 129–33.

37. Edward N. Siguel and Robert H. Lerman, "Role of Essential Fatty Acids: Dangers in the U.S. Department of Agriculture Dietary Recommendations ('Pyramid') and in Low-Fat Diets," *The American Journal of Clinical Nutrition* 60 (1994): 973–79.

38. W. Willet, et al., "Intake of Trans Fatty Acids and Risk of Coronary Heart Disease among Women," *Lancet* 341 (1993): 581–85.

39. Ray Delgado, "McFries to Get Healthier Grease," *San Francisco Chronicle* (3 September 2002), A5.

40. W. Willet, et al., op. cit.

41. D. Kromhout, E. Bosschieter, and C. Coulander, "The Inverse Relation Between Fish Consumption and 20-Year Mortality from Coronary Heart Disease," *The New England Journal of Medicine* 312 (1985): 1205–9.

42. Clemens Von Schacky, "Prophylaxis of Atherosclerosis with Marine Omega-3 Fatty Acids," *Annals of Internal Medicine* 107 (1987): 890–99.

43. Cynthia Ripson, et al., "Oat Products and Lipid Lowering: A Meta-Analysis," *Journal of the American Medical Association* 267 (1992): 3317–25.

44. D. Hunninghake, et al., "Hypocholesterolemic Effects of a Dietary Fiber Supplement," *American Journal of Clinical Nutrition* 59 (1994): 1050–54.

45. J. J. Cerda, et al., "The Effects of Grapefruit Pectin on Patients at Risk for Coronary Heart Disease Without Altering Diet or Lifestyle," *Clinical Cardiology* 11 (1988): 589–94.

46. T. Wolever, et al., "Method of Administration Influences the Serum Cholesterol-Lowering Effect of Psyllium," *American Journal of Clinical Nutrition* 59 (1994): 1055–59.

47. S. M. Potter, "Overview of the Proposed Mechanisms for the Hypocholesterolemic Effect of Soy," *Journal of Nutrition* 125 (1995): 606S.

48. D. Kritchevsky, et al., *Nutrition in Cardio-Cerebrovascular Diseases* (15 March 1993): 180–214.

49. M. Stampfer, et al., "Vitamin E Consumption and the Risk of Coronary Disease in Women," *The New England Journal of Medicine* 328 (1993): 1444–49.

50. J. Jandak and S. Richardson, "Alpha-Tocopherol and Effective Inhibition of Platelet Adhesion," *Blood* 72 (1989): 141–49.

51. J. Hallfrisch, et al., "High Plasma Vitamin C Associated with High Plasma HDL- and HDL-2 Cholesterol," *American Journal of Clinical Nutrition* 60 (1994): 100–5.

52. A. Kardinaal, et al., "Antioxidants in Adipose Tissue and Risk of Myocardial Infarction: The EURAMIC Study," *Lancet* (1993): 1379–84.

53. JoAnn Munson, M.D., presented to American Heart Association, Anaheim, CA, 1991.

54. Susan Peterson, "Beta Carotene, Vitamin E Cut Women's Heart Risk," *The Orange County Register* (14 Nov. 1991), 26.

55. Lars Brattstrom, Bjorn Hultberg, and Jan Erik Hardebo, "Folic Acid Responsive Postmenopausal Homocysteinemia," *Metabolism* 34 (1985): 107–77.

56. Meir Stampfer and Walter Willet, "Homocysteine and Marginal Vitamin D Deficiency: The Importance of Adequate Vitamin Intake," *Journal of the American Medical Association* 270 (1993): 2726–27.

57. G. P. Littarru, et al., "Deficiency of Coenzyme Q10 in Human Heart Disease Part II," *International Journal of Vitamin and Nutrition Research* 42 (1972): 413.

58. Yoshiro Nakamura, et al., "Protection of Ischemic Myocardium with Coenzyme Q10," *Cardiovascular Research* 16 (1982): 132–37.

59. E. Baggio, et al., "Italian Multicenter Study on the Safety and Efficacy of Coenzyme Q10 as Adjunctive Therapy in Heart Failure," *Molecular Aspects in Medicine*, suppl. (1994): S287–94.

60. K. Folkers, et al., "Biochemical Rationale and Myocardial Tissue Data on the Effective Therapy of Cardiomyopathy with Coenzyme Q10," *Procedures of the National Academy of Sciences* 82 (1985): 901–4.

61. Stephen Sinatra, M.D., "Coenzyme Q10: Truly a Miracle in Our Midst," *HeartSense* 2.7 (19 July 1996): 1–2.

62. Ibid.

CHAPTER 10

1. Mortimer Zuckerman, ed., "Battling Breast Cancer," *U.S. News and World Report* (23 November 1992).

2. S. W. Fletcher and G. A. Colditz, "Failure of Estrogen plus Progestin Therapy for Prevention," *Journal of the American Medical Association* 288 (2002): 366–68.

3. Catherine Schairer, et al., "Menopausal Estrogen and Estrogen-Progestin Replacement Therapy and Breast Cancer Risk," *Journal of the American Medical Association* 283 (2000): 485–91.

4. Morris Notelovitz, M.D., and Diana Tonnessen, *Menopause and Midlife Health* (New York: St. Martin's Press, 1993), 380.

5. D. Lindsey Berkson, *Hormone Deception* (Chicago, IL: Contemporary Books, 2000), 173.

6. G. A. Colditz, "Review: Relationship Between Estrogen Levels, Use of Hormone Replacement Therapy, and Breast Cancer," *Journal of the National Cancer Institute* 90 (1998): 814–23.

7. E. Dewailly, P. Ayotte, and S. Dodin, "Could the Rising Levels of Estrogen Receptors in Breast Cancer Be Due to Estrogenic Pollutants?" *Journal of the National Cancer Institute* 89 (1997): 888.

8. K. Steinberg, et al., "A Meta-Analysis of the Effect of Estrogen Replacement Therapy on the Risk of Breast Cancer," *Journal of the American Medical Association* 265 (1991): 1985–90.

9. Gina Kolata, "Brief Hormone Use Not Proven Safe," *San Francisco Chronicle* (24 October 2002): A6.

10. John R. Lee, M.D., "The Breast Cancer Profile in Saliva Hormone Level Testing," *The John R. Lee, M.D., Medical Letter* (August 2002), 5–6.

11. A. H. Follingstad, "Estriol: The Forgotten Estrogen?" *Journal of the American Medical Association* 239 (1978): 29–30.

12. Ronald Watson and Tina Leonard, "Selenium and Vitamins A, E, and C: Nutrients with Cancer-Prevention Properties," *Journal of the American Dietetic Association* 86 (1986): 505.

13. Henry Dreher, *Your Defense Against Cancer* (New York: Harper and Row, 1988), 8.

14. David J. Hunter, Donna Spiegelman, and Hans-Olov Adami, "Cohort Studies of Fat Intake and the Risk of Breast Cancer: A Pooled Analysis," *New England Journal of Medicine* 334 (1996): 356–61.

15. P. Buell, "Changing Incidence of Breast Cancer in Japanese-American Women," *Journal of the National Cancer Institute* 51 (1973): 1479–83.

16. L. Kinlen, "Meat and Fat Consumption and Cancer Mortality: A Study of Strict Religious Orders in Britain," *Lancet* (1982): 946–49.

17. H. P. Lee, et al., "Dietary Effects on Breast Cancer Risk in Singapore," *Lancet* 337 (1991): 1197–1200.

18. Ibid.

19. R. E. Hughes, "Hypothesis: A New Look at Dietary Fiber in Human Nutrition," *Clinical Nutrition* 406 (1986): 81–86.

20. John R. Lee, M.D., David Zava, Ph.D., and Virginia Hopkins, *What Your Doctor May Not Tell You about Breast Cancer* (New York: Warner Books, 2002), 133.

21. A. H. Wu, M. C. Pike, and D. O. Stram, "Meta-Analysis: Dietary Fat Intake, Serum Estrogen Levels, and the Risk of Breast Cancer," *Journal of the National Cancer Institute* 91 (1999): 529–34.

22. Alicja Wolk, et al., "A Prospective Study of Association of Monounsaturated Fat and Other Types of Fat with Risk of Breast Cancer," *Archives of Internal Medicines* 158 (1998): 41–45.

23. A. P. Simpoulos, "Summary of the NATO Advanced Research Workshop on Dietary Omega-3 and Omega-6 Fatty Acids: Biologic Effects and Nutritional Essentials," *Journal of Nutritional Medicine* 119 (1989): 521–28.

24. Julie Corliss, "Seafood Fatty Acids May Lower Cancer Risk," *Journal of the National Cancer Institute* 81 (1989): 1530–31.

25. L. A. Cohen, M. E. Kendall, E. Zang, C. Meschter, and D. P. Rose, "Modulation of N-Nitrosomethylurea-Induced Mammary L-Tumor Promotion by Dietary Fiber and Fat," *Journal of the National Cancer Institute* 83 (1991): 496–501.

26. Nicholas Petrakis and Eileen King, "Cytological Abnormalities in Nipple Asperates of Breast Fluid from Women with Severe Constipation," *Lancet* (28 Nov. 1981): 1204.

27. W. J. Blot, et al., "Nutrition Intervention Trials in Linxian, China: Supplementation with Specific Vitamin/Mineral Combinations, Cancer Incidence, and Disease-Specific Mortality in the General Population," *Journal of the National Cancer Institute* 85 (1993): 1483–92.

28. D. Hunter, et al., "A Prospective Study of the Intake of Vitamins C, E, and A and the Risk of Breast Cancer," *New England Journal of Medicine* 329 (1993): 234–40.

29. Ibid.

30. H. Stahelin, K. Gey, and E. Ludin, "Beta-Carotene and Cancer Prevention: The Basal Study," *American Journal of Clinical Nutrition* 53 (1991): 265S–69S.

31. K. F. Gey, G. B. Brubacher, and H. B. Stahelin, "Plasma Levels of Antioxidant Vitamins in Relation to Ischemic Heart Disease and Cancer," *American Journal of Clinical Nutrition* 45 (1987): 1368–77.

32. Gladys Block, "Vitamin C and Cancer Prevention: The Epidemiologic Evidence," *American Journal of Clinical Nutrition* 53 (1991): 270S–282S.

33. S. G. Jenkinson, "Oxygen Toxicity," *Journal of Intensive Care Medicine* 3 (1988): 137–52.

34. P. Knekt, et al., "Vitamin E and Cancer Prevention," *American Journal of Clinical Nutrition* 53 (1991): 283S–286S.

35. N. J. Walt, et al., *British Journal of Cancer Research* 49 (1984): 321.

36. Jeffrey Bland, "Safety Issues Regarding Supplements," *Preventive Medicine Update* 13.3 (March 1993): 211.

37. Jukka Salonen, et al., "Risk of Cancer and Vitamin A and E: Matched Case-Control Analysis of Prospective Data," *British Medical Journal* 290 (1985): 417.

38. G. N. Schraucer, et al., *Japanese Journal of Cancer Research* 76 (May 1985): 374.

39. Larry C. Clark and Gerald Combs, "Selenium Compounds and the Prevention of Cancer: Research Needs and Public Health Implications," *Journal of Nutrition* 116 (1986): 170.

40. H. P. Lee, et al., "Dietary Effects on Breast-Cancer Risk in Singapore," *Lancet* 337 (1991): 1197–200.

41. Mark Messina, et al., "Phyto-oestrogens and Breast Cancer," *Lancet* 350 (1997): 971–72.

42. Marc Goodman, et al., "Association of Soy and Fiber Consumption with the Risk of Endometrial Cancer," *American Journal of Epidemiology* 146 (1997): 294–306.

43. J. Michnovicz and H. Bradlow, "Altered Estrogen Metabolism and Excretion in Humans Following Consumption of Indole-3 Carbonol," *Nutrition and Cancer* 16 (1991): 59–66.

44. *Journal of the National Cancer Institute* (1994).

45. Christiane, Northrup, M.D., *The Wisdom of Menopause* (New York: Bantam Books, 2001), 412.

46. C. C. Chen, et al., "Adverse Life Events and Breast Cancer: Case-Control Study," *British Medical Journal* 311 (1995): 1527–29.

47. D. Spiegel, H. Kraemer, J. Bloom, and E. Gottheil, "Effect of Psychosocial Treatment on Survival of Patients with Metastatic Breast Cancer," *The Lancet* (October 1989): 889–91.

CHAPTER 11

1. J. B. Schmidt, et al., "Treatment of Skin Aging with Topical Estrogens," *International Journal of Dermatology* 35 (1996): 669–74.

2. Morris Notelovitz, M.D., and Diana Tonnessen, *Menopause and Midlife Health* (New York: St. Martin's Press, 1993), 158.

3. Emrika Padus, *The Woman's Encyclopedia of Health and Natural Healing* (Emmaus, PA: Rodale Press, 1981), 271.

4. Richard A. Kunin, M.D., *Mega-Nutrition for Women* (New York: McGraw-Hill, 1983), 46.

CHAPTER 12

1. Susan E. Hankinson, R.N., Graham A. Colditz, M.D., JoAnn E. Manson, M.D., and Frank E. Speizer, M.D., eds., *Healthy Women, Healthy Lives* (New York: Simon and Schuster Source, 2001), 293.

2. E. Cheraskin, M.D., and W. M. Ringdorf, Jr., with Arline Brecher, *Psychodietetics: Food as Key to Emotional Health* (New York: Bantam Books, 1981), 30.

3. Jane Brody, "Research Suggests Pulling the Strings on Yo Yo Dieting," *The New York Times* (27 June 1991).

4. Pamela Peeke, M.D., M.P.H., *Fight Fat after Forty* (New York: Penguin Books, 2001), 12.

5. Ibid., 32.

6. K. Raikkonon, et al., "Anger, Hostility, and Visceral Adipose Tissue in Healthy Postmenopausal Women," *Metabolism* 48 (1999): 1146–51.

7. Barbara Edelstein, M.D., *The Woman Doctor's Medical Guide for Women* (New York: William Morrow, 1982), 146.

8. W. Insull, et al., "Results of a Randomized Feasibility Study of a Low-Fat Diet," *Archives of Internal Medicine* 150 (1990): 421–27.

CHAPTER 13

1. Sharie Miller, "Getting Started, Staying Fit," *Vogue* 175 (April 1985): 340.

2. Philip Elmer-Dewitt, "Extra Years for Extra Effort," *Time* (17 March 1986): 66.

3. Richard A. Kunin, M.D., *Mega-Nutrition for Women* (New York: McGraw-Hill, 1983), 150.

4. Morris Notelovitz, M.D., and Diana Tonnessen, *Menopause and Midlife Health* (New York: St. Martin's Press, 1993), 329.

5. Kenneth H. Cooper, M.D., *The New Aerobics* (New York: Bantam Books, 1981), 16.

6. Covert Bailey, *Smart Exercises: Burning the Fat, Getting Fit* (Boston, MA: Houghton Mifflin Company, 1994), 42.

7. Covert Bailey, *The Fit or Fat Woman* (Boston, MA: Houghton Mifflin Company, 1989), 28.

8. J. F. Aloia, D. M. McGowan, A. N. Vaswani, et al., "Relationship of Menopause to Skeletal Muscular Mass," *American Journal of Clinical Nutrition* 53 (1991): 1378–83.

9. Notelovitz and Tonnessen, *Menopause and Midlife Health*, 102.

10. Bob Anderson, *Stretching* (Bolinas, CA: Shelter Publications, 1980).

CHAPTER 14

1. Henry Beiler, *Food Is Your Best Medicine* (New York: Random House, 1965), 34.

2. U.S. Department of Health and Human Services, *Ten Leading Causes of Death in the U.S., 1977* (Washington, DC: Government Printing Office, 1980).

3. Select Committee on Nutrition and Human Needs, U.S. Senate, *Dietary Goals for the United States* (Washington, DC: Government Printing Office, 1977).

4. *Journal of the American Dietetic Association* (September 1994).

5. Gladys Block, "Dietary Guidelines: The Results of Food Consumption Surveys," *American Journal of Clinical Nutrition* 53 (1991): 356S–357S.

6. *Benefits of Nutritional Supplementation,* Council for Responsible Nutrition (Washington, DC: 1990).

7. R. S. Murphy and G. A. Muhad, "Methodologic Considerations of the National Health and Nutrition Examination Survey," *American Journal of Clinical Nutrition*, 35, suppl. (May 1982).

8. Ibid.

9. Sherwood L. Gorbach, M.D., David R. Zimmerman, and Margo Woods, *The Doctor's Anti-Breast Cancer Diet* (New York: Simon and Schuster, 1984), 15.

10. Weston Price, *Nutrition and Physical Degeneration* (Santa Monica, CA: Price-Potter Foundation, 1970).

11. M. de Lorgeril, et al., "Mediterranean Diet, Traditional Risk Factors, and the Rate of Cardiovascular Complications after Myocardial Infarction," *Circulation* 99 (1999): 779–85.

12. R. H. Fletcher, and K. M. Fairfield, "Vitamins for Chronic Disease Prevention in Adults," *Journal of the American Medical Association* 287 (2002): 3127–29.

13. Richard A. Kunin, M.D., *Mega-Nutrition for Women* (New York: McGraw-Hill, 1983), 12.

CHAPTER 15

1. National Research Council, "Diet and Health Implications for Reducing Chronic Disease Risk," (Washington, DC: National Academy Press, 1980).

2. Walter Willet, "Diet and Health: What Should We Eat?" *Science* 264 (1994): 532–37.

CHAPTER 16

1. "Pesticides in 61 Percent of Fruits, Vegetables," *Associated Press* (April 1994).

2. M. S. Biskind, "Nutritional Deficiencies in the Etiology of Menorrhagia, Cystic Mastitis and Premenstrual Tension, Treatment with Vitamin B Complex," *Journal of Clinical Endocrinology and Metabolism* 3 (1943): 227.

3. Niels H. Lauersen, M.D., and Eileen Stukane, *Listen to Your Body: A Gynecologist Answers Women's Most Intimate Questions* (New York: Berkley Books, 1983), 120.

4. Peter W. Curatolo, M.D., and David Robertson, M.D., "The Health Consequences of Caffeine," *Annals of Internal Medicine* 98 (1983): 641–53.

5. Lynn Rosenberg, et al., "Breast Cancer and Alcoholic Beverage Consumption," *Lancet* (30 January 1982): 267–69.

6. Jeffrey Bland, Ph.D., *Nutraerobics* (New York: Harper and Row, 1983), 214.

CHAPTER 17

1. Jeffrey Bland, Ph.D., *Nutraerobics* (New York: Harper and Row, 1983), 68.

2. *American Journal of Clinical Nutrition* 24 (1971): 269.

CHAPTER 18

1. Patricia Hausman, *The Right Dose: How to Take Vitamins and Minerals Safely* (Emmaus, PA: Rodale Press, 1987).

2. "Is This the Right Way to Test Supplements?" *University of California, Berkeley, Wellness Letter* 16.12 (12 September 2000): 1.

3. "Yes, but Which Supplement," *Tufts University Health and Nutrition Letter* (May 2001): 1.

4. Sheldon Saul Hendler, M.D., *The Doctor's Vitamin and Mineral Encyclopedia* (New York: Simon and Schuster, 1990), 428.

GLOSSARY

Adipose (fat)—commonly used in describing the part of the body where fat is stored.

Adrenal glands—small, pyramid-shaped glands situated on top of each kidney that secrete various substances, among which are the steroid hormones androgen, estrogen, and progestogen.

Adrenal cortex—outer part of the adrenal gland that secretes cortisone-like hormones.

Adrenaline—neurotransmitter produced by the adrenal gland, released in response to fear, heightened emotion, or physiological stress.

Amenorrhea—failure to menstruate.

Amino acid—organic compound of carbon, hydrogen, oxygen, and nitrogen; the building blocks of protein.

Amphetamine—drug used as a stimulant for people in tired or depressed states; also used to decrease nasal congestion and to decrease appetite.

Androgen—male sex hormones (for example, testosterone).

Androstenedione—weak androgen abundantly secreted by menopausal ovaries as well as the adrenal glands; a major source of estrogen during and after menopause.

Anovulatory cycle—menstrual cycle without ovulation or the release of an egg.

Antiestrogenic—a substance that can oppose the effects of estrogens.

Antihypertensive—medication used to lower high blood pressure.

Antioxidant—a substance that prevents oxidation or inhibits reactions promoted by oxygen. These chemicals prevent free oxygen radicals from harming the body; for example, they can prevent formation of cholesterol plaques within blood vessels. Examples of common antioxidants are vitamins E and C.

Arteriosclerosis—a group of diseases characterized by thickening and loss of elasticity of artery walls; may be due to an accumulation of fibrous tissue, fatty substances, or minerals.

Atherosclerosis—a type of arteriosclerosis in which the inner layer of the artery wall is made thick and irregular by deposits of the fatty substance plaque.

Atrophy—withering of an organ that had previously been normally developed.

Basal metabolic rate (BMR)—temperature of the body at the time of awakening each morning.

Beta-carotene—compound in plants that the body converts into vitamin A.

Bioflavonoid—constituent of the vitamin C complex.

Blood-sugar control mechanism—regulates the amount of sugar in the bloodstream; includes the pancreas, insulin, glucagon, and adrenaline.

Blood-sugar level—amount of glucose (sugar) circulating in the bloodstream (normal levels are between 80 and 120 mg).

Calcitonin—calcium-sparing hormone released primarily by the thyroid gland; acts to slow the breakdown of bone.

351

Calcium balance—net processes in which calcium enters the body (through the diet) and leaves the body (through sweat, urine, and feces).

Carotid arteries—large arteries on either side of the neck that supply blood to the head.

Catecholamines—breakdown products of adrenaline.

Cellulose—carbohydrate found in the woody part of plants and trees; provides fiber to the body.

Cervix—narrow lower end of the uterus that extends into the vagina.

Chelation—process of covering a mineral with an amino acid to enhance its absorption rate.

Cholesterol—a fatlike substance found in the cell walls of all animals, including humans; some cholesterol is manufactured in the body and some comes from foods of animal origin.

Collagen—protein that is the supportive component of bone, connective tissue, cartilage, and skin.

Corpus luteum—yellow body seen in the ovary after ovulation, the cells of which produce progesterone, estrogen, and other hormones.

Corticosteroids—drugs that resemble the adrenal hormones.

Cortisone—adrenal hormone that can be harmful to bones; also a drug that resembles the adrenal hormone.

Cysteine—sulfur-containing amino acid.

Daidzein—an isoflavone found in soy that has been shown to have anticancer properties.

Deoxyribonucleic acid (DNA)—the fundamental component of living matter.

Diuretic—agent that promotes the excretion of urine.

Dopamine—important brain neurotransmitter that plays a role in body movement, motivation, primitive drives, sexual behavior, emotions, and immune-system function.

Double-blind study—study in which neither the experimenter nor the subjects know who is getting what treatment.

Dysmenorrhea—painful or difficult menstruation.

Edema—excessive accumulation of fluid in tissues, causing swelling.

Endocrine glands—glands that manufacture hormones and release them into the bloodstream (such as adrenal glands, ovaries, and pancreas).

Endorphins—natural opiate-like substances in the brain that control pain, among other things.

Enzyme—protein capable of producing or accelerating a specific biochemical reaction at body temperature.

Epidemiological study—study of the occurrence and prevalence of disease.

Estradiol—form of estrogen found in the blood of premenopausal women.

Estriol—form of estrogen found in the blood of pregnant women.

Estrogen—class of female sex hormones found in both men and women, but in larger proportions in women; primarily responsible for the development and maintenance of female sex characteristics and reproductive functions in women.

Estrone—weaker form of estrogen; found in the blood of menopausal women.

Fibroids—fibrous, noncancerous growths most commonly found in or on the uterus.

Follicle—small, round sac; in the ovary, each egg is contained in a follicle.

Follicle-stimulating hormone (FSH)—hormone secreted by the pituitary gland that stimulates the follicles in the ovary to grow and mature.

Free radicals—highly reactive molecular fragments, generally harmful to the body.

Gammalinolenic acid (GLA)—poly-unsaturated fat used by the body to produce certain prostaglandins that control several important body processes.

Genistein—an isoflavone found in soy that has very strong estrogenic effects as compared to other plant estrogens. It has a strong anticancer effect on the body.

Glucose—simple sugar that is the usual form in which the carbohydrate exists in the bloodstream.

Glucose tolerance factor (GTF)—a chromium compound that aids insulin in the control of blood sugar.

Glycogen—principal form in which a carbohydrate is stored in the body for ready conversion into energy; found in the liver and muscle tissue in particular.

Hemoglobin—protein in the blood that contains iron and carries oxygen from the lungs to the tissues.

High density lipoprotein (HDL)—the smallest lipoprotein, which removes cholesterol from LDL and cells and transports it back to the liver, where cholesterol is broken down into bile acids and excreted into the intestine; high levels are associated with low risk of heart disease.

Histamine—compound found in many tissues that is responsible for the increased permeability of blood vessels and plays a major role in allergic reactions.

Homeostasis—body's tendency to maintain a steady state of equilibrium despite external changes.

Hormone—chemical substance produced in one part of the body and carried in the blood to another part of the body, where it has specific effects.

Hydrogenation—addition of hydrogen to any unsaturated compound (oils are changed to solid fats by this process).

Hypoglycemia—low or falling concentration of glucose in the bloodstream, often caused by an excessive intake of refined carbohydrates in the diet.

Hypothalamus—part of the brain containing groups of nerve cells that control temperature, sleep, water balance, and other chemical and visceral activities.

Hysterectomy—surgical removal of the uterus (a radical hysterectomy includes removal of the uterus, cervix, ovaries, egg tubes, and sometimes lymph nodes near the ovaries).

Incontinence—inability to control urine retention.

Insulin—protein hormone secreted by the pancreas into the blood; regulates carbohydrate, fat, and protein metabolism.

Isoflavones—compounds found in some plant products that have estrogenic properties; genistein and daidzein are examples of isoflavones.

Labia majora—major lips or folds of skin of the female external genitals, located on either side of the entrance to the vagina.

Labia minora—the inner flaps of skin located under the labia majora.

Lactase—intestinal enzyme that breaks down lactose (a sugar) into easily digested compounds.

Lactobacillus acidophilus—class of friendly bacteria found in yogurt and other milk products; also found in both the intestines and the vagina, where it controls the growth of yeast.

Lactose—sugar found in milk and other dairy products.

Lactose intolerance—deficiency of the lactase enzyme, which results in uncomfortable gastrointestinal symptoms when foods containing lactose are eaten.

Lecithin—waxlike substance with emulsifying and antioxidant properties, found in animals and plants.

Lipoprotein—a complex particle consisting of lipid (fat), protein, and cholesterol molecules bound together to transport fat through the blood.

Low-density lipoprotein (LDL)—particles that are rich in cholesterol; high levels in the blood are associated with the premature development of atherosclerosis and an increased risk of heart disease.

Luteinizing hormone (LH)—hormone produced by the pituitary (a large surge of this hormone in each menstrual cycle precedes ovulation by twelve to twenty-four hours).

Menarche—beginning of menstruation.

Menorrhagia—excessive bleeding during menstruation.

Metabolism—sum of chemical changes; the building up or destruction of cells that takes place in the body.

Monounsaturated fat—a fat chemically constituted to be capable of absorbing additional hydrogen; these fats have been shown to lower blood cholesterol levels (olive oil, for example).

Neurotransmitter—substance that transmits nerve impulses across a synapse; brain chemicals that are involved in carrying messages to and from the brain.

Oophorectomy—removal of the ovaries (also called ovariectomy).

Osteopenia—lower than normal bone mass.

Ovary—one of two female organs containing the eggs and the cells that produce the female hormones estrogen and progesterone.

Ovulation—process during which a mature egg is released from the ovary.

Oxalates—compounds that can interfere with the absorption of calcium; found in some leafy green vegetables, such as spinach.

Oxidation—process of combining with oxygen.

Pancreas—large glandular organ, extending across the upper abdomen close to the liver, that secretes digestive juices into the intestinal tract; it contains enzymes that act upon protein, fat, and carbohydrates; also secretes the hormone insulin directly into the blood.

Phytates—phosphorus-containing compounds that can interfere with the absorption of calcium; found in the outer husk of cereal grains.

Phytohormones—plant substances that are structurally and functionally similar to human hormones; their effects on the body are weak compared to those of human hormones.

Pituitary gland—small, oval organ at the base of the brain that produces many important hormones (particularly FSH and LH) and has been called "the master gland."

Placebo—pill having no medicinal value, often used as a control in an experimental situation.

Plaque—a deposit of fatty (and other) substances in the inner lining of the artery wall, characteristic of atherosclerosis.

Platelets—substances in the blood that help form blood clots.

Progesterone—hormone produced by the ovary during the second half of the menstrual cycle; promotes the growth of the uterine lining prior to menstruation and, in pregnancy, the growth of the placenta.

Progestins—synthetic version of the female hormone progesterone.

Progestogens—group of synthetic steroid hormones that includes progesterone and other hormones that have similar effects.

Prostaglandin—one of several compounds formed from essential fatty acids and whose activities affect the nervous, circulatory, and reproductive systems and metabolism; research indicates that a type of prostaglandin is implicated in muscular contractions and menstrual cramps.

Ribonucleic acid (RNA)—compound of nucleic acid responsible for the transmission of inherited traits.

Serotonin—substance present in many tissues (especially the blood and nerve tissue) that stimulates a variety of smooth muscles and nerves and is believed to function as a neurotransmitter.

Syndrome—set of symptoms that occur together.

Testosterone—strongest of the male sex hormones, found in both women and men, but in much greater proportions in men.

Thyroid gland—organ at the base of the neck primarily responsible for regulating the rate of metabolism.

Tinctures—powdered herbs that are added to a fifty-fifty solution of alcohol and water.

Triglyceride—the main type of lipid (fatty substance) found in the fat tissue of the body and also the main type of fat found in food; high levels in the blood are associated with a greater risk of coronary atherosclerosis.

Uterus—complex female organ composed of smooth muscle and glandular lining; the womb.

Vagina—muscular canal in the female that extends from the vulva to the cervix.

Vasodilation—enlargement or dilation of blood vessels.

Vulva—external female sex organ, composed of the major and minor lips (labia majora and minora), the clitoris, and the opening of the vagina.

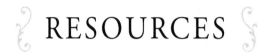

RESOURCES

BOOKS

Arthritis

Judith Horstman, *The Arthritis Foundation's Guide to Alternative Therapies* (Atlanta, GA: Arthritis Foundation, 1999).

Jason Theodosakis, M.D., Brenda Adderly, and Barry Fox, *Maximizing the Arthritis Cure* (New York: St. Martin's Press, 1998).

Depression

Alice Miller, *The Truth Will Set You Free* (New York: Basic Books, 2001).

Deborah Sichel, M.D., and Jeanne Watson Driscoll, R.N., *Women's Moods* (New York: William Morrow and Company, Inc., 1999).

Diet and Nutrition

Jean Carper, *Food, Your Miracle Medicine: How Food Can Prevent and Cure Over 100 Symptoms and Problems* (New York: HarperPerennial, 1994).

Lissa DeAngelis and Molly Siple, *Recipes for Change: Cooking for Health and Vitality at Menopause* (New York: Dutton, 1996).

Ann Louise Gittleman, *Super Nutrition for Women* (New York: Bantam Doubleday Dell Publishers, 1991).

Dr. Lana Liew, with Linda Ojeda, Ph.D., *The Natural Estrogen Diet and Recipe Book: Healthy Recipes for Perimenopause and Menopause* (Alameda, CA: Hunter House Publishers, 2003).

Mark Messina, Ph.D., and Virginia Messina, with Ken Setchell, Ph.D., *The Simple Soybean and Your Health* (Garden City Park, NY: Avery Publishing Group, 1994).

Carol Ann Rinzler, *The Healing Power of Soy* (Rocklin, CA: Prima Publishing, 1998).

Nina Shandler, *Estrogen the Natural Way: Over 250 Easy and Delicious Recipes for Menopause* (New York: Villard, 1997).

Elizabeth Somer, M.D., *Nutrition for Women* (New York: Owl Books, Henry Holt and Company, 1995).

Debra Waterhouse, *Outsmarting the Midlife Fat Cell: Winning Weight-Control Strategies for Women Over 35 to Stay Fit Through Menopause* (New York: Hyperion, 1998).

Andrew Weil, M.D., *Eating Well for Optimum Health: The Essential Guide to Food, Diet, and Nutrition* (New York: Alfred A. Knopf, 2000).

Ruth Winter, *Super Soy: The Miracle Bean* (New York: Crown Trade Paperbacks, 1996.

Exercise

Denise Austin, *Jump Start* (New York: Simon and Schuster, 1996).

Covert Bailey, *The Ultimate Fit or Fat* (Boston, MA: Houghton Mifflin Company, 1999).

Covert Bailey and Lea Bishop, *The Fit or Fat Woman* (Boston, MA: Houghton Mifflin Company, 1989).

Joanie Greggains, *Fit Happens* (New York: Villard Books, 2000).

Lisa Hoffman, *Better than Ever: The 4-Week Workout Program for Women Over Forty* (New York: Contemporary Publishing, 1997).

Miriam E. Nelson, Ph.D., with Sarah Wernick, Ph.D., *Strong Women Stay Young* (New York, Bantam Books, 2000).

(Video) Kathy Smith, *Moving Through Menopause.*

Charlene Torkelson, *Get Fit While You Sit* (Alameda, CA: Hunter House Publishers, 1999).

Hormones and Health

D. Lindsey Berkson, *Hormone Deception* (Chicago, IL: Contemporary Books, 2000).

Ellen Brown and Lynn Walker, *Menopause and Estrogen: Natural Alternatives to Hormone Replacement Therapy* (Berkeley, CA: Frog, Ltd., 1996).

Sandra Coney, *The Menopause Industry: How the Medical Establishment Exploits Women* (Alameda, CA: Hunter House Publishers, 1994).

Susan Lark, M.D., *The Estrogen Decision* (Los Altos, CA: Westchester Publishing Company, 1994).

Marcus Laux, N.D., and Christine Conrad, *Natural Woman, Natural Menopause* (New York: HarperCollins Publishers, Inc., 1997).

John R. Lee, M.D., with Virginia Hopkins, *What Your Doctor May Not Tell You about Menopause* (New York: Warner Books, 1996).

John R. Lee, M.D., Jesse Hanley, M.D., and Virginia Hopkins, *What Your Doctor May Not Tell You about Premenopause* (New York: Warner Books, 1999).

Susan M. Love, M.D., with Karen Lindsey, *Dr. Susan Love's Hormone Book* (New York: Random House, 1997).

Susan Rako, M.D., *The Hormone of Desire* (New York: Three Rivers Press, 1996).

Carol Ann Rinzler, *Estrogen and Breast Cancer: A Warning to Women* (New York: Macmillan Publishing Company, 1993).

Lorilee Schoenbeck, N.D., with Cheryl A. Gibson, M.D., and M. Brooke Barss, M.D., *Menopause: Bridging the Gap Between Natural and Conventional Medicine* (New York: Kensington Publishing Corp., 2002).

Erika Schwartz, M.D., *The Hormone Solution* (New York: Warner Books Inc., 2002).

Shawn Talbott, Ph.D. *The Cortisol Connection: Why Stress Makes You Fat and Ruins Your Health—and What You Can Do about It* (Alameda, CA: Hunter House Publishers, 2002).

Elizabeth Lee Vliet, M.D., *Screaming to Be Heard: Hormonal Connections Women Suggest...and Doctors Ignore* (New York: M. Evans and Company, 1995).

Jonathan V. Wright, M.D., and John Morgenthaler, *Natural Hormone Replacement: For Women Over 45* (Petaluma, CA: Smart Publications, 1997).

Midlife Health

Lonnie Barbach, Ph.D., *The Pause: Positive Approaches to Menopause* (New York: Penguin Books, 2000).

Alan R. Gaby, M.D., *Preventing and Reversing Osteoporosis* (Rocklin, CA: Prima Publishing, 1994).

Ann Louise Gittleman, *Before the Change: Taking Charge of Your Perimenopause* (San Francisco, CA: Harper, 1998).

Bernadine Healy, M.D., *A New Prescription for Women's Health: Getting the Best Medical Care in a Man's World* (New York: Viking Penguin, 1995).

George J. Kessler, D.O., P.C., with Colleen Kapklein, *Bone Density Diet: 6 Weeks to a Strong Body and Mind* (New York: Ballantine Books, 2000).

Christiane Northrup, M.D., *The Wisdom of Menopause* (New York: Bantam Books, 2001).

Morris Notelovitz, M.D., and Diana Tonnessen, *Menopause and Midlife Health* (New York: St. Martin's Press, 1993).

Pamela Peeke, M.D., *Fight Fat after Forty* (New York: Penguin Books, 2000).

Midlife Issues

William Bridges, *Transitions: Making Sense of Life's Changes* (Reading, MA: Addison-Wesley Publishing Company, 1980).

Allan B. Chinen, M.D., *Once upon a Midlife: Classic Stories and Mythic Tales to Illuminate the Middle Years* (New York: Jeremy P. Tarcher/Perigee, 1992).

Clarissa Pinkola Estes, Ph.D., *Women Who Run with the Wolves* (New York: Ballantine Books, 1992).

Lawrence C. Katz, Ph.D., and Manning Rubin, *Keep Your Brain Alive* (New York: Workman Publishing Company, 1999).

Sue Monk Kidd, *When the Heart Waits: Spiritual Direction for Life's Sacred Questions* (San Francisco, CA: Harper San Francisco, 1990).

Alice Miller, *The Drama of the Gifted Child: The Search for the True Self* (New York: Basic Books, 1997).

Letty Cottin Pogrebin, *Getting Over Getting Older* (New York: Berkley Books, 1997).

Gail Sheehy, *The Silent Passage: Menopause* (New York: Random House, 1992).

Dena Taylor and Amber Coverdale Sumrall, eds., *Women of the 14th Moon: Writings on Menopause* (Freedom, CA: The Crossing Press, 1991).

Judith Viorst, *Necessary Losses: The Loves, Illusions, Dependencies and Impossible Expectations That All of Us Have to Give Up in Order to Grow* (New York: Fawcett Gold Metal, 1986).

Women's Health

Debbie DeAngelo, RNC, BSN, *Sudden Menopause: Restoring Health and Emotional Well-Being* (Alameda, CA: Hunter House Publishers, 2001).

Ann Louise Gittleman, M.S., *How to Stay Young and Healthy in a Toxic World* (Los Angeles, CA: Keats Publishing, 1999).

Ann Louise Gittleman, M.S., with Melissa Diane Smith, *Why Am I Always So Tired?* (New York: HarperCollins Publishers, 1999).

Tori Hudson, N.D., *Women's Encyclopedia of Natural Medicine: Alternative Therapies and Integrative Medicine* (Lincolnwood, IL: Keats, 1999).

John R. Lee, M.D., David Zava, Ph.D., and Virginia Hopkins, *What Your Doctor May Not Tell You about Breast Cancer* (New York: Warner Books Inc., 2002).

Marianne J. Legato, M.D., and Carol Colman, *The Female Heart: The Truth about Women and Coronary Artery Disease* (New York: Simon and Schuster, 1992).

Michael Murray, N.D., and Joseph Pizzorno, N.D., *Encyclopedia of Natural Medicine* (Rocklin, CA: Prima Publishing, 1991).

Miriam E. Nelson, Ph.D., with Judy Knipe, *Strong Women Eat Well* (New York: G.P. Putnam's Sons, 2001).

Christiane Northrup, M.D., *Women's Bodies, Women's Wisdom: Creating Physical and Emotional Health and Healing* (New York: Bantam Books, 1998).

Linda Ojeda, Ph.D., *Her Healthy Heart: A Woman's Guide to Preventing and Reversing Heart Disease* Naturally (Alameda, CA: Hunter House Publishers, 1998).

Elizabeth Plourde, C.L.S., M.A., *Hysterectomy and Ovary Removal* (Irvine, CA: New Voice Publications, 2002).

Richard L. Shames, M.D., and Karilee Halo Shames, R.N., Ph.D., *Thyroid Power* (New York: A HarperResource Book, 2002).

NEWSLETTERS

Berkeley Wellness Newsletter, University of California at Berkeley, P.O. Box 10922, Des Moines, IA 50340.

Dr. Andrew Weil's Self Healing: Creating Natural Health for Your Body and Mind, edited by Andrew Weil, M.D., c/o Thorne Communications, Inc., 42 Pleasant St., Watertown, MA 02472.

Dr. Christiane Northrup's Health Wisdom for Women, edited by Christiane Northrup, M.D., c/o Phillips Publishing, 7811 Montrose Road, Potomac, MD 20854.

Health and Nutrition Letter, Tufts University, P.O. Box 2465, Boulder, CO 80322.

Hot Flash: Newsletter for Midlife and Older Women, edited by Jane Porcino, Ph.D., School of Allied Health Professionals, State University of New York, Box 816, Stony Brook, NY 11790.

The Lark Letter, Susan Lark, M.D., Phillips Publishing, Inc., 7811 Montrose Road, Potomac, MD 20859.

Women's Health Watch, Harvard Medical School, 164 Longwood Ave., Boston, MA 02115.

NATURAL HORMONES

Bajamar Women's Health Care (800) 255-8025

FemGest (Women's Wisdom Nutritional) (800) 705-5559

Progest (Transitions for Health) (800) 888-6814

Women's International Pharmacy (800) 279-5708

SOY PRODUCTS

(Information) U.S. Soyfoods Directory; www.soyfoods.com

Revival Soy (800) 500-2055; www.revivalsoy.com

SALIVA HORMONE TESTING

Aeron LifeCycles Clinical Laboratory (800) 631-7900; www.aeron.com

ZRT Laboratory (503) 466-2445; www.salivatest.com

WEBSITES FOR MENOPAUSE AND WOMEN'S HEALTH

Hot Flash!: www.families-first.com/hotflash

Power Surge: www.power-surge.com

Dr. John Lee: www.johnleemd.com

Dr. Susan Lark: www.drlark.com

Women's health: www.ivillage.com

Dr. Erika Schwartz (Natural Hormone Pharmacy): www.hormonesolution.com

North American Menopause Society: www.menopause.org

LOCATE A COMPOUNDING PHARMACY IN YOUR AREA

International Academy of Compounding Pharmacists (IACP)
PO Box 1365, Sugar Land TX 77487
(800) 927-4227
E-mail: iacpinfo@iacprx.org   Website: www.iacprx.org

LOCATE A PHYSICIAN IN YOUR AREA

American Association for Advancement in Medicine (ACAM)
23121 Verdugo Dr., Ste. 204, Laguna Hills CA 92653
Fax: (949) 455-9679   Website: www.acam.org

INDEX

9 781630 267872